PLACE IN RETURN BOX to remove this checkout from your record.
TO _____ on or before date due.

DEVELOPMENTAL NEUROBIOLOGY

Developmental Neurobiology

Editors

Philippe Evrard
Professor of Pediatric Neurology
Hôpital Universitaire Saint-Luc
Brussels, Belgium

Alexandre Minkowski
Professor of Pediatrics
Centre de Recherche de Biologie du
Développement Foetal et Néonatal
Paris, France

Nestlé Nutrition
Workshop Series
Volume 12

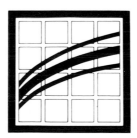

NESTLÉ NUTRITION

RAVEN PRESS ■ NEW YORK

Nestec Ltd., Avenue Nestlé, 1800 Vevey, Switzerland
Raven Press, Ltd., 1185 Avenue of the Americas, New York,
New York 10036

Made in the United States of America

Library of Congress Cataloging-in Publication Data

Developmental neurobiology / editors, Philippe Evrard, Alexandre
  Minkowski.
      p.   cm.—(Nestlé Nutrition workshop series ; v. 12)
    Papers presented at a Nestlé Nutrition workshop.
    Includes bibliographies and index.
    ISBN 0-88167-544-X (Raven Press)
    1. Developmental neurology—Congresses.   I. Evrard, Philippe,
  Prof.   II. Minkowski, Alexandre.   III. Nestlé Nutrition S.A.
  IV. Series.
      [DNLM: 1. Brain—growth & development—congresses.   2. Nervous
  System—growth & development—congresses.   3. Nutrition—congresses.
  W1   NE228 v. 12 / WL 300 D4886]
  QP363.5.D484   1989
  612.6'40181—dc20
  DNLM/DLC
  for Library of Congress   89-8333
                                                                  CIP

The material contained in this volume was submitted as previously
unpublished material, except in the instances in which credit has been given to
the source from which some of the material was derived.
    Great care has been taken to maintain the accuracy of the information
contained in the volume. However, neither Nestec nor Raven Press can be held
responsible for errors or for any consequences arising from the use of the
information contained herein.

9 8 7 6 5 4 3 2 1

Preface

Our understanding of the normal and abnormal development of the central nervous system (CNS) has long been deficient in comparison with other fields of biomedical research. Human malformations were considered "vagaries of nature" so mysterious as to be unavoidable. Over the last two decades, advances in developmental neurobiology have revolutionized our understanding of neurodevelopmental disorders. In addition, the analysis of these disorders has raised basic neurobiological questions about mammalian development and has prompted new experimental approaches.

Developmental neurobiology covers an extended period from fecundation to advanced adult age and is of crucial interest to many clinicians.

Obstetricians, neonatologists, pediatric neurologists, pediatricians, and gynecologists involved in *in vitro* fertilization confront daily the dangers of the prenatal period and have to cope with the consequences of prenatal problems. Antenatal loss and mortality is around 70% of all conceptions. Postnatal problems, both major and minor, resulting from prenatal disturbances afflict nearly 10% of those who survive embryonic and fetal life. The nervous system is often a target. Statistical data suggest that 25% of conceptions are affected by developmental disturbances of the CNS and that these embryonic and fetal neurological disorders account for a high percentage of fetal deaths. These prenatal disorders often jeopardize postnatal survival and functional perspectives: 40% of infant deaths occurring during the first year of postnatal life seem to be related in some way to prenatal malformations of the CNS, and the subsequent achievement potential for those who survive depends in part on their prenatal neural development. Furthermore, recent studies demonstrate that postnatal neurological handicaps result more frequently from prenatal etiologies than classically reported and that neonatal problems often can be provoked or encouraged by prenatal factors (1).

Augmenting further the importance of prenatal neuropathology and of the nascent field of developmental imaging, "minor" cortical dysgeneses, subtle and quantitative cytoarchitectonic disturbances, and defective neuronal growth and differentiation have been implicated recently as causative factors or as anatomical witnesses for dyslexia, autism, partial epilepsy, fetal alcohol syndrome, and mental deficiency of unknown etiology.

The care and protection of the developing CNS and neurological prognosis at birth are among the priorities of neonatal medicine. Postnatal development depends to a great extent on the appropriate decisions taken at this critical point of human life.

Pediatric neurology and the entire fields of pediatrics, education, learning, and rehabilitation deal daily with postnatal central nervous system development and plasticity.

The biological and environmental factors interfering with the successive developmental steps seem to be unequally distributed in the various socioeconomic levels and add an important sociological dimension to the developmental problems (for a review, see ref. 2).

We hope this book paves the way for a cooperative effort between scholars in neurobiological research and clinicians, and that knowledge will be exchanged between human developmental pathology—where knowledge is still humble and demands are huge—and basic research approaches.

REFERENCES

1. Evrard P, de Saint-Georges P, Kadhim HJ, Gadisseux JF. Pathology of prenatal encephalopathies. In: *Child neurology and developmental disabilities*. Baltimore: Brookes Publishing Co, 1989.
2. Hamburg DA. Reducing the casualties of early life: a preventive orientation. Annual Report, Carnegie Corporation of New York, 1985.
PHILIPPE EVRARD

This is the first time that Nestlé has undertaken the organization of a workshop on the subject of developmental neurobiology. The aim of the workshop was to bring together neuroscientists, pediatricians, and neurologists, in order to override the gap existing between clinicians (mainly pediatric neurologists and perinatologists) and basic scientists of the developing brain. Indeed, although our understanding of the developing brain has evolved very rapidly during the last 20 years, mainly owing to the recent development of molecular genetics, the brain still seems to be a "black box" for many clinicians.

This objective, to obtain a common wavelength that can be used by clinicians and basic scientists, has been achieved. We consider this event a promising new avenue for the future. Nestlé should be congratulated for considering the suggestions made by Professor Evrard and myself and for accepting the organization of this workshop.

ALEXANDRE MINKOWSKI

Acknowledgments

We have to thank Professor Alexandre Minkowski. After having founded modern French neonatology and making critical contributions to European and world neonatology, he has supported developmental neuropathology and neurobiology with the same enthusiasm. Dr. Pierre Guesry has generously supported our symposium and, more importantly, was an exigent intellectual leader for the organization, the discussions, and the publications. Dr. Hazim J. Kadhim and Dr. Jean-François Gadisseux devoted much of their research time to the difficult editorial work. We wish to thank the authors for their patience with the delay of the publication due to reasons beyond our, Nestlé's, and the publisher's control. Important papers resist the erosion of time over decades.

PHILIPPE EVRARD

Foreword

Everyone will agree that the brain is the noblest among noble organs in the human species and that everything should be done to protect it during pregnancy, delivery, and infancy. Such protection is essential in order to potentially improve the learning ability during infancy and childhood, and to slow down the involution which should match the life span prolongation. This protection should guard not only against traumatism (physical, vascular, or anoxic) but also against biochemical disturbances.

During the 1970s the dogma was that the brain was very resistant to biochemical disturbances (except oxygen) and that, for example, malnutrition had very little impact on brain development. It now appears that this may not be the case, and that some fatty acids essential for brain development control can only be partially synthesized. Their lack in food during pregnancy and lactation or in artificial feeding could have consequences on myelination, as already shown in animal experiments.

This renewal of interest for nutritional problems in developmental neurobiology led Nestlé to warmly accept Professor Minkowski's proposal to organize a Nestlé Nutrition Workshop gathering the most knowledgeable experts in the field. The subjects were sometimes difficult for nonspecialists, but always fascinating. We hope that the readers of this book will feel the fascination more than the difficulty.

PIERRE R. GUESRY, M.D.
Vice President
Nestlé Products Technical Assistance Co. Ltd.

Contents

Contributors

Angel Ballabriga*
Hospital Infantil Vall d'Hebron
Universidad Autónoma
Paseo Vall d'Hebron S/N
Barcelona 08035, Spain

Gilles Barbin*
INSERM Unité 114
Collège de France
Chaire de Neuropharmacologie
11 Place Marcelin Berthelot
75231 Paris Cédex 05, France

J. Belmar
Department of Cell Biology
Catholic University of Chile
Santiago 11, Chile

S. Bourgoin
INSERM Unité 288
Neurobiologie Cellulaire et Fonctionnelle
Faculté de Médecine Pitié-Salpêtrière
91 Boulevard de l'Hôpital
75634 Paris Cédex 13, France

Jean-Marie Bourre*
INSERM Unité 26
Hôpital Fernand Widal
200 Rue du Faubourg St. Denis
75475 Paris Cédex 10, France

Anthony T. Campagnoni*
Mental Retardation Research Center
Neuropsychiatric Institute
UCLA Center for Health Sciences
760 Westwood Plaza
Los Angeles, California 90024

C.W. Campagnoni
Mental Retardation Research Center
Neuropsychiatric Institute
UCLA Center for Health Sciences
760 Westwood Plaza
Los Angeles, California 90024

Verne S. Caviness, Jr.*
Division of Pediatric Neurology
Massachusetts General Hospital
and Harvard Medical School
115 Fruit Street
Boston, Massachusetts 02114

C. Chanez*
INSERM Unité 29
Centre de Recherches de Biologie
du Développement Foetal et Néonatal
123 Boulevard de Port Royal
75674 Paris Cédex 14, France

Michael E. Charness
Ernest Gallo Clinic and Research Center
Department of Neurology
University of California
San Francisco General Hospital
San Francisco, California 94110

Philippe de Saint-Georges
Service de Neurologie Pédiatrique et
Laboratoire de Neurologie du
Développement
Hôpital Universitaire Saint-Luc
Avenue Hippocrate 10
Boîte UCL 10/1303
B-1200 Brussels, Belgium

F. De Vitry
Groupe de Neuroendocrinologie
Cellulaire
ER CNRS 89
Collège de France
11 Place Marcelin Berthelot
75231 Paris Cédex 05, France

L. De Vries
Department of Pediatrics and Neonatal
Medicine
Royal Postgraduate Medical School
Hammersmith Hospital
Du Cane Road
London W12 OHS, England

*Authors who attended the workshop.

Ivan Diamond
Ernest Gallo Clinic and Research Center
Department of Neurology
University of California
San Francisco General Hospital
San Francisco, California 94110

Jean-Pierre Draye
International Institute of Cellular
* and Molecular Pathology (ICP)*
* and Department of Pediatric Neurology*
Catholic University of Louvain (UCL)
75 Avenue Hippocrate
B-1200 Brussels, Belgium

Lilly M.S. Dubowitz*
Department of Pediatrics and Neonatal
* Medicine*
Royal Postgraduate Medical School
Hammersmith Hospital
Du Cane Road
London W12 OHS, England

Philippe Evrard*
Service de Neurologie Pédiatrique et
* Laboratoire de Neurologie du*
* Développement*
Hôpital Universitaire Saint-Luc
Avenue Hippocrate 10
Boîte UCL 10/1303
B-1200 Brussels, Belgium

Jean-François Gadisseux*
Service de Neurologie Pédiatrique
Université Catholique de Louvain
Avenue Hippocrate 10
Boîte UCL 10/1303
B-1200 Brussels, Belgium

André M. Goffinet
Service de Neurologie Pédiatrique
Hôpital Universitaire Saint-Luc
Avenue Hippocrate 10
Boîte UCL 10/1303
B-1200 Brussels, Belgium

Sidney L. Goldfischer*
Department of Pathology
Albert Einstein College of Medicine
1300 Morris Park Avenue
The Bronx, New York 10461

Adrienne S. Gordon
Ernest Gallo Clinic and Research Center
Department of Neurology
University of California
San Francisco General Hospital
San Francisco, California 94110

Jean-Louis Guénet*
Institut Pasteur
25 Rue du Dr Roux
75724 Paris Cédex 15, France

Michel Hamon*
INSERM Unité 288
Neurobiologie Cellulaire et Fonctionnelle
Faculté de Médecine Pitié Salpêtrière
91 Boulevard de l'Hôpital
75634 Paris Cédex 13, France

A. Hernández
Institute of Nutrition and Food
* Technology (INTA)*
University of Chile
Santiago 11, Chile

N. Herschkowitz*
Department of Pediatrics
Universitäts Kinderklinik
Freiburgstrasse 23
3010 Bern 4, Switzerland

M. Hunkeler
Department of Chemistry
University of Maryland
College Park, Maryland 20742

Hazim J. Kadhim
Service de Neurologie Pédiatrique
Hôpital Universitaire Saint-Luc
Avenue Hippocrate 10
Boîte UCL 10/1303
B-1200 Brussels, Belgium

Norman Kretchmer
Department of Nutritional Sciences
University of California
College of Natural Resources
Agricultural Experiment Station
Berkeley, California 94720

Isabelle Labrique
International Institute of Cellular
  and Molecular Pathology (ICP)
Catholic University of Louvain
75 Avenue Hippocrate
B-1200 Brussels, Belgium

Hans Lou*
John F. Kennedy Institut
Department of Neuropediatrics
G1. Landevej 7
2600 Glostrup, Denmark

Manuela Martìnez*
Autonomous University of Barcelona
Hospital Infantil Vall d'Hebron
Paseo Vall d'Hebron S/N
Barcelona 08035, Spain

Alexandre Minkowski*
INSERM Unité 29
Centre de Recherches de Biologie
  du Développement Foetal et Néonatal
123 Blvd. de Port-Royal
75674 Paris Cédex 14, France

J. Mushin
Department of Pediatrics and Neonatal
  Medicine
Royal Postgraduate Medical School
Hammersmith Hospital
Du Cane Road
London W12 OHS, England

H. Pérez
Institute of Nutrition and Food
  Technology (INTA)
University of Chile
Santiago 11, Chile

P.J. Pretorius
Department of Chemistry
University of Maryland
College Park, Maryland 20742

H.J. Roth
Department of Chemistry
University of Maryland
College Park, Maryland 20742

S. Ruiz
Institute of Nutrition
  and Food Technology (INTA)
University of Chile
Santiago 11, Chile

C. Sotelo*
INSERM Unité 106
Histologie Normale et Pathologique
  du Système Nerveux
Hôpital de la Salpêtrière
47 Boulevard de l'Hôpital
75651 Paris Cédex 13, France

Rubén Soto-Moyano*
Institute of Nutrition and Food
  Technology (INTA)
University of Chile
Casilla 15138
Santiago 11, Chile

Martin H. Teicher*
Department of Psychiatry
Harvard Medical School
Mailman Research Center and McLean
  Hospital
115 Mill Street
Belmont, Massachusetts 02178

Joseph Vamecq
International Institute of Cellular
  and Molecular Pathology (ICP)
Catholic University of Louvain
75 Avenue Hippocrate
B-1200 Brussels, Belgium

François Van Hoof
International Institute of Cellular
  and Molecular Pathology (ICP)
  and Service de Neurologie Pédiatrique
Hôpital Universitaire Saint-Luc
Avenue Hippocrate 10
Boîte UCL 10/1303
B-1200 Brussels, Belgium

Joseph Volpe*
Division of Neurology
Departments of Pediatrics, Neurology,
and Biological Chemistry
Washington University School of Medicine
St. Louis Children's Hospital
400 South Kingshighway Boulevard
P.O. Box 14871
St. Louis, Missouri 63178

Roger S. Williams*
Department of Neurology
The Billings Clinic
2512 Irving Place
Billings, Montana 59101

Invited Attendees

Manuel Nieto Barrera / *Seville, Spain*
Béchir Hamza / *Tunis, Tunisia*
Manuel Moya Benavent / *Alicante,*
  Spain
Juan Brines Solanes / *Valencia, Spain*
Ching-Siang-Chi / *Taichung, Taiwan*
Emilio Fernández Alvarez /
  Barcelona, Spain
Carmen Roche Ferrero / *Madrid,*
  Spain
E.A. Haan / *Parkville, Australia*
S.K. Hendarto / *Jakarta, Indonesia*

Krishnan / *Kuala Lumpur, Malaysia*
M.T. Lahrech / *Rabat, Morocco*
A.H. Markum / *Jakarta, Indonesia*
Carlos Martì Henneberg / *Barcelona,*
  Spain
Fernando Mulas Delgado / *Valencia,*
  Spain
Ignacio Pascual Castroviejo / *Madrid,*
  Spain
José Quero Jiménez / *Madrid, Spain*
Manuel Roig Quillis / *Barcelona,*
  Spain

Nestlé Participants

Pierre R. Guesry
Vice President
Nestec Ltd.
Vevey, Switzerland
Philippe Goyens
Nestec Ltd.
Vevey, Switzerland

Carlos Conill Forcadell
Sociedad Nestlé A.E.P.A.
Barcelona, Spain
Antonio Quesada Marco
Sociedad Nestlé A.E.P.A.
Barcelona, Spain

Nestlé Nutrition Workshop Series

Developmental Neurobiology, edited by
Philippe Evrard and Alexandre Minkowski.
Nestlé Nutrition Workshop Series, Vol. 12.
Nestec Ltd., Vevey/Raven Press, Ltd.,
New York © 1989.

Normal Development of Cerebral Neocortex

Verne S. Caviness, Jr.

Division of Pediatric Neurology, Massachusetts General Hospital and Harvard Medical School, Boston, Massachusetts 02114

The mammalian central nervous system develops through a series of complex cellular processes which may be grouped into two broad phases (1,2). The first, cytogenesis and histogenesis, is a phase in which neurons are formed, move to their correct positions, and elaborate the primary neuritic processes which contribute to emerging dendritic fields and axon fascicles. The second, differentiation and growth, is a phase in which neurons increase in overall size and with respect to the complexity of their structural and molecular organization. During this phase they elaborate terminal dendritic and axonal arborizations and form connections.

It is important to realize that the incremental processes, cell generation and growth and synaptogenesis, are not definitive morphogenetic events. The fine details of neuronal structure and organization of circuitry depend upon regressive events which occur terminally during development (3–5). Depending upon the part of the nervous system in question, these include cell death as well as axonal pruning and synaptic elimination. It is probable that these regressive processes serve to optimize the final configuration of projections, both quantitatively and with respect to patterns of divergence or convergence. They probably add substantially to the potential of the developing nervous system to adapt to injury.

Although not emphasized in this chapter, the events of neural development depend upon and are closely coordinated with the development of nonneuronal cell populations (6,7). These include the intrinsic neuroglial elements—astrocytes and oligodendroglia. The former play critical structural, supportive, and metabolic roles in the nervous system throughout life. The latter form the myelin investments of axons which are essential to electrical conduction.

The cellular events of development unfold through an extended segment of the life of the organism. In man they continue through intrauterine life and well into postnatal life (6–9). The phase of cytogenesis and histogenesis is, relatively speaking, quickly accomplished. With respect to the human central nervous system, and in particular the forebrain, the cytogenetic and histogenetic events are largely completed during the first half of gestation. They proceed well into the first postnatal year in the cerebellum. The phase of differentiation and growth proceeds most rapidly during the second half of gestation and in the first 6 to 12 months of postnatal life. However, it continues at a slower rate much longer. Thus it may continue to shape the structure and adaptive potential of the nervous system of the child through the early school years and even beyond into postpubertal life.

It is a corollary of the complexity of developmental events that they are associated with an unrivaled level of risk to the organism (10). In humans the risk of mortality may be as high as 30% during the first trimester of gestation and remains high, as much as eight times that of the general population, through the first six postnatal months. Grossly evident malformation, functionally or cosmetically significant, is characteristic of 3% to 5% of live births, and malformation of the central nervous system is conspicuous among these. The gravest structural anomalies, in general, result from disorders that disrupt cytogenetic or histogenetic events. Among these survival is improbable, and where it occurs, functional disability is grave.

Substantial disability may result from disorders of development which do not lead to deformities that are grossly evident at birth. Large numbers of these lesser disturbances may be ascertained only by their functional consequences, such as disturbances of learning, language disorders, autism, and recurrent seizures. It is probable that these milder disorders reflect, in most instances, disturbances of the processes of growth and differentiation.

CYTOGENESIS AND HISTOGENESIS

Neurogenesis

The central nervous system is a vast community of neurons, numbering more than 12 billion in man (9,11). The majority of neurons and many glial cells are generated in a specialized pseudostratified columnar epithelium which lines the ventricular cavities. At the ventricular surface, adjacent cells are bound together by specialized intercellular junctions. The subventricular aspect of each cell is free to move to and fro with respect to the plane of fixation at the ventricular surface. During the phase of DNA synthesis, the cell is elongated with the nucleus in an extreme subventricular position. As the DNA cycle enters the G_2-phase, the cell constricts to become spherical at the ventricular surface where mitosis occurs.

As development proceeds, additional populations of cells undergo their terminal divisions in a subventricular zone, located just distal to the ventricular zone. It is probable that most, perhaps all, cells generated in the subventricular zone are glial. Certain other well-recognized zones of cell generation are located more superficially in the wall of the developing brain. An extensively studied example in the cerebellum is the external granular layer, a subpially located generative zone which gives rise to the granule cells, interneurons of the molecular layer, and certain glial species of the cerebellar cortex. In humans and other primates, a subpial germinal layer (Brunn) arises transiently in the rostrolateral region of the developing cerebrum. The fate of cells arising in this zone is unknown. Additional populations of neurons, exceptional in their place of origin, include the granular pyramids of the dentate gyrus of the hippocampal formation and the granule cells of the olfactory bulb. Both these cell classes undergo their terminal divisions within the cortical structures that they inhabit. Their terminal divisions thus occur in positions remote from the periventricular germinal zones which give rise to other neurons of the same cortical structures.

Cell Class Determination

The neuronal populations of the nervous system are composed of multiple classes, each class distinctive by virtue of its morphology, namely, its general size and patterns of dendritic and axonal arborization (4,9,12). Each class is further distinctive because of its patterns of afferent and efferent connections. Finally, each has a distinctive set of transmitter substances as well as other molecular properties. Within the cerebrum and cerebellum and, perhaps, widely in the central nervous system, determination of cell class is probably completed and irreversible as a consequence of molecular-genetic events occurring within the generative zone rather than subsequently in the life history of the cell. The antecedent molecular genetic events are probably region-specific. Thus, the generative zone of origin of cerebral neocortical neurons gives rise to entirely different neuronal classes than the zone of origin of cerebellar cortical neurons.

It is unclear when the molecular events of determination occur with respect to generation order in a given lineage, and this may differ from cell class to cell class. Determination of astrocytic lineage, at least insofar as it is expressed by the synthesis of glial fibrillary acidic protein (GFAP), appears to occur with a terminal division in the ventricular zone (13). With respect to the cerebral neocortex, the principal classes are generated in a set sequence. Possibly each class is an "obligatory" product of a terminal division within a given generative sequence (14). Thus cell division in a given sector of the generative zone will form successively the polymorphic, large pyramidal, stellate, medium and small pyramidal cells, that is, the principal neuronal classes of the neocortex. Factors extrinsic to the dividing cells may have little influence on the determination of class as generation sequences continue. Thus the neuron classes which issue from a region of generative epithelium may in some instances be produced even if cell division proceeds *in vitro*. This is certainly the case for the granular cells of the cerebellar cortex. Multiple neuronal classes of the cerebral neocortex are able to achieve their distinctive class-characteristic morphologies even when they differentiate in subcortical locations at only a short remove from the ventricular zone (12).

It is possible that certain neuronal classes are committed even prior to their terminal division. For example, the number of Purkinje cells surviving in the cerebellar cortex of normal mouse-lurcher mutant chimeras is variable but always an integral multiple of 10,000 (15). By extrapolation from the length of the generative cycle and the time of the terminal division, determination of this cell class would occur as early as the seventh to eighth embryonic day, that is, about the time of neurulation and well before the Purkinje cells undergo their terminal divisions.

Cell Deployment

The majority of neurons of the central nervous system are generated in epithelia removed, variably, from the positions they will occupy in the adult nervous system. Once their divisions are completed, the young neurons must travel substantial distances to reach their definitive positions. Particularly where long migrations are involved, the young neurons move as freely motile elements, crossing a terrain of great complexity. The task seems particularly challenging for the neurons of the cerebral neocortex of the primate which arise during late stages of cytogenesis. These young cells must travel distances that are hundreds of times their own diameters (9).

The final positions that the neuron will come to occupy in the neocortex may be predicted from the position in the generative zone and the time at which the cell undergoes its terminal mitosis. Its position with respect to the tangential coordinates of the cortex appears to depend upon the tangential coordinates of its position in the ventricular zone at the time it undergoes its terminal division (14). Thus, the mechanism of cell migration is such that it provides for an orderly topologic transformation of the generative zone upon the cortex, apparently with minimal lateral mixing. The final position in the radial dimension of the cortex, on the other hand, depends upon the point in the sequence of cell divisions that gives rise to the cell. Thus there is a systematic inside-out relationship between cell generation order and cell position in the cortex. That is, the earliest formed cells will inhabit the deepest cortical layer, layer VI, whereas progressively later formed cells will occupy positions at progressively more superficial layers.

The radially outward migratory movements of the cell are guided by close apposition to the surface of specialized glial elements, the radial glial cells of the forebrain, and the Bergmann glial cells of the cerebellar cortex (9). In the case of the forebrain, the cell body of the glial cell is located deep in the cerebral wall, in or close to the ventricular zone. A centrally directed process is attached to the periventricular basal lamina. A radially ascending process continues upward from the cell body to cross the full width of the cerebral wall. The ascending process branches only within the marginal zone where the terminal branches become integral with the limiting glial membrane.

The ascent of the young neuron along the radial glial fiber appears to depend principally upon an interaction between the young neuron and the glial cell and may be independent of interactions with other tissue elements. Thus the phenomenon has been observed to proceed relatively normally in isolation within a teratoma removed surgically in the perinatal period from a human brain (16). It may occur in explants of tissue from experimental animals maintained *in vitro* (17). The neuronal–glial interaction is probably implemented by a highly selective molecular affinity between neuronal and glial surfaces.

Its ascent completed, the young neuron appears to become detached from the glial fiber and instead becomes adherent to other postmigratory elements in its milieu. Despite substantial subsequent expansion of the cortex in the process of growth and cellular differentiation, young postmigratory cells maintain their position with respect to other migratory cohorts (14). Although the glial fiber provides guidance to the young neuron in its ascent across the cerebral wall, it may not provide the clues which direct the cell to its laminar destination within the cortex. Other structures, quite separate from the radial glial fiber, may dictate the radial level at which the cell terminates its migration.

The molecular layer itself, acting as a mechanical barrier, may determine the point of arrest of migration (18). It is a zone of densely packed, tangentially aligned axons, among other classes of neurites. One observes, in support of this possibility, that young neurons of the neocortex uniformly continue their migrations until they reach the molecular layer, where they stop. Further, in certain developmental disorders in man which are associated with disruption of the molecular layer with formation of a mesenchymal–glial scar between superficial cortex and leptomeninges, young neurons may continue their outward movement through the breach in the molecular layer barrier. They may actually continue their movements beyond the confines of the cerebrum and establish viable ectopic colonies in the extracerebral subarachnoid compartment (18).

GROWTH AND DIFFERENTIATION

After the young neuron has completed its last mitotic division, it undergoes molecular transformations which are expressed in dramatic enlargement of cell soma, neurite outgrowth, and progressive elaboration of its dendritic surfaces and axonal systems. The greater part of this explosive change is delayed until after the cell has completed its migration and achieved its position relative to other elements. However, for certain populations of cells, for example the large projection neurons of neocortical layers V and VI and the cerebellar granular cells, axonal elaboration may proceed concurrently with migration (19).

Neuritic outgrowth, both axonal and dendritic, is directed by a terminally expanded specialized organelle referred to as the growth cone (4,20). It is a principal locus of cell membrane addition during the process of axonal elongation. The membranous surface of the growth cone is replete with receptors of multiple classes, and the growth cone appears to release transmitter substances in its movements. Probing filapodial and laminar extensions issue transiently from the growth cone as the structure "feels its way along." The directed growth behavior of the elongating neurite, led by its growth cone, has been shown *in vitro* to be strongly directed by substances in its microenvironment. With regard to outgrowing neurites of anterior horn cells or peripheral sensory ganglia, the neurite responds to undefined substances from either nerve or muscle condition media or to nerve growth factor. The outgrowing neurites will grow selectively on surfaces impregnated with such trophic factors. They will turn actively in the direction of and grow toward trophic factors delivered into the culture medium in soluble form as a jet.

No such direct evidence establishes trophic control over neurite growth within the central nervous system, although circumstantial evidence for it is strong. With regard to the developing pyramidal cells of the neocortex, elaboration of apical and basal dendritic systems appears to occur in reciprocal relation to contact with axonal components of the molecular and subplate layers (14). Where the positional relationship of the neuronal soma and the axonal plexuses is anomalous, as for example in the neocortex and cerebellar cortex of the reeler mutant mouse, the pattern of primary dendritic branching may be anomalous. As under normal circumstances, however, the direction of outgrowth is toward adjacent axonal plexuses, and branching occurs only within these plexuses (14).

A host of soluble and membrane-bound substances might act with variable selectivity to direct the growth behavior of neurites in the central nervous system. Within the neocortex the noradrenergic and GABAergic projection systems are both candidates. Axons which synthesize and contain these transmitters ascend from brain stem sources to ramify richly as components of the earliest axonal plexuses of the molecular and subplate layers of the neocortex (21). Receptors for the adrenergic transmitters are co-localized on cellular processes from the earliest time of entry of the axonal systems (22).

Axons of long projection tend to grow together in a common fascicle toward a projection target and may do so for great distances, depending upon the specific system. Collateral branches may arise from the fascicle along its length. Only terminally, however, do the axons defasciculate as they direct their terminal arborizations toward their selected synaptic targets. Homophilic binding of axon to axon by cell adhesion molecules may be the molecular mechanism providing for such fasciculation. Antibodies against one of these neuronal cell adhesion molecules (NCAM) have been shown to disrupt fasciculation of the retinofugal projection of chicks (5). As might be predicted, NCAM is not expressed on the terminal portions of the axons, beyond the point of defasciculation which gives rise to the final arborizations.

The trajectory followed by an axonal fascicle may be determined by interactions between "pioneer" axonal processes and other possibly non-axonal and even non-neuronal elements stationed along the way. Initial decussation of fibers of the corpus callosum, for example, appears to depend upon guidance over the surface of an interhemispheric bridging glial platform ("glial sling"). An acallosal forebrain results when this sling is disrupted surgically or fails to develop as a consequence of autosomal recessive mutation (2).

The pattern of distribution of terminals of a projection beyond the point of defasciculation is probably governed by multiple factors. With regard to those projections that are topologically ordered, as with the retinotectal projection, the process of matching source to target appears to be simplified somewhat by the fact that the relative positions of cells of origin generally anticipate the relative positions of axons in the optic nerve and tract. That is, axons which are side by side in the axon fascicle come from and go to neighboring cells.

Molecular complementarity of axon and target structures probably also acts to assure conjunction of the appropriate structures. Thus, from a limited series of studies in the developing retinotectal projection of the chick, it appears that there are certain antigens expressed at graded concentrations on the cell membranes of both retinal and tectal cells (23). The alignment of these gradients with respect to the coordinates of the retina corresponds to a retinotopic order as projected upon the tectum, suggesting that the antigens could play a role in the alignment mechanism. It should be noted, however, that the pattern of termination of projections is in some measure flexible. Thus the entirety of the retinal projection is able to contract in orderly topologic fashion upon a substantially reduced target where the tectal surface has been partially ablated (24).

Synaptogenesis

Synaptogenesis, quantitatively speaking, is a relatively late event in the course of neural growth and differentiation (25,26), although a trivial proportion of the full synaptic complement does appear early in histogenesis. Widely dispersed synapses may, for example, be identified in the molecular and subplate layers of the neocortex from the earliest events of neocortical histogenesis. Much later in development, as dendritic arbors of neurons approach their definitive sizes and shapes and spines appear on spiney neurons, there is a surge of synaptogenesis. Throughout the nervous system, type I asymmetric synapses are the most precocious and predominant. Their distribution is principally upon dendritic spines, where present, and smaller, relatively distal segments of a given dendritic arbor. Type II symmetric synapses are less numerous, appear relatively late in the course of neural development, and are principally distributed on the soma and proximal dendritic trunks of target neurons.

The synapses of a given projection tend to have a highly characteristic distribution in the terminal field—selective with respect to target cell class and relatively uniform with respect to pattern and density of distribution upon the target cells. Further, the morphologic characteristics of the synaptic junction, for example its length and degree of curvature, may be highly characteristic of the contact between a projection and cell class. These attributes of the synaptic pattern characteristic of a projection may be characteristic only if the projection in question develops normally. Quite uncharacteristic or "plastic" modifications may be obtained under abnormal conditions of development. Thus, where the cerebellar Purkinje cell develops in isolation from the parallel fiber axons of granular cells, it may accept heterotopic synapsis from incoming mossy fibers (27). Further, the pattern of distribution as well as the pre- and postsynaptic membrane specializations may be dramatically unlike anything encountered under conditions of normal development. Thus both spines and membranous densities may be grotesquely enlarged and the latter may persist in isolation from synaptic junctions (28).

Regressive Events

Regressive events (cell death, axonal pruning, and synaptic elimination) appear to be characteristic of many, perhaps all, regions of the central nervous system (3). They occur as terminal mechanisms of development and are generally delayed until projections approach their final configurations. The degree of change in a system occurring with these regressive processes may be substantial in scale. Thus as many as 50% of anterior horn cells and retinal ganglion cells may be eliminated by "naturally programmed cell death" (29). Programmed death appears to eliminate neurons from the superficial neocortical layers, although the impact of this process upon connectivity is uncertain.

Regressive processes appear to be influenced profoundly by the integrity and functional state of the neural system in question as well as by metabolic properties of the milieu. With regard to the anterior horn cells of the spinal cord, the portion of cells to die may be diminished by a limb graft, which increases the size of the target field of projection of this cell class (29). Reciprocally, the number to die may be heightened by removal of the target field. Somewhat paradoxically, the process of death may be substantially delayed by blocking synaptic conduction with curare.

Axonal pruning has been demonstrated to be a vigorous phenomenon with respect to multiple neocortical projections and occurs without death of the cell of origin (30). Presumably, the cell chooses another principal target of projection at the same time that it prunes back the axon to be lost. A particularly dramatic example of this phenomenon is the loss of callosal axons linking the temporal visual field representations of neocortical area 17, which occurs in a wide range of mammalian species (31,32). As another example thus far recognized only in rodents, a massive projection from occipital and temporal neocortical fields, present at birth, is subsequently entirely eliminated by axon pruning (3). Further, as much as 50% of a neonatal/neocortical-to-spinal projection, arising in the primary somatosensory cortical representation (SI) cortex of the mouse, is lost by axon pruning (33).

Similarly, there is a terminal overshoot in the number and density of synapses. In the visual cortex of the human cerebral hemisphere, for example, the overshoot may be 30% to 40% (25). Peak synaptic complement is achieved in the first 6 to 12 months of postnatal life and sustained for approximately 1 to 2 years. Subsequent regression to adult levels occurs between 5 and 10 years of age. The noradrenergic projection appears to be one of multiple regulators of the synaptic elimination phenomenon. It has been demonstrated in rodents that destruction of this projection is associated with a terminal delay in pruning of synapses, although the normal complement is eventually achieved (34). Where the system has been destroyed in developing kittens, the normal adaptive functional plasticity of the visual system has been found to be impaired. Thus under conditions of monocular deprivation, the majority of neurons of the visual cortex normally become responsive principally to visual stimulation from the sighted and not the deprived eye (35). This does not occur after destruction of the noradrenergic projection; instead, approximately half remain responsive to stimuli delivered to the deprived eye (36). This plastic potential for a shift in ocular dominance after monocular deprivation may be restored by infusion of noradrenalin (36).

In man these terminal regressive phenomena, particularly synaptic elimination, occur in late gestation and in the early postnatal period. This is a time when the nervous system is critically governed in its development by environmental determinants. Thus in early postnatal life, eye occlusion or uncorrected strabismus may profoundly affect visual acuity for life. Cognitive and more broadly ranging social and perceptual potentialities may be shaped irrevocably by the quality of the environment. It is of substantial importance in this regard that certain teratogenic substances to which the fetus may be exposed (37–39), in particular alcohol, appear to depress the strength of the noradrenergic projection (40,41). Such exposure may be followed in postnatal life by substantial cognitive and memory deficits.

REFERENCES

1. Caviness VS Jr, Williams RS. Cellular patterns in developmental malformations of neocortex: neuron–glial interactions. In: Arima M, Suzuki Y, Yabuuchi H, eds. *The developing brain and its disorders*. Tokyo: University of Tokyo Press, 1984:43–67.
2. Silver J, Lorenz SE, Wahlsten D, Coughlin J. Axonal guidance during development of the great cerebral commissures: descriptive and experimental studies *in vivo* on the role of preformed glial pathways. *J Comp Neurol* 1982;210:10–29.
3. Cowan WM, Fawcett JW, O'Leary DDM, Stanfield BB. Regressive events in neurogenesis. *Science* 1984;225:1258–65.
4. Purves D, Lichtman JW. *Principles of neural development*. Sunderland, MA: Sinauer Associates, 1984;433.
5. Edelman GM. Cell-adhesion molecules: a molecular basis for animal form. *Sci Am* 1984;250:118–29.
6. Gilles FH, Leviton Λ, Dooling EC, eds. *The developing human brain*. Boston: John Wright, 1983; 349.
7. Lemire RJ, Loeser JD, Leech RW, Alvord EC Jr. *Normal and abnormal development of the human nervous system*. New York: Harper & Row, 1975;421.
8. Hamilton WJ, Boyd JD, Mossman HW. *Human embryology*. Baltimore: Williams & Wilkins, 1962;493.
9. Sidman RL, Rakic P. Development of the human central nervous system. In: Haymaker W, Adams RD, eds. *Histology and histopathology of the nervous system*. Springfield, IL: Charles C Thomas, 1982:3–145.
10. Niswander KR, Gordon M, eds. *The women and their pregnancies*. Philadelphia: WB Saunders, 1972;540.
11. Jacobson M. *Developmental neurobiology*. 2nd Ed. New York: Plenum Press, 1978;562.
12. Caviness VS Jr, Williams RS. Cellular pathology of developing human cortex. In: Katzman R, ed. *Congenital and acquired cognitive disorders*. New York: Raven Press, 1979:69–89.
13. Levitt P, Cooper MLM, Rakic P. Early divergence and changing proportions of neuronal and glial precursor cells in the primate cerebral ventricular zone. *Dev Biol* 1983;96:472–84.
14. Caviness VS, Pinto-Lord MC, Evrard P. The development of laminated pattern in the mammalian cortex. In: Brinkley LL, Carlson BM, Connelly TG, eds. *Morphogenesis and pattern formation*. New York: Raven Press, 1981:103–26.
15. Wetts R, Herrup K. Cerebellar Purkinje cells are descended from a small number of progenitors committed during early development: quantitative analysis of lurcher chimeric mice. *J Neurosci* 1982;2:1494–8.
16. Landrieu P, Goffinet A, Caviness VS, Lyon G. Formation of neocortex in a congenital human teratoma. *Acta neuropathol* 1981;55:35–8.
17. Hatten ME, Liem RKH, Mason CA. Defects in specific associations between astroglia and neurons occur in microcultures of weaver mouse cerebellar cells. *J Neurosci* 1984;4:1163–72.
18. Caviness VS Jr, Evrard P, Lyon G. Radial neuronal assemblies, ectopia and necrosis of developing cortex: a case analysis. *Acta Neuropathol (Berlin)* 1978;41:67–72.
19. Shoukimas GM, Hinds JW. The development of the cerebral cortex in the embryonic mouse: an electron microscopic serial section analysis. *J Comp Neurol* 1978;179:795–830.

20. Gundersen RW, Park KHC. The effects of conditioned media on spinal neurites: substrate-associated changes in neurite direction and adherence. *Dev Biol* 1984;104:18–27.
21. Caviness VS Jr, Korde MG. Monaminergic afferents to the neocortex. A developmental histofluorescence study in normal and reeler mouse embryos. *Brain Res* 1981;209:1–9.
22. Goffinet AM, Hemmendinger LM, Caviness VS Jr. Autoradiographic study of beta-1 adrenergic receptor development in the mouse forebrain. *Dev Brain Res* 1986;24:187–91.
23. Trisler CD, Schneider MD, Nirenberg M. A topographic gradient of molecules in retina can be used to identify neuron position. *Proc Natl Acad Sci USA* 1981;78:2145–9.
24. Schneider GE, So KF, Jhaveri S, Edwards MA. Regeneration, re-routing and redistribution of axons after early lesions: changes with age and functional impact. In: Dimitrijevic M, Eccles JC, eds. *Recent advances in restorative neurology, upper motorneuron function and disfunction*. New York.Karger, 1985.295–310.
25. Huttenlocher PR. Synapse elimination and plasticity in developing human cerebral cortex. *Am J Ment Defic* 1984;88:488–96.
26. Lund RD. *Development and plasticity of the brain*. New York: Oxford University Press, 1978;370.
27. Wilson L, Sotelo C, Caviness VS Jr. Heterologous synapses upon Purkinje cells in the cerebellum of the reeler mutant mouse: an experimental light and electron microscopic study. *Brain Res* 1981;213:63–82.
28. Mariani J, Crepel F, Mikoshiba K, Changeux J-P, Sotelo C. Anatomical, physiological and biochemical studies of the cerebellum from reeler mutant mouse. *Philos Trans R Soc London* 1977;281:1–28.
29. Oppenheim RW, Chu-Wang I-W. Aspects of naturally occurring motorneuron death in the chick spinal cord during embryonic development. In: Burnstock G, Vrbova G, eds. *Somatic and autonomic nerve–muscle interactions*. New York: Elsevier, 1983:57–107.
30. Innocenti GM. Development of interhemispheric cortical connections. *Neurosci Res Program Bull* 1982;20:532–40.
31. Innocenti GM. Growth and reshaping of axons in the establishment of visual callosal connections. *Science* 1981;212:824–7.
32. Ivy GO, Akers RM, Killackey HP. Differential distribution of callosal projection neurons in the neonatal and adult rat. *Brain Res* 1979;173:532–7.
33. Crandall JE, Whitcomb JM, Caviness VS Jr. Development of the spinal-medullary projection from the mouse barrel field. *J Comp Neurol* 1985;239:205–15.
34. Blue ME, Parnavelas JG. The effect of neonatal 6-hydroxydopamine treatment on synaptogenesis in the visual cortex of the rat. *J Comp Neurol* 1982;205:199–205.
35. Wiesel TN. The postnatal development of the visual cortex and the influence of environment. Nobel lecture, 8 December 1981. Stockholm: Norstedts Tryckeri, 1982.
36. Kasamatsu T, Pettigrew JD, Ary M. Restoration of visual cortical plasticity by local microperfusion of norepinephrine. *J Comp Neurol* 1979;185:163–82.
37. Clarren SK, Smith DW. The fetal alcohol syndrome. *N Engl J Med* 1978;298:1063–7.
38. Streissguth AP, Herman CS, Smith DW. Intelligence, behavior and dysmorphogenesis in the fetal alcohol syndrome: a report on 20 patients. *J Pediatr* 1978;92:363–7.
39. Streissguth AP, Landesman-Dwyer S, Martin JC, Smith DW. Teratogenic effects of alcohol in humans and laboratory animals. *Science* 1980;209:353–61.
40. Lichtensteiger W, Schlumpf M, Davis MD. Catecholamines and nicotine in early neuroendocrine organization. *Monogr Neurol Sci* 1983;9:213–24.
41. Shoemaker WJ, Baetge G, Azad R, Sapin V, Bloom FE. Effect of prenatal alcohol exposure on amine and neurotransmitter systems. *Monogr Neural Sci* 1983;9:130–9.

Developmental Neurobiology, edited by
Philippe Evrard and Alexandre Minkowski.
Nestlé Nutrition Workshop Series, Vol. 12.
Nestec Ltd., Vevey/Raven Press, Ltd.,
New York © 1989.

Cerebral Malformations Arising in the First Half of Gestation

Roger S. Williams

Eunice Kennedy Shriver Center, Waltham, Massachusetts 02154

The brain evolves through a series of temporally overlapping stages. Brain malformations may be analyzed in the context of the stage or stages during which the pathologic process was judged to be initially and maximally active.

Cytogenesis is the stage of maximal proliferation of neurons and glia. Most neurons of the spinal cord and brain stem are generated by 10 weeks (menstrual age). Most neurons of the forebrain including the cerebral hemispheres are generated by 20 weeks (1,2). Known exceptions include the granule cells of the dentate gyrus and cerebellum, which continue to proliferate postnatally. The proliferation of astrocytes and oligodendroglia also extends into the postnatal period. In contrast to neurons, glial cells retain the ability to proliferate throughout the life of the individual.

The definitive structure of the brain arises during the stage of histogenesis (1–4). Histogenesis occurs as postmitotic brain cells move, differentiate, and interact with each other and surrounding non-neural tissues in a series of sequential steps. Neurulation is an early, brief step in the process of histogenesis. The neural tube closes at 28 to 30 days gestation. Neurulation is mediated in part by the interaction of neuroectoderm and surrounding structures, especially the notocord and prechordal mesoderm. Development of optic and olfactory structure is "induced" by interaction with adjacent mesoectoderm. The cerebral vesicles evaginate and are "cleaved" into two hemispheres, probably because they are constrained at the midline by the relatively more inert anterior wall (lamina terminalis) of the third ventricle. Postmitotic young neurons migrate from their birthplace in the germinal tissue adjacent to ventricles to their definitive positions. Many neurons seem to require an interaction with the processes of specialized astrocytes, the radial glia, to complete long-distance migration through an increasingly complicated terrain. The "end-foot" specializations of radial glial processes also interact with the pia and its underlying basement membrane to form a trilaminate envelope that, in conjunction with the dura and skull, constrains the developing brain. The hydraulic forces generated by the formation of cerebrospinal fluid from the choroid plexus within the ventricles and the amniotic fluid surrounding the fetus are also critical determinants of the integrity and final form of the developing brain. Specialized cytoplasmic processes (axons and dendrites) grow and differentiate from young neurons. These are the structural basis for the intercellular connections characteristic of the mature nervous system. Axons converge on the anterior wall of the third ventricle, guided perhaps by a sling-like mat of glial processes, and cross the midline in selected areas to form the major forebrain commissures. Growing axons fasciculate together and seek out their targets selectively. The growing processes seem to be genetically preprogrammed with hierarchical preferences for surface molecules on target cells with which they can interact. For most if not all brain areas, the number of nerve cells generated is greatly in excess of the number surviving to maturity. Presumably nerve cells of the same type must compete with each other for available postsynaptic connections. The least successful competitors will die. Similarly, synaptic connections are initially more exuberant and are ultimately pruned to more efficient densities. The phenomena of natural cell death (5) and synaptic remodeling (6) may provide a safety factor that ensures normal brain development over a wide range of environmental stresses.

Disruption of the above mechanisms can be expected to result in substantial structural abnormalities of the developing brain. A number of characteristic syndromes have been identified (3,7–9). Fortunately, most are relatively uncommon. With few exceptions, the etiologic agents and their pathological mechanisms of action are largely unknown. In general, the structural abnormalities take three basic forms: true malformations, tissue deformations secondary to abnormal mechanical factors, and tissue destruction. In the following brief discussion, selected examples will be discussed in light of the developmental stage and epoch when the pathological process seemed to be initially and maximally active. Table 1 lists classical examples of cerebral malformations along with the timetable of normal developmental events (10).

DISORDERS OF CYTOGENESIS

Although there are no well-defined malformations of the human brain known to result from abnormal cytogenesis, extreme microcephaly is a plausible candidate (7). The number of neurons formed in any brain region is determined by at least three factors (4): duration of the proliferative period as a whole, which depending on the brain region, may vary from a few days to several months; duration of the cell cycle, which may vary from a few hours to several days and may vary over time among cells of the same region and between cells of different regions; and total number of precursor cells from which a neural population is derived.

In experimental animals, microcephaly can be produced by extreme malnutrition, toxins such as alcohol and antimetabolites, and by X-radiation during the critical period of cytogenesis. Infectious agents, such as rubella viruses, cause microcephaly in humans. Presumably these agents reduce the total number of precursor cells. The frequent occurrence of microcephaly in familial syndromes with multiple congenital anomalies and in chromosomal disorders suggests that genetic factors are also important.

TABLE 1. *Summary of developmental events in the human central nervous system*

Gestational age in weeks	Important developmental events[a]	Behavioral correlates[b]	Malformations
3rd	Neural folds close to form neural tube, begining in cervical region, and progressing rostrally and caudally Cranial and cervical flexures appear Spinal and cranial motor nuclei develop		Rachischisis
4th	Paired optic vesicles evaginate Spinal and cranial motor nerves emerge Spinal ganglia develop and axons enter CNS Closure of neural tube		Myelomeningocele Exencephaly-anencephaly
5th	Diencephalic nuclei develop Pineal and hypophysis evaginate from diencephalon Evagination of telencephalic (cerebral) vesicles Orbit and lens induced by the optic primordia Choroid plexus develops and CSF fills neural tube Basal ganglia and amygdala develop Major cerebral arteries form Canalization and development of the caudal spinal cord Posterior commissure develops Germinal cells appear in rhombic lip (primordia for the cerebellum and cerebellar relay nuclei) Thinning of the roof of the 4th ventricle (posterior membranous area) allows egress of CSF		Holoprosencephaly-cyclopia "Caudal regression syndrome" Dandy-Walker syndrome
6th	Neural retina develops Olfactory nerves grow through ethmoid to base of brain Secretory vesicles appear in choroid plexus Allocortical (hippocampus, olfactory) primordia appears		Anophthalmia retinal colobomas
7th	Neocortical primordia appears Olfactory bulb evaginates Formation of pigmented retinal epithelium and ciliary body	Aversive movement of head to perioral stimulation	Arrhinencephaly (absence of olfactory structures) Aniridia
8th–11th	Cortical plate appears in neocortex First synapses appear in the mo-	Stimulation of face—lids close, head and trunk turn aver-	Cerebral, cerebellar, and brain stem heterotopias

(continued)

TABLE 1. *(continued)*

Gestational age in weeks	Important developmental events[a]	Behavioral correlates[b]	Malformations
	lecular layer and subplate regions of neocortex	sively, and pelvis rotates	Arthrogryposis
	Neurons migrate from the rhombic lip	Stimulation of lips—ventral flexion of head toward stimulus, mouth opens	Hydrocephalus
	Retinogeniculate (optic nerve) pathways form		
	Germinal zone of 3rd ventricle is exhausted	Flexion of fingers to palmar stimulation	
	Cortical plate of cerebellum appears	Flexion of leg with genital stimulation	
	Anterior commissure develops	Plantar flexion with stimulation of the sole	
	Cortical plate of the hippocampus develops		
	Hippocampal commissure appears		
	Sylvian and hippocampal fissures form		
	Skeletal muscle (including spindles) innervated and joint cavities differentiate		
	Basal foramina and subarachnoid spaces open		
12th–15th	Corpus callosum forms	Stimulation of face—eyes move, facial "sneer", mouth opens	Agenesis of corpus callosum (and Probst bundle)
	Cavum septum pellucidum formed		Lissencephaly-pachygyria
	Migration of neurons to neocortex in full swing; cortical wall triples in thickness	Swallowing reflex and tongue movements appear	Walker-Warburg syndrome
	Corticospinal fibers decussate		Zellweger syndrome
	Purkinje cell migration complete; inward migration of external granule cells begins	Palmomental reflex appears	
		Individual finger movements	
		Babinski reflex appears	
16th–20th	Germinal zones of lateral ventricles are depleted	Mature tactile grasp reflex	Extreme microcephaly
	Last wave of neocortical migration	Pursing of lips to oral stimulation	Hydrocephalus may cause syrinx, aqueductal stenosis, encephalocele, posterior fossa (Chiari) malformations, and excessive gyration
	Prominence of subventricular germinal zone and first wave of glial migration		
	Thalamocortical afferents invade the depths of the cortical plate, synapses appear, and large pyramidal neurons begin to differentiate		Megalencephaly (?)
	Cerebral subarachnoid spaces are open to the sagittal sinus		
	Active phase of natural nerve cell death		
20th–24th	Neuronal migration to neocortex	Respiratory move-	Classical (4 layer)

TABLE 1. *(continued)*

Gestational age in weeks	Important developmental events[a]	Behavioral correlates[b]	Malformations
	complete Granule cells of cerebellum and dentate gyrus of hippocampus continue to proliferate and migrate Radial glial cells release ventricular attachments and migrate into cortex as protoplasmic astrocytes Primary gyri and sulci form Myelination begins: retinogeniculate, brain stem auditory and visual motor, and sensory lemniscal pathways are among the first	ments and phonation Sucking reflex develops Sneeze with nasal stimulation	polymicrogyria Porencephaly Hydranencephaly Subarachnoid ectopias "White matter hypoplasia"
25th–term	Granule cell migration continues Glial proliferation continues Appearance of glial fibrils and acidic glial fibrillary protein signal increasing capacity for glial response to injury Secondary gyri and sulci form, maturation of supragranular neocortical layers begins Myelination of internal capsule begins Robust growth of dendrites and axons, and synaptogenesis	Glabellar reflex Rooting and sucking reflexes combine Traction grasp response Cremasteric reflex appears	Matrix hemorrhages Telencephalic leukoencephalopathy Cystic perinatal encephalomalacia Status marmoratus Kernicterus

[a]From refs. 1–3.
[b]From ref. 10.

DISORDERS OF HISTOGENESIS

Disorders of Neurulation

Malformations presumed to be due to failure of normal neural tube closure are among those most commonly encountered in humans, and include anencephaly, exencephaly, and spinal myelomeningocele. The incidence of these dysraphic states varies from 0.1% to 0.5% of all live births and is much higher among aborted and stillborn fetuses (7). Neural tube defects can be produced in experimental animals by the introduction of a variety of teratogens during the stage of closure of the anterior and posterior neuropores, corresponding to the fourth week of pregnancy in humans (1). Epidemiologic studies suggest that abnormal genetic and environmental factors may be causative, but in most instances the etiologic agent is never identified. Usually there are also abnormalities of the adjacent skull, face, or vertebrae. Diagnosis can be suspected when risk factors are high, and can usually be confirmed with ultrasound and elevated concentrations of alpha fetoprotein in the amniotic fluid.

Disorders of Forebrain Induction

In the fifth week the diencephalic nuclei develop, and the optic vesicles evaginate and interact with overlying mesoectodermal structures to form the orbits and lenses (1). Fibers grow from the olfactory placode toward the base of the brain through a perforant zone (cribriform plate) in the developing ethmoid bone. In the sixth week the neural retina forms, and retinal axons grow through the optic stalk toward the brain supradjacent to the developing sphenoid bone. The olfactory vesicle evaginates from the base of the brain, and as it contacts in-growing olfactory fibers, the olfactory bulbs and tracts differentiate. The major forebrain axonal commissures develop in a specialized region above the lamina terminalis in the anterior wall of the third ventricle between 10 and 12 weeks of gestation. Pathological insults occurring in this region between 5 and 12 weeks of gestation result in a spectrum of abnormalities that may include absence of fusion of the eyes (anophthalmia, cyclopia), deformity of the face and skull, partial absence and fusion of anterior diencephalic and telencephalic nuclei, failure of the developing forebrain to cleave into two hemispheres (holoprosencephaly), and absence of the forebrain commissures (agenesis of corpus callosum).

Disorders of Cerebrospinal Fluid Circulation

Encephaloceles are often included among the dysraphic conditions, but these seldom arise from regions adjacent to the seam of neural tube closure. In over 75% of cases encephalocele occurs through a defect in the occipital bone and includes relatively well-differentiated structures of the posterior cerebral hemispheres or posterior fossa. They may result from defective interaction of neuroectoderm with adjacent mesoderm, but most seem to arise from hydrocephalus and herniation of brain and leptomeninges through a locus of least resistance in the developing skull (11). Other malformations and deformations of the brain presumed to result from hydrocephalus include hydromyelia, syringomyelia, syringobulbia, the Dandy-Walker and Chiari malformations, and excessive convolution of the cerebral hemispheres (polygyria) (12). Congenital hydrocephalus is a significant problem in pediatric neurology and regrettably little is known about its pathogenesis. Congenital hydrocephalus can be produced in experimental animals by transplacental infection with certain viruses (13) and the administration of antigen–antibody complexes (14).

Disorder of Neuronal Migration

A critical step in normal histogenesis is the long-distance migration of neurons in conjunction with radial glial processes. In many regions the length of the migratory pathway is exceptionally long and migration occurs over a protracted time period. Pathological conditions that are below the threshold for tissue destruction may result in disordered neuronal migration during this period. The most characteristic of these is lissencephaly-pachygyria, a condition in which the brain has no or only a few abnormally broad gyri (7,15). The malformed cortex is abnormally thick and consists of 4 layers: a molecular layer and incompletely formed true cortex (layers 1 and 2) are separated from a broad field of heterotopic neurons (layer 4) by a thin cell-sparse zone (layer 3). The subcortical heterotopia consists of well-differentiated neurons typical of those found normally in the neocortex, and pyramidal cells are aligned normally with their apical shafts directed radially outward toward the cortical surface. Presumably cortical development proceeds normally until about 13 to 15 weeks gestation, when migration of neurons along radial glial processes is interrupted, nearly completely. Heterotopic neurons survive and differentiate normally, but do not segregate normally by cell class into recognizable tangential laminae. Other neuronal groups migrating over long distances at the same time are also affected. Heterotopic Purkinje cells are found laterally in the cerebellar hemispheres and heterotopias are present in the pons and medulla. Brain structures that develop prior to and after 13 to 15 weeks gestation have a more normal appearance. Most cases of lissencephaly-pachygyria are sporadic and the etiology is not known. In typical cases the malformation is localized to cortical regions that are at the border zones of perfusion of the major cerebral arteries. This peculiar topographic localization suggests that ischemic factors may be etiologically important in some cases, but there is no experimental support for this hypothesis. Lissencephaly-pachygyria may be seen also in conjunction with multiple facial and somatic anomalies such as the Miller-Dieker syndrome. This syndrome has been reported in siblings, and recent cytogenetic studies suggest an abnormality on chromosome 17 (16).

Two other familial syndromes are associated with abnormalities of neuronal migration. These are the Zellweger and Walker–Warburg syndromes (17,18). In Zellweger syndrome there is a characteristic abnormality of cerebral convolutions, and heterotopic neurons are found in the cerebrum, cerebellum, and brain stem. The appearance is different from that of classical lissencephaly-pachygyria. In addition to the abnormalities of migration stemming from the first half of gestation, infants with the Zellweger syndrome have abnormalities of myelination, increased numbers of reactive astrocytes, and abnormalities of kidney and liver. The absence of recognizable peroxisomes in electron micrographs and reduced peroxisomal enzyme activity suggest that the Zellweger syndrome may be a hereditary metabolic disorder affecting the development of the brain and other organs over several epochs (19). In the Walker-Warburg malformation there is retinal dysgenesis, hydrocephalus, obliteration of the subarachnoid space with reactive connective and glial tissue, multifocal necrosis at the brain surface, agyria and subcortical neuronal heterotopias in the cerebrum, and polymicrogyria of the cerebellum. Many cases have occipital encephaloceles. Although the syndrome is familial and said to exhibit an autosomal recessive pattern of inheritance (20), the neuropathological findings are more consistent with meningoencephalitis (18). However, to date attempts to isolate known infectious agents have been unsuccessful.

Disorders of Natural Cell Death

Little is known about the biological mechanisms that govern natural nerve cell death and reductive synaptic remodeling in the normal brain (5,6). There are no human cerebral malformations known to result from abnormalities of these processes. A form of anophthalmia in genetically mutant mice seems to result from failure of a normally transient population of glial cells to degenerate as retinal axons grow into the optic stalk. Extreme degrees of macrocephaly (megalencephaly) could theoretically result from a defective natural cell death. Extreme macrocephaly is rare and it is not yet clear whether these brains have excessive numbers of nerve cells or glia, abnormally exuberant synaptic connections, or some combination of both features (7). In a case studied personally (*unpublished*), the size of individual nerve cells and astrocytes seemed normal in routine and Golgi preparations.

Disorders of the Pial–Glial Barrier

Defective development of or damage to the pial–glial membrane at the surface of the brain results in abnormal passage of neural cells and processes into the subarachnoid compartment. When this occurs at the cerebral surface, the normal laminar pattern of the underlying cortex is distorted and the subarachnoid neural ectopias have a wartlike appearance (21). In some instances the defect seems to occur after the normal migration of neurons is largely complete, that is, after 20 weeks gestation, and the breech is bridged by the processes of radial glia. Subjacent neurons, which are still immature, appear to have the capacity to resume migration again and move out into the subarachnoid compartment where they survive and differentiate. Extreme examples of neuronal ectopia have been reported in infants with presumed fetal alcohol syndrome (22), but may occur also in infants without alcohol exposure.

Disorders of Cerebral Gyration

The principal gyri form on the medial surfaces of the cerebrum before 20 weeks, and on the lateral surfaces, after 24 weeks gestation in humans (23). The migrational disorders noted above cause abnormal gyration. Severe destructive processes will leave large defects in the cerebrum (hydranencephaly, porencephaly), especially if they occur before the stage of glial maturation at about 30 to 35 weeks gestation (23). By contrast, destructive lesions that cause subtotal (laminar) necrosis of the cortex result in disordered gyration (24). When these occur before 30 to 35 weeks gestation, the cortex is anomalously thin and hyperconvoluted (polymicrogyria). When they occur after 30 to 35 weeks gestation, the primary and secondary gyral architecture is established and astrocytes have the capacity to repair focal tissue damage with a glial scar. The surface appearance of shrunken gliotic gyri may also be hyperconvoluted (ulegyria) (7).

SUMMARY

Pathoanatomic analysis of these congenital malformations provides important clues to the stages of brain development that were interrupted, and hence, when the pathological process was maximally active. In some cases, the histological characteristics of the lesions also suggest plausible pathogenetic mechanisms. Armed with these clues, hypotheses can be developed regarding etiologic factors that can be tested with appropriate animal models, or in the future with improved epidemiological and neuropathological analyses of human cerebral malformations.

ACKNOWLEDGMENT

This work was supported in part by NIH grants MH 34079 and HD 04147.

REFERENCES

1. Sidman RL, Rakic P. Development of the human central nervous system. In: Haymaker W, Adams RD, eds. *Histology and histopathology of the nervous system.* Springfield, IL: Charles C Thomas, 1982:3–145.
2. Jacobson M. *Developmental neurobiology.* 2nd ed. New York: Plenum Press, 1978.
3. Lemire RJ, Loeser JD, Leech RW, et al. *Normal and abnormal development of the human nervous system.* New York: Harper & Row, 1975.
4. Cowan WM. The development of the brain. *Sci Am* 1979 Sep:57–67.
5. Oppenheim RW. Neuronal cell death and some related phenomena during neurogenesis: a selective historical review and progress report. In: Cowan WM, ed. *Studies in development neurobiology.* New York: Oxford University Press, 1981:74–133.
6. Cowan WM, Fawcett JW, O'Leary DDM, Stanfield BB. Regressive events in neurogenesis. *Science* 1984;225:1258–65.
7. Friede RL. *Developmental neuropathology.* New York: Springer, 1975.
8. Caviness VS Jr, Williams RS. Cellular pathology of developing cortex: In: Katzman R, ed. *Congenital and acquired cognitive disorders.* New York: Raven Press, 1979: 69–89.
9. Williams RS, Caviness VS Jr. Normal and abnormal development of the brain. In: Tartar RE, Goldstein G, eds. *Advances in clinical neuropsychology.* New York: Plenum, 1984:1–62.
10. Humphrey T. Some correlations between the appearance of human fetal reflexes and development of the nervous system. *Prog Brain Res* 1964;4:93–135.
11. Caviness VS Jr, Evrard P. Occipital encephalocele: a pathologic and anatomic analysis. *Acta Neuropathol* 1975;32:245–55.
12. Caviness VS Jr. The Chiari malformations of the posterior fossa and their relation to hydrocephalus. *Dev Med Child Neurol* 1976;18:103–16.
13. Adeloye A, Warkany J. Experimental congenital hydrocephalus. *Child's Brain* 1976;2:325–60.
14. Duckett S, Brent RL, Jensh RP. The morphology of immunologically induced hydrocephalus in the newborn rat. *J Neuropathol Exp Neurol* 1974;33:365–73.

15. Stewart RM, Richman DP, Caviness VS Jr. Lissencephaly and pachygyria: an architectonic and topographical analysis. *Acta Neuropathol* 1975;31:1–12.
16. Dobyns WB, Stratton RF, Parke JT, Greenberg F, Nussbaum RL, Ledbetter DH. Miller-Dieker syndrome: lissencephaly and monosomy 17p. *J Pediatr* 1983;102:552–8.
17. Evrard P, Caviness VS Jr, Prats-Vinas J, Lyon G. The mechanism of arrest of neuronal migration in the Zellweger malformation: an hypothesis based upon cytoarchitectonic analysis. *Acta Neuropathol* 1978;41:109–17.
18. Williams RS, Swisher CN, Jennings M, Ambler M, Caviness VS Jr. Cerebro-ocular dysgenesis (Walker-Warburg syndrome): neuropathologic and etiologic analysis. *Neurology* 1984;34:1531–41.
19. Moser AE, Inderjit Singh AB, Brown FR, et al. The cerebrohepatorenal (Zellweger) syndrome. *New Engl J Med* 1984;310:1141–6.
20. Pagon RA, Chandler JW, Collie WR, et al. Hydrocephalus, agyria, retinal dysplasia, encephalocele (HARD ± E) syndrome: an autosomal recessive condition. *Birth Defects* 1978;14(6B):233–41.
21. Caviness VS Jr, Evrard P, Lyon G. Radial neuronal assemblies, ectopia and necrosis of developing cortex: a case analysis. *Acta Neuropathol* 1978;41:67–72.
22. Clarren SK, Smith DW. The fetal alcohol syndrome. *New Engl J Med* 1978;298:1063–7.
23. Gilles FH, Leviton A, Dooling EC. *The developing human brain: Growth and epidemiologic neuropathology*. Boston: J Wright, 1983.
24. Williams RS, Ferrante RJ, Caviness VS Jr. The cellular pathology of microgyria: a golgi analysis. *Acta Neuropathol* 1976;36:269–83.

Developmental Neurobiology, edited by
Philippe Evrard and Alexandre Minkowski.
Nestlé Nutrition Workshop Series, Vol. 12.
Nestec Ltd., Vevey/Raven Press, Ltd.,
New York © 1989.

Abnormal Development and Destructive Processes of the Human Brain During the Second Half of Gestation

Philippe Evrard, Hazim J. Kadhim, Philippe de Saint-Georges, and Jean-François Gadisseux

Pediatric Neurology Service and Laboratory of Developmental Neurology, Hôpital Universitaire Saint-Luc, B-1200 Brussels, Belgium

Most viable developmental brain disorders occurring during the second half of gestation lead to neurological defects that can range from minimal learning or motor deficits to major motor and cognitive handicaps. These disorders are of great public health significance since the affected individuals require special attention or education as well as long-term medical care for their motor, epileptic, and intellectual handicaps.

ABNORMAL HISTOGENETIC EVENTS DURING THE SECOND HALF OF GESTATION IN THE HUMAN FOREBRAIN

Most neural cyto- and histogenetic events in the human forebrain occur during the first half of gestation. Most developmental steps in the second half of gestation launch growth and differentiation that persist long into the postnatal life (1,2) (Table 1). Residual, but important, histogenetic activities continue during the last 20 weeks of pregnancy (Table 2). Their disturbances will be reviewed in this section.

Precocious Exhaustion of the Telencephalic Germinative Activity in Microcephalia Vera

Systematic measurements of the germinative zone in the human fetal brain support the hypothesis of precocious exhaustion of germinative zone mitotic activity in typical cases of genetic microcephalia vera (3). In the normal forebrain, the absolute volume of the germinative layer reaches its maximum around the 26th week of gestation, after the end of neuronal production. In fetal microcephalia vera from our

TABLE 1. *Prenatal developmental steps with examples of abnormal development*

Cytogenesis and histogenesis (first half of gestation[a])	
Main steps	Disturbances in the developmental program[b]
1. Separation of the main embryonic sheets 2. Neurulation 3. Neuronal multiplication 4. Neuronal migration 5. Regional development of the cerebral vesicles	Errors of the program Disturbances in the performance of the program Role of aleatory aspects during execution of developmental program

Growth and differentiation (second half of gestation[c])	
Developmental features	Main lesional mechanisms[d]
Growth and arborization Connections and synaptogenesis Myelination Gliogenesis	1. Disturbances of "residual" histogenesis 2. CSF hypertension: prenatal hydrocephalus 3. Perfusion failures—hypoxias[e] 4. Infections[e] 5. Trauma[e] 6. "Minor" disturbances Intrauterine steric hindrance Minor cortical disturbances during growth and differentiation period

[a]Cyto- and histogenesis not fully completed at mid-gestation.
[b]Growth and differentiation program can be disturbed by the same mechanisms.
[c]Growth and differentiation continue during postnatal life.
[d]Role of metabolic disturbances is not detailed in this table but is discussed elsewhere in the chapter.
[e]These etiological aspects can also interfere with cytogenesis and histogenesis.
Reprinted from Evrard et al. (11), with permission of Paul H. Brookes Publishing Company.

TABLE 2. *Main histogenetic events during the second half of human gestation*

Continued neuronal production for the cerebellum and allocortex
Residual neuronal production in the telencephalic germinal layer
Migration of late-generated neurons
Brun's layer histogenesis
Glial transformation (transformation of RGCs into astrocytes)
Glial production in the germinative zone

collection,* the ventricular zone was completely lacking at the 26th week (Fig. 1). This early exhaustion of the germinative zone which dates back to the last stages of neuron production precludes the normal production of the last migrating neurons destined for layers 3 and 2. This precocious germinative exhaustion gives, therefore, a pathogenic explanation for the severe neuronal depletion in those superficial neocortical layers which characterizes the cytoarchitectonic pattern of microcephalia vera described by Williams (4). The quantitative estimate of the neuronal complement in the vertical cortical dimension performed with a method modified from Rockel's (5,6) supports this pathogenic explanation (Fig. 1). The study of younger fetal specimens of microcephalia vera would permit one to determine the fetal age at which the germinative activity fails in this disease.

Disturbances of Glial Transformation

The glycogen staining method combining reduced osmium postfixation with a modified Thiéry staining technique allows the unequivocal identification of radial glial cells (RGCs) throughout gestation and of radial glial fascicles (7,8). This method permits at the electron microscope level the identification and quantitative study of radial glial fibers (RGFs) and their relationships with migrating neurons and other neuronal elements. Moreover, it permits the study of the transformation of the RGCs into astrocytes during the second half of gestation through a process of nuclear migration (Fig. 2) and autophagy of glial processes (Fig. 3) (7,8). The application of this method in studying human abnormal neuronal patterns enabled us to describe a severe depletion of RGFs or an early glial transformation in holoprosencephaly (9) and to suggest the existence of abnormal radial glial fascicles in the Potter syndrome (10) with total renal dysplasia (11). In fetal Hunter disease, the glycogen staining method showed the distribution of storage material between glial and neuronal phases at early prenatal stages of the process (12).

Disturbances of Late Neuronal Migration

Subpial ectopias are cellular masses containing neurons that either did not normally discontinue or abnormally resumed their migration at the junction between the cortical plate and the plexiform zone and "overmigrated" into the extraneural compartment. Scars between adjacent plexiform zones and discontinuities of the subpial basal membrane are often associated with such subpial ectopias which suggests that normal arrest of migration is dependent on the integrity of the pial–glial interface. Massive neuronal ectopias are fairly common in fetal alcohol syndrome (FAS)

---

*The human brains used for this study were collected in accordance with the ethical rules of our laboratory. Human fetal brains are obtained for neuropathological and neuroanatomical studies from cases involving miscarriage, abortion, and deceased premature infants. In cases of abortion, we accept specimens only if the obstetrician submitting the specimen formally certifies that the ethical rules applicable in his department were respected.

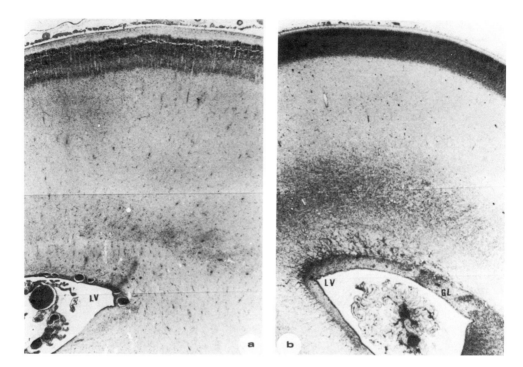

FIG. 1. Premature exhaustion of the germinative zone in microcephalia vera. **a:** Microcephalia vera, human fetal forebrain, 26th week of gestation. **b:** Normal human fetal forebrain, 26th week, same cortical region, for comparison. In microcephalia vera the germinative zone is exhausted at this age, and the intermediate zone is almost devoid of late migrating glial and neuronal cells. In the neocortex the number of neurons calculated in the vertical columns by a modified Rockel's method is 20% less than in the control; layers 6 to 4 are normal, whereas the two superficial layers are almost missing. LV, lateral ventricle; GL, germinative zone. (From ref. 11, with permission of Paul H. Brookes Publishing Company.)

(Fig. 4) without being pathognomonic for this syndrome. Subpial ectopias are also encountered in a heterogeneous group of malformations and can occasionally be present in the normal brain (13–18). In our fetal material, subpial neuronal ectopias prevail between 20 and 25 weeks of gestation, suggesting that they are a late migratory event.

Abnormalities of the Subpial Granular Layer

Brun's layer, a transitory subpial granular layer characteristic of the human fetal brain, is generated from the postolfactory germinative zone. Its volume increases until the 20th week of gestation and finally disappears around the 34th week (19,20). The fetal case of microcephalia vera shown in Fig. 1 was devoid of the subpial granular layer; this feature is in line with a precocious generalized exhaustion of the germinative zones, including that of the ganglionic eminence and postolfactory

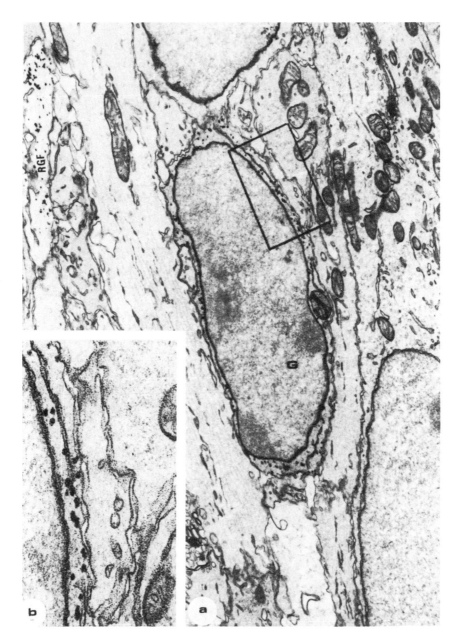

FIG. 2. Appearance of glial cell bodies within the cortical plate at the end of the period of neuronal migration. **a:** Glycogen labeling according to Gadisseux and Evrard (7). These glial nuclei appear within the cortical plate from 21st week in the human fetal neocortex and from embryonic day 18 in the mouse. **b:** Insert from **a**. G, Glial cell body, with cytoplasm containing glycogen. RGF, isolated radial glial fiber.

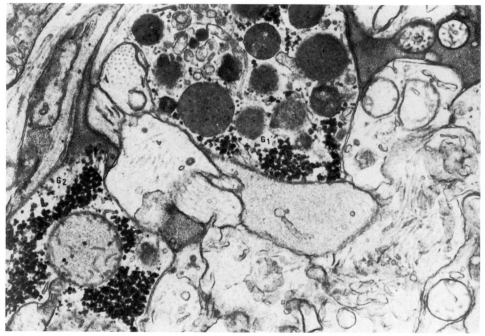

FIG. 3. Lysosomal proliferation in glial processes of radial glial cells. Human fetal molecular layer, 24th week of gestation. Glycogen staining according to ref. 8. G1 and G2, glial profiles filled with glycogen. Lysosomal proliferation in glial profile G1. Proliferation of the lysosomal apparatus and autophagy become intense, after the period of neuronal migration, in segments of RGFs during the RGC transformation into astrocytes.

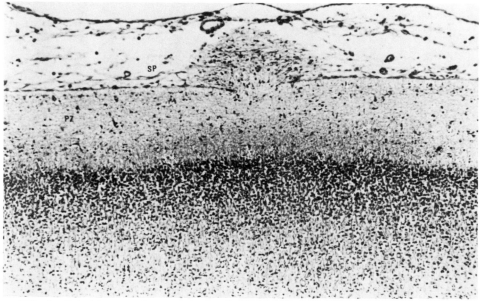

FIG. 4. Subpial neuronal ectopia. Human fetal neocortex, 24th week of gestation. Discontinuity of basal membrane and subpial neuronal ectopia. Beneath these ectopias, the laminar pattern of underlying cortex is often distorted and, less frequently, perfectly preserved, especially in the fetal alcohol syndrome (FAS). The subpial granular layer (Brun's layer) is absent in this case of FAS. PZ, molecular layer; SP, subpial space.

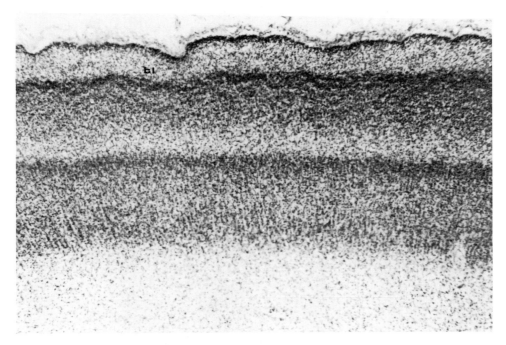

FIG. 5. Brun's layer in Neu's syndrome. Neocortex from a premature newborn with Neu's syndrome. Brun's layer is very overdeveloped and abnormally persistent in this case of Neu's syndrome. In contrast, Brun's layer is absent in cases of microcephalia vera at the 26th week of gestation (Fig. 1) and of FAS at the 24th week of gestation (Fig. 4). bl, subpial granular layer.

region. By contrast, we observed cases of microcephaly associated with Neu's syndrome displaying an abnormally conspicuous and persistent Brun's layer as well as severe disturbances of the neocortical laminar organization (Fig. 5).

PRENATAL HYPERTENSION OF THE CEREBROSPINAL FLUID

We recently completed the analysis of 124 cases of fetal hydrocephalus collected in a Multicenter Study Program organized by the Société Européenne de Neurologie Pédiatrique (21) (Table 3). The following briefly summarizes the results of the pathological and clinical observations, including prenatal ultrasound.

Most cases of prenatal hydrocephalus are secondary to hemorrhages, infections, and resorption of damaged nervous tissue causing obstructions in the cerebrospinal fluid (CSF) pathway (Table 4). The following prenatal disorders are examples of such mechanisms: (a) Membranous stenosis of the aqueduct of Sylvius is due to obliteration and subsequent thinning of the aqueductal plug under CSF pressure. The obliteration is not a consequence of a disturbance in the developmental program but can be provoked by intercurrent infections, such as mumps during the last trimester of pregnancy, which seems to have been the cause in one of our cases. (b) In

TABLE 3. *Multicenter collaborative study of prenatal abnormal brain development[a]*

Abnormality	Number of observations[b]
Anencephaly	130
Hydrocephalus	124
Meningomyelocele	59
Nondestructive microcephaly	34
Encephalocele	23
Holoprosencephaly	11
Hydranencephaly	6
Multicystic encephalomalacia	4
Intracranial tumor	4
Microgyria	3
Porencephaly	3
Megalencephaly	3
Craniostenosis	3
Acardia-acephaly	2
Primary intracerebral hemorrhage	1
Total	*410*

[a]Collaborative study program, Société Européenne de Neurologie Pédiatrique, Branch of the European Federation of Child Neurology Societies. The original data summarized in this table have been partly reported in Evrard et al. (21) and Van Lierde and Evrard (22).
[b]As of 1984.

the disorders hydranencephaly and holoprosencephaly, stenosis of the aqueduct, a frequent finding, seems to be caused by obstruction resulting from brain tissue resorption. (c) Our clinicopathological material supports the view that aqueductal stenosis in familial X-linked hydrocephalus (Bickers' and Adams' type) can be secondary to prenatal compression of the mesencephalon by the dilated lateral ventricles (23). The Multicenter Collaborative Program provided a large collection of Bickers' and Adams' cases that had been followed prenatally by ultrasound. Analysis of this material permitted two clear conclusions about the natural history of this

TABLE 4. *Prenatal hydrocephalus*

"Primary" hydrocephalus (?)
　　Non-opening of Magendie's and Luschka's foramina
　　Inadequate permeability of subarachnoid space
　　Other
"Secondary" hydrocephalus
　　Hemorrhage
　　Infections
　　Brain tissue resorption

syndrome: first, this type of hydrocephalus is usually more acute than the other types of prenatal hydrocephalus, and the acute exacerbation seems to coincide with the secondary aqueductal obliteration; and second, of major diagnostic importance, its onset and detection are comparatively late (Fig. 6).

Prenatal primary hydrocephalus is rare. It is due either to the non-opening of Magendie's and Luschka's foramina, to an abnormally low permeability of subarachnoid spaces and areas of CSF resorption, or possibly to other, more hypothetical mechanisms. In a case of occipital ventriculocele described by Evrard and Caviness (24), obliteration or a lack of opening of Magendie's and Luschka's foramina was observed. Examination of the serial sections showed that the neural tube was perfectly closed. On the basis of the morphological and topological observations, we conclude that the ventriculocele had extruded under CSF hypertension after the 5th month of fetal life. In our ultrasound prenatal material, cases of severe hydrocephalus detected around the 20th week seem to have exploded in encephaloceles or ventriculoceles at approximately the 25th week of gestation, thus confirming our hypothesis based on neuroanatomical evidence for some of these cases (24,25).

The ultrasound diagnosis of prenatal hydrocephalus by measuring the biparietal diameter is usually made only very late (mean fetal age: 30.5 weeks) (Fig. 7). An earlier diagnosis can be obtained by observing the dislocation of the choroid plexus in the lateral ventricles and the evolution of the ratio between the diameter of the lateral ventricle and the thickness of the cerebral mantle (26,27). Unfortunately, except in highly specialized multidisciplinary centers, mistaken sonographic diagnoses of prenatal hydrocephalies are innumerable along with their serious consequences

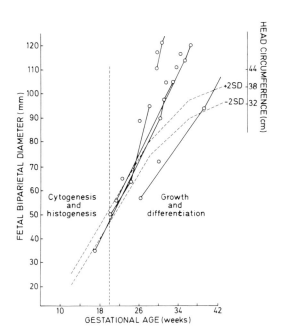

FIG. 6. Prenatal growth of biparietal diameter estimated by repeated ultrasonic examinations in fetuses with hydrocephalus secondary to X-linked aqueductal stenosis (12 cases).

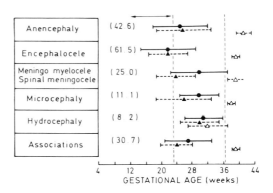

FIG. 7. Age of prenatal diagnosis in five groups of prenatal CNS malformations. |- - - -|, percentage of cases diagnosed before the 24th week of gestation; -●-, age at diagnosis (mean + SD); -▲-, age at delivery in cases of interrupted pregnancy (mean + SD); -△-, age at delivery in cases of pregnancy to term (mean + SD). (Modified from ref. 21.)

(Fig. 7) (21,28). During fetal life, several CNS malformations should be differentiated from hydrocephalus: for example, partial callosal "agenesis" (where reduction of the posterior callosal radiation and tapetum causing a dilation of the posterior horns of the lateral ventricles is often confused with posterior hydrocephalus); cystic and reversible dilation of the choroid plexuses; papillomas of choroid plexuses and other prenatal intracranial tumors; holoprosencephalies; and "physiological" dilation of the lateral ventricles.

Knowledge of CSF circulation during human development is still very incomplete. The literature yields no definitive information concerning the time of estab-

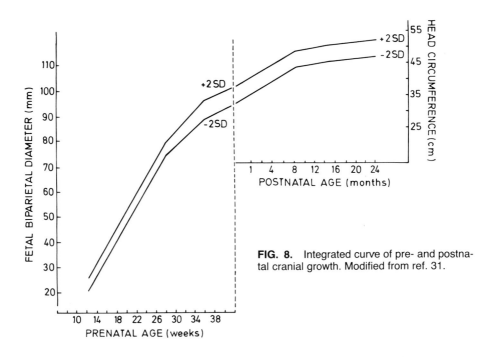

FIG. 8. Integrated curve of pre- and postnatal cranial growth. Modified from ref. 31.

lishment of CSF circulation. Our Collaborative Study Program did not add any data concerning the time of onset; in several specimens at early stages of CSF circulation, there seems to be some CSF accumulation with a transitory dilation of pericerebral spaces during a period limited to a part of the second half of gestation. This period sometimes extends into the first year of postnatal life and could lead to a clinical syndrome of postnatal external hydrocephalus (29).

With M. Van Lierde, we recently developed a cranial growth curve integrating prenatal and postnatal life. This curve proved to be useful for the study of the natural history and treatment of prenatal brain disorders, including antenatal hydrocephalus (Fig. 8) (30,31).

PERFUSION FAILURE—HYPOXIA DURING THE SECOND HALF OF GESTATION

Perfusion failures and hypoxias of the fetal brain are frequent causes of viable human malformations and are probably responsible for a large part of the neurodevelopmental disturbances occurring during the last two trimesters of gestation (32,33). The involvement of this mechanism has been clearly demonstrated in cases of maternal shock and hypoxia, maternal hypo- and hypertension, maternal thrombophlebitis, fetomaternal and fetofetal transfusions, premature placental separation or excessive infarction, and circulatory disturbances (by systemic hypotension or arteritis) due to viral infection (e.g., cytomegalovirus). Arterial embolism has also been incriminated (Table 5). In the Multicenter Collaborative Program (Table 3) sequential ultrasound studies were carried out in several cases from the time of occurrence of the prenatal perfusion disturbance until birth. These observations confirmed the pathogenesis of cerebral lesions in these cases (21,31).

Despite such progress, the nature and pathogenesis of ischemic disturbances affecting prenatal development of the nervous system often remains unknown. This area of investigation deserves greater priority in research programs, as a better understanding in this area is essential for the prevention of neurological handicaps. Few statistical data regarding perfusion failure and hypoxia responsible for human fetal brain damage are presently available. Ornoy (34) reported that one third of mothers having newborns with brain abnormalities presented with genital blood losses during pregnancy, a percentage much higher than in the control population. According to Ornoy (34), these bleedings are associated in most cases either with perfusion failures of the fetal brain or with fetal malnutrition. These interesting data need to be reproduced and expanded.

As in postnatal life, brain ischemias in the second half of gestation can display a vascular territorial distribution and, in cortical areas not completely destroyed, may produce cortical laminar necrosis. Unfortunately, *a posteriori* diagnosis of prenatal brain ischemias is sometimes made difficult by the later appearance of dense glial scars and the developmental characteristics of brain vascularization during fetal life (Table 6).

TABLE 5. *Main known causes of fetal brain perfusion failure*

Fetal origin
  Circulatory disturbances due to an infection (arteritis, systemic hypotension)
  Hydrops fetalis, thrombocytopenia
  Embolism (placental and others) with arterial occlusion
  Multiple monochorial pregnancies with placental vascular anastomoses
  Feto-fetal transfusion
Placental and cord origin
  Premature placental separation
  Possibly excessive infarction
  See above
Maternal origin
  Maternal shock, e.g., toxic, anaphylactic
  Maternal hypoxia, e.g., CO-intoxication, butane intoxication
  Extreme maternal stress (?)
  Abdominal trauma
  Maternal hypo- and hypertension
  Maternal thrombophlebitis
  Feto-maternal transfusion

The above cited etiologies concern certain neuropathologically proven fetal brain perfusion failures. Many other causes of fetal brain hypoxia have been reported or suggested.
Reprinted from Evrard et al. (11), with permission of Paul H. Brookes Publishing Company.

Polymicrogyria, hydranencephaly, porencephaly, and multicystic encephalopathies exemplify the main categories of perfusion disturbances of the fetal brain (Tables 3 and 6).

The basic lesion in microgyrias or polymicrogyrias is cortical laminar necrosis predominating in layer 5, due to perfusion failure with vascular topography (Table 7) (31,33,35). The cortical laminar destruction enhances the prenatal growth differ-

TABLE 6. *Examples of perfusion failure—hypoxia*

During the period of cytogenesis—histogenesis
  Lissencephaly type I (?)
  Onset of rare microgyric variants
  Others
During the period of growth and differentiation
  From 6th month on
    Microgyria
    Porencephaly
    Hydranencephaly
  Last months and perinatal period
    Hydranencephaly
    Multicystic encephalomalacias
    Ulegyria

Translated and modified from Evrard et al. (1).

TABLE 7. *Neocortical topography of select developmental lesions*

Targets	Main pattern of cytoarchitectonic lesions
Glial guides	Radial
Germinative zone	Laminar
Postmigratory neurons (hypoxias)	Vascular and/or laminar territories

This table summarizes a few frequent patterns; other abnormal neuronal patterns are discussed in the chapter (for a more comprehensive survey, see also ref. 11).

ences between inner and outer cortical layers. This results in a reduction of the wave length of the cortical folding with multiplication of the convolutions (36). While clinical and neuropathological studies of many cases of polymicrogyria suggested prenatal cytomegalovirus (CMV) infection, we also observed other causes of perfusion failure that have been reported in the literature, such as carbon monoxide intoxication, toxoplasmosis, and syphilis (37–40). On the basis of the neuropathological analysis, most prenatal perfusion failures causing microgyria appear to occur after the end of neuronal migration and before the establishment of the gyration (i.e., 20–30 weeks of gestation). When diagnosed by prenatal sequential ultrasound, most fetal accidents or diseases resulting in polymicrogyria take place during the same period, confirming the neuropathological dating (Fig. 9). There are, however, rare

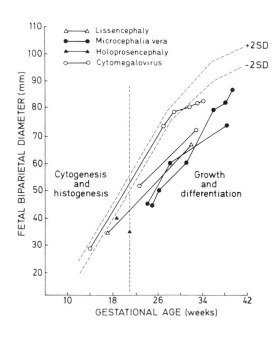

FIG. 9. Prenatal growth of biparietal diameter measured by sequential ultrasound examinations in fetuses with different types of microcephaly. The two cases secondary to cytomegalovirus infections were associated with polymicrogyria. The original data summarized in this figure were collected in part in the Collaborative Study Program, Société Européenne de Neurologie Pédiatrique, Branch of the European Federation of Child Neurology Societies, and reported in part in refs. 21 and 22.

cases of polymicrogyria occurring at the migratory period. These variants are reviewed by Evrard et al. (11). After birth, using computerized tomography (CT) scanning or nuclear magnetic resonance (NMR) imaging, the abnormal folding can be diagnosed in many microgyric brains.

In hydranencephaly, perfusion failure is considerably extensive with destruction of brain territories irrigated by the internal carotid arteries (33,41). The vertebrobasilar territory is usually preserved, with remnants of temporal and occipital cortex. Some compensatory circulation also develops in the basal ganglia. In the Multicenter Collaborative Study, we investigated sequential prenatal ultrasound findings and clinicopathological specimens of six cases of hydranencephaly that occurred at around 30 weeks of gestation, which is later than has usually been reported (Table 3) (21,31). Three conclusions can be drawn: (a) These cases are the consequence of either maternal shock (especially of toxic origin) or a sudden fetal illness with transitory, but complete, disappearance of fetal movements without maternal problems (42) (Table 8). (b) Two patterns of evolution of the lesions during the last 10 weeks of gestation are observed in our material: either a massive hemorrhage during the days following the initial perfusion failure or a progressive and slow resorption of the hemispheres without hemorrhage. These two different patterns of evolution can be described as follows: In one of our cases, fetal movement ceased abruptly after 30 weeks of normal gestation. At that time, the cortical mantle was thick. Ultrasound examinations demonstrated progressive resorption of the brain regions irrigated by both internal carotid arteries (Fig. 10). The baby, born at term, was admitted to our department with hydranencephaly, which was later confirmed by postmortem examination. In other cases, after severe maternal shock around 30 weeks of gestation, the mothers recovered fully and the fetuses were followed up by repeated ultrasound examination until birth. The day after the maternal shock, the fetal brain was shown to have had a massive hemorrhage. When ultrasound had been routinely performed before perfusion failure, brain growth was recorded as normal until the accident. Perfusion failure was then followed by a period of relative

TABLE 8. *Length of prenatal aggressions to CNS*

Single impact
  Acute hypoxic accident
  Trauma
Impacts at different periods
  Rubella
  Alcohol
Protracted Action
  Extraneural defect associated with certain "dysraphisms" (?)
  Hydrocephalus
  Alcohol
  Walker-Warburg (virus or metabolic) (?)
  Septo-optic dysplasia (??)

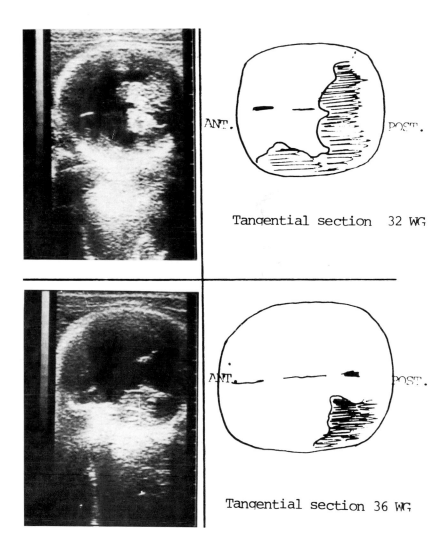

FIG. 10. Ultrasound examination of fetal brain with hydranencephaly at the 32nd and 36th week of gestation. Sequential ultrasonic examination demonstrated progressive resorption of brain regions irrigated by both internal carotid arteries.

microcephaly due to tissue destruction, and later by a progressive macrocephaly due to development of secondary hydrocephalus (Fig. 11).

Porencephalies are focal cerebral defects due to destructive processes also occurring during the second half of gestation in areas perfused by major cerebral arteries. Their clinical manifestations may include cerebral palsy and epilepsy. Intellectual

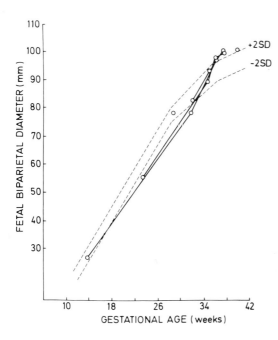

FIG. 11. Prenatal development of biparietal diameter measured by successive ultrasound examinations in fetuses with hydranencephaly. This pattern has been observed in six cases.

function is often preserved. As previously described, porencephalies can expand further and still remain treatable during postnatal life (43). The appearance of porencephaly following perfusion failure and its expanding character during prenatal life have been illustrated by sequential ultrasound studies in an observation from the Multicenter Study Program (31).

Our observations suggested that certain multicystic encephalomalacias could be due to prenatal, possibly chronic, perfusion failure starting from the 26th week of fetal life (Table 8).

Ulegyrias and cerebral cortical sclerosis are due to hypoxias occurring much later including the perinatal period (33).

PRENATAL INFECTIONS

Virtually all types of infectious agents can invade the fetal CNS during periods of cytogenesis-histogenesis and of growth and differentiation (44,45). The main viral agents incriminated in prenatal disturbances of the development of the human CNS are listed in Table 9, as modified from Johnson (45). During the cytogenesis-histogenesis period infectious agents, especially viral, can inhibit neuronal multiplication. This is assumed to be one of the effects of prenatal rubella (Tables 8 and 9). During the growth and differentiation period infectious agents can provoke men-

TABLE 9. *Main viral infections of the human fetal brain*

Demonstrated agents	Suspected agents
Arbovirus	Antirubella vaccine
Cytomegalovirus	Coxsackievirus
Epstein-Barr virus	Echovirus
Hepatitis B	Hepatitis A
Herpes simplex	Influenza
Polio virus	Measles
Rubella	Mumps
Varicella-Zoster virus	HTLV3

Modified from Johnson (44,45).

ingitis or inflammatory encephalitis with focal or multifocal destructions (Table 10). Hydrocephalus and secondary microcephaly can result from such processes.

Observations concerning prenatal infections led to the following conclusions: First, fetal brain growth curves recorded by sequential ultrasound observations permit differentiation between destructive microcephalies and microcephalies resulting from a precocious derangement of neuronal production and migration (e.g., microcephalia vera, lissencephaly) (Fig. 9). (For an overview of the developmental mechanisms in the different types of microcephalies, see ref. 11.) Second, the prenatal diagnosis of the different classes of multicystic lesions can be approached by ultrasound; for example, the walls of the necrotic cysts in toxoplasmosis appear irregular in shape and in density in contrast with ischemic multicystic lesions (Fig. 12).

TABLE 10. *Possible effects of viral infections on the developing CNS*

Indirect
    Constitutional effect on mother
    Infection of placenta
Direct fetal infection
    Generalized encephalitis with necrotic or inflammatory lesions
    Chromosomal damage
    Mitotic inhibition
    Partial or complete destruction of selected cell populations altering embryogenesis
    Possible metabolic disturbances in certain cell populations
    Localized ependymitis
    Circulatory disturbances

Most items of this table derive from Johnson (45), with modifications.

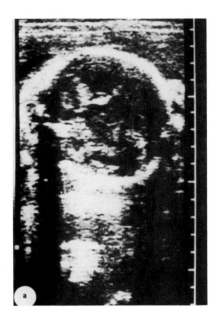
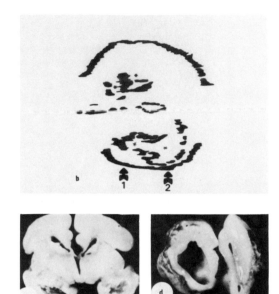

FIG. 12. Multicystic lesion secondary to prenatal toxoplasmosis infection. **a:** Prenatal ultrasound examination of the multicystic brain. **b:** Schematic drawing of the ultrasound examination. The asterisks indicate the multiple necrotic lesions in the fetal brain secondary to the toxoplasmosis infection. **c** and **d:** Spontaneous abortion occurred one week after the ultrasound examination. Neuropathological examination of the brain confirmed the widespread cortico-subcortical necrotic lesions.

MINOR CORTICAL DYSGENESES, INTRAUTERINE CONSTRAINTS, AND OTHER NEURODEVELOPMENTAL PROBLEMS

Prenatal neurology is a vast field of paramount clinical importance. The clinico-pathological data given above provide guidelines for approaching this new domain. Many other avenues open in the fetal neurology of the second half of gestation. They are cited in this section but will not be covered in detail.

Minor developmental brain abnormalities including minor cortical dysgeneses and defects in neuronal growth and differentiation of the second half of gestation are now identified as anatomical witnesses or as causative factors in several neuro-psychological disturbances, in mental deficiency, and in other neurological conditions (46). Neuronal ectopias, discussed above, are one example. Several other types of minor developmental brain abnormalities and their clinicopathological significance are reviewed and discussed by Evrard et al. (11). Prenatal sexual brain differentiation and its possible disturbances provoking certain minor cortical dysgeneses are reviewed by Geschwind and Galaburda (47) and by Kelly (48).

Craniostenoses are sometimes suspected in our material from the 15th week of gestation; at early stages, the differential diagnosis with microcephaly is difficult. Certain forms of craniostenosis may be secondary to or favored by intrauterine constraints (6,49,50). Intrauterine pressure and steric hindrance also have an influence on brain growth during the second half of gestation (51).

Szliwowski (52) discussed fetal epilepsy; in the Multicenter Collaborative Study Program, epileptic fits subsequent to brain perfusion failure have been recorded with ultrasound between the 30th and 35th gestational week. Other fetal motor and behavioral data will not be discussed here and are reviewed by Awoust and Levi (53).

CONCLUSIONS

In this chapter, we have discussed and given examples of conceptual and methodological approaches to abnormal brain development during the second half of gestation. Several new tools have led to significant progress in this field: the application of advances in basic developmental neurobiology to the understanding of human brain malformations, multicenter and multidisciplinary cooperation to collect and study the pertinent neuropathological specimens, and the application in fetal neurology of clinicopathological correlations including prenatal sequential ultrasound. In a field still poorly explored, any progress can have important consequences for public health and clinical medicine. The basic neurobiological questions raised about mammalian development by the analysis of the human brain malformations add to the critical importance of this field.

ACKNOWLEDGMENTS

This work was supported in part by the generous support of Mrs. Albert Froehlich and by grants of the Action Concertée Gouvernementale, the Fonds de la Recherche Scientifique Médicale, the Fondation Roi Baudouin, and the Fondation Médicale Reine Elisabeth.

This chapter owes much to the close collaboration over the last 16 years between Dr. Verne S. Caviness, Jr. (Boston, Massachusetts), Dr. Philippe Evrard, and Dr. Gilles Lyon (UCL, Brussels, Belgium). We thank Dr. Joëlle Awoust (U.L.B., Brussels), Dr. Georges Boog (Brest, France), Dr. Martha Denckla (Baltimore, Maryland), Dr. A. Henocq (Rouen, France), Dr. Bernard Le Marec (Rennes, France), Dr. Salvatore Levi (U.L.B., Brussels), Dr. Jean-Paul Misson (Liège, Belgium), Dr. Dominique Parain (Rouen), Dr. Cecilia Pinto-Lord (Dover, New Hampshire), Dr. Michel Van Lierde (UCL, Brussels), and Dr. Roger Williams (Billings, Montana) for their stimulating discussions. We are especially grateful to all those who participated in the collaborative study and referred material. Ms. P. Debluts, Ms. C. Defat, Ms. A.M. Rona, Ms. A. Stefanovic, and Ms. Ch. Vynckier provided very valuable and agreeable help during this work.

REFERENCES

1. Evrard P, Lyon G, Gadisseux JF. Le développement prénatal du système nerveux et ses perturbations: mécanismes généraux. *Progrès en néonatologie,* vol 4. Basel, NY: Karger, 1984:63–9.
2. Williams RS, Caviness VS. Normal and abnormal development of the brain. In: Tarter RE, Goldstein G, eds. *Advances in clinical neuropsychology,* vol 2. New York: Plenum, 1984:1–62.
3. Lyon G, Evrard P, Gadisseux JF. Les anomalies du développement du télencéphalie humain pendant la période de cytogenèse-histogenèse (première moitié de la grossesse), *Progrès en néonatologie,* vol 4. Basel, NY: Karger, 1984:70–84.
4. Williams RS. Golgi and routine microscopic analysis of congenital microcephaly ("microcephalia vera"). *Ann Neurol* 1979;6:173.
5. Rockel AJ, Hiorns RW, Powel TPS. The basic uniformity in structure of the neocortex. *Brain* 1980;103:221–44.
6. Evrard P, Gadisseux JF, Lyon G. Les malformations du système nerveux. In: P. Royer. *Naissance du cerveau.* Paris: Nestlé, 1982;49–74.
7. Gadisseux JF, Evrard P. Glio-neuronal relationship in the developing central nervous system: a histochemical-electron microscope study of radial glial cell particulate glycogen in normal and reeler mice and the human fetus. *Dev Neurosci* 1985;7:12–37.
8. Kadhim HJ, Gadisseux JF, Evrard P. Topographical and cytological evolution of the glial phase during the prenatal development of the human brain: a histochemical and electron microscopic study. *J Neuropathol Exp Neurol* 1988;47(n°.2):166–88.
9. de Saint-Georges P, Della Giustina E, Kadhim HJ, Evrard P. Etude du développement foetal du cortex holopresencephalique. *Rev Neurol* 1989.
10. Lammens M, de Saint-Georges P, Kadhim HJ, Gosseye S, Awoust J, Levi S, and Evrard P. Developmental brain lesions in Potter syndrome: a light microscopic and ultrastructural study. *Clin Neuropathol* 1988;7(4):181.
11. Evrard P, de Saint-Georges P, Kadhim H, Gadisseux J-F. Pathology of prenatal encephalopathies. In: *Child neurology and developmental disabilities,* Baltimore: Paul H. Brookes, 1989;153–76.
12. Kadhim HJ, Gadisseux JF, de Saint-Georges P, Della Giustina E, and Evrard P. Methodological progress in studying normal and pathological human fetal brain. *Rev Neurol,* 1989; abstract (*in press*).
13. Abel EL, Jacobson S, Sherwin BT. *In utero* alcohol exposure: functional and structural brain damage. *Neurobehav Toxicol Teratol* 1983;5:363–6.
14. Borges S, Lewis PD. Effects of alcohol on the developing nervous system. *Trends Neurosci* 1981;4:13–15.
15. Clarren SL, Alvord EC, Sumi JM, Streissguth AP, Smith DW. Brain malformations related to prenatal exposure to ethanol. *J Pediatr* 1978;92:64–67.
16. Clarren SK, Smith DW. The fetal alcohol syndrome. *New Engl J Med* 1978;298:1063–7.
17. Caviness VS, Evrard P, Lyon G. Radial neuronal assemblies, ectopia and necrosis of developing cortex. *Acta Neuropathol* 1978;41:67–72.
18. Steissguth AP, Landesmandwyer S, Martin JS, Smith DW. Teratogenic effects of alcohol in humans and laboratory animals. *Science* 1980;209:353–61.
19. Gadisseux JF, Lyon G, Goffinet AM. The subpial granular layer of human embryonic cortex: a cytological analysis. *Neuroscience* 1984;10:47, abstract.
20. Brun A. The subpial granular layer of the foetal cerebral cortex in man. *Acta Path Microbiol Scand Sect A Suppl* 1965;179(7):3–98.
21. Evrard P, Belpaire MC, Boog G, et al. Apport de l'échotomographie à la neurologie prénatale. Résultats d'une étude multicentrique organisée par la SNI. *J Fr Echograph* 1985;2:123–6.
22. Van Lierde M, Evrard P. Conclusions d'une étude multicentrique européene sur les anomalies du tube neural. *J Génét Hum* 1986;34:343–65.
23. Landrieu P, Ninane J, Ferrière G, Lyon G. Aqueductal stenosis in X-linked hydrocephalus: a secondary phenomenon? *Dev Med Child Neurol* 1979;21:637–52.
24. Evrard P, Caviness VS. Extensive developmental defect associated with posterior fossa ventriculocele. *J Neuropathol Exp Neurol* 1974;33:385–99.
25. Caviness VS, Evrard P. Occipital encephalocele: a pathologic and anatomic analysis. *Acta Neuropathol* 1975;32:245–55.
26. Denkhaus H, Winsberg F. Ultrasonic measurement of the fetal ventricular system. *Radiology* 1979;131:781–7.

27. Chervenak F, Berkowitz RL, Tortora M, Chitkara U, Hobbins JC. Diagnosis of ventriculomegaly before fetal viability. *Obstet Gynecol* 1984;64:652–6.
28. Fiske CE, Filly RA, Callen PW. Sonographic measurement of lateral ventricular width in early dilatation. *J Clin Ultrasound* 1981;9:303–10.
29. Alvarez LA, Maytal J, Shinnar S. Idiopathic external hydrocephalus: natural history and relationship to benign familial macrocephaly. *Pediatrics* 1986;77:901–7.
30. Chef E. Problèmes posés par la construction et l'utilisation d'une courbe de croissance intra-utérine. *J Gynécol Obstet Biol Reprod* 1979;8:613–23.
31. Evrard P, Lyon G, Gadisseux JF. Les processus destructifs agissant durant la seconde moitié de la grossesse, durant la période de croissance et de différenciation du tissu nerveux. *Progrès en Néonatologie*, vol 4, Basel, NY: Karger, 1984:85–106.
32. Evrard P, Lyon G, Caviness VS. A new look on cerebral malformations. *Neuropediatrics* 1977;8:506–7.
33. Lyon G, Robain O. Encéphalopathies circulatoires prénatales et périnatales. *Acta Neuropathol* 1967;9:79–98.
34. Ornoy A, Benady S, Kohen-Raz A. Association between maternal bleeding during gestation and congenital anomalies in the offspring. *Am J Obstet Gynecol* 1976;124:474–8.
35. Richman DP, Stewart RM, Caviness VS. Cerebral microgyria in a 27 weeks fetus: an architectonic and topographic analysis. *J Neuropathol Exp Neurol* 1970;139:227–44.
36. Richman DP, Stewart RM, Hutchinson JW, Caviness VS. Mechanical model of brain convolutional development. *Science* 1975;189:18–21.
37. Marques Dias MJ, Harmant-Van Rijckevorsel G, Landrieu P, Lyon G. Prenatal cytomegalovirus disease and cerebral microgyria: evidence for perfusion failure, not disturbance of histogenesis, as the major cause of fetal cytomegalovirus encephalopathy. *Neuropediatrics* 1984;15:18–24.
38. Kalter H, Warkany J. Congenital malformations. Etiologic factors and their role in prevention, 2 parts. *New Engl J Med* 1983;308:424–31.
39. Friede EL, Mikolasek J. Postencephalitic porencephaly, hydranencephaly or polymicrogyria. A review. *Acta Neuropathol* 1978;43:161–8.
40. Ferrer I. A Golgi analysis of unlayered polymicrogyria. *Acta Neuropathol* 1984;65:69–76.
41. Lyon G. Les encéphalopathies non évolutives. *Louvain Méd* 1970;89:341–73.
42. Ong BY, Ellison PH, Browning C. Intrauterine stroke in the neonate. *Arch Neurol* 1983;40:55–6.
43. Tardieu M, Evrard P, Lyon G. Progressive expanding congenital porencephalies: a treatable cause of progressive encephalopathy. *Pediatrics* 1981;68:198–202.
44. Johnson RT. Problems in relating viral infections to malformations in man. *Contrib Epidemiol Biostatistics* 1979;1:138–46.
45. Johnson RT, *Viral infections of the nervous system*. New York: Raven Press, 1982.
46. Purpura DP. Dendritic differentiation in human cerebral cortex: normal and aberrant developmental patterns. In: Kreutzberg GW, ed. *Advances in Neurology*, vol 12. New York: Raven Press, 1975:91–116.
47. Geschwind N, Galaburda AM. *Cerebral lateralization: biological mechanisms, associations, and pathology*. Cambridge, MA: Massachusetts Institute of Technology Press, 1987.
48. Kelly DD. Sexual differentiation of the nervous system. In: Kandel E, Schwartz JH, eds. *Principles of neural science*, New York: Elsevier, 1985:771–83.
49. Higginbottom MC, Jones KL, James HE. Intrauterine constraint and craniosynostosis. *Neurosurgery* 1980;6:39–43.
50. Graham JM, Badura RJ, Smith DW. Coronal craniostenosis: fetal head constraint as one possible cause. *Pediatrics* 1980;65:995–1002.
51. Mamelle N, Lazar P. Etude allométrique de la croissance relative de la tête et du corps chez le foetus et le nouveau-né. *J Gynécol Obstet Biol Reprod* 1979;8:703–9.
52. Szliwowski HB, Paquot E, Wacquez M, Avni EF, Awoust J, Flament-Durand J. Respiratory arrest during pregnancy, intrauterine convulsions and repercussions on the fetus. In: *4th International Child Neurology Congress*, 1986: 222, abstract.
53. Awoust J, Levi S. New aspects of fetal dynamics with a special emphasis on eye movements. *Ultrasound Med Biol* 1984;10:107–16.

Developmental Neurobiology, edited by
Philippe Evrard and Alexandre Minkowski.
Nestlé Nutrition Workshop Series, Vol. 12.
Nestec Ltd., Vevey/Raven Press, Ltd.,
New York © 1989.

Discussion for Chapters by Caviness, Williams, and Evrard

Dr. Sotelo: I should like Dr. Evrard and Dr. Caviness to speculate about the mechanism of the formation of the gyri. According to Dr. Williams it appears that cytogenetic problems may be responsible for the absence of gyri, but in your chapter, Dr. Evrard, it seems that problems in brain vascularization may actually induce the formation of gyri. Thus my general question is as follows: Is the physiological mechanism of the formation of gyri related to cell division, blood vessel formation, change in the basal membranes, or something else?

Dr. Evrard: Dr. Caviness proposed a few years ago a mechanism involving differential growth of the inner and outer part of the cortex. This hypothesis seems to be very useful and satisfactory in explaining micropolygyria, lissencephaly, abnormalities of gyration in Zellweger's syndrome and other malformations. I think we should be looking at problems of growth and differentiation when considering such malformations, rather than neuronal multiplication, especially when you consider the condition of radial microbrain, as we now call this entity, where there is a gross reduction in neuronal multiplication but a normal vertical composition (with a reduction in the number of adjacent vertical columns). In this condition the gyrations are almost perfect — so much so that if I make a photographic enlargement of such a brain, weighing, say, 16 g at term, you would think that it was a normal neonatal brain of 300 g. I believe that the events at the end of migration and during growth and differentiation are most likely to modify gyration.

Dr. Caviness: The basic seed for the idea to which Dr. Evrard refers grew out of a conversation at a cocktail party with a geologist named Hutchison and Dave Richman, a neurologist and topologist who was working with me on pathologic specimens at the time! You begin with the observation that in the course of gyration there are certain fissures which bear a constant relation to other structures in the brain, and many which are more or less randomly distributed among them. The constant fissures are the central and sylvian fissures from the outset, to which are later added the temporal gyri as gyral formation progresses. The hypothesis about the formation of the gyri is a geological one, that is, that convolutions occur due to surface buckling when there is differential expansion of an outer layer with respect to an inner layer. In the case of the cerebral cortex, I am referring specifically to greater growth in the supragranular than in the infragranular layers, giving rise to the buckling that accounts for the more or less randomly distributed gyri. The constantly distributed gyri would occur because of certain specific and constant restraints in the developing brain, perhaps related to connections.

Specific malformations occur in various ways. One is where gyral formation more or less approximates that of the normal brain but the gyri have been badly damaged. This usually reflects pathologic processes which have been set in motion after the establishment of the primary pattern; an apt example would be perinatal encephalopathy with consequent ulegyria. Other types of malformation are associated with too few gyri (lissencephaly or pachygyria) or too many (polymicrogyria, in which the gyral pattern bears no resemblance to the normal pattern). In lissencephalic malformations one reproducibly observes that the lower range of layers is better constituted than the upper range of layers, for example layers 5 and 6 developing in the near absence of supragranular layers in microcephaly vera or lissencephaly. In polymicrogyria all five of the cellular layers are formed but the infragranular layer is badly disrupted by pseudolaminar necrosis, occurring presumably as a result of perfusion failure. Thus there is differential expansion of the superficial zone giving rise to excessive nontopological buckling.

Dr. Kretchmer: Two questions for Dr. Caviness: You discussed migration at the beginning of your talk. Migration is a typical phenomenon of cellular development. Do you have any idea of the mechanism of the movement of cells in the brain? Is it ATP-dependent? Is myosin involved? Second, how does pruning of synapses occur? Is it just cell death, and if it is, what might be causing it?

Dr. Caviness: Cellular movement must be considered separately from the guiding mechanism. We have a cellular model for the latter, but we have no direct observations on the former, so we must extrapolate back to studies of movement in motile organisms and *in vivo* preparations. We expect to learn more from such studies, but we have no direct information about events within the intact brain.

The pruning of synapses is a reduction phenomenon where both pruning and synaptic elimination occur. We need to separate the phenomena of axonal pruning and synaptic elimination on the one hand from cell death on the other. Cell death seems to proceed independently of axon pruning and synaptic elimination, which are regressive events involving cells that will ultimately survive and contribute to the cerebral circuitry. We have very little information on the events that determine the final synaptic complement and distribution. We tend to accept generally in neurobiology that it has to do with competition, with the stabilization of synapses as a result of functional validation.

Dr. Kretchmer: Dr. Williams stated that microcephaly in experimental animals can be produced by extreme malnutrition and by toxins such as alcohol and antimetabolites. Is this true microcephaly, or is it just associated with generally reduced body size? And do all these adverse stimuli, malnutrition, toxins, antimetabolites, radiation, etc., work in the same way?

Dr. Williams: With respect to malnutrition and probably alcohol, the effects on the brain occur only after more severe effects on overall body growth. The brain is privileged in this respect, and conservatory mechanisms preserve brain growth at the expense of virtually all other growth. It is only after malnutrition reaches a certain threshold that brain growth is also retarded. The small brain that is seen in malnutrition is not necessarily a malfunctioning brain though in many cases it may be.

With alcohol other brain abnormalities occur as well, including ectopia of the brain and cytoarchitectural abnormalities in the underlying cortex. Malformations of the brain produced by pulses of low intensity X-rays are caused by damage to the germinal cells and perhaps the RGCs exclusively. Postmitotic cells are unaffected. Death of germinal cells results in too few nerve cells in the cortex. Cells that were beginning to migrate may become disordered, so that subcortical heterotopias may appear. The mechanism of these various forms of damage is thus quite different depending on which etiologic agent is involved.

Dr. Gadisseux: It is possible to produce lissencephaly in the ferret with methylazoxymethanol. When this occurs there is a rarification in the upper layers of the cortical plate, just as occurs in microcephaly. It is very clear that in this experimental model there is a loss of neurons.

Dr. Krishnan: Would Dr. Caviness please let us know how the number of synapses is determined?

Dr. Caviness: This is one of the important unanswered questions. We really do not know what constitutes the optimum number of synapses in the interaction of an afferent system with its target neuron, and we do not even have a useful theory about it. What we do observe is that the number changes, and there are two qualities of change: the number of neurons that a given afferent axon may contact and the number of synapses that this axon may have on a given cell. The factors that influence these qualities are likely to have more to do with competition between converging systems and the activity that these systems support than they are to be related to molecular specificity. In relation to the projection of the climbing fibers upon the cerebellum, we know for example that a given climbing fiber may contact two or three or perhaps more Purkinje cells and that in the course of normal development this drops back to a single fiber. However, if the normal innervation of the Purkinje cells by parallel fibers does not occur, this reduction in convergence is lost, and multiple fibers continue to be projected. Dr. Mariani may have more to say about this.

Dr. Mariani: I agree that we do not know the mechanism involved in the quantitative regulation of the number of synaptic contacts made by one fiber, but it is probably linked to a physiological function of the afferent fiber. I believe that the quantitative regulation of the number of synaptic contacts made by one fiber on its target is linked in a major way to its physiology, for example, the change in calcium concentration in the target due to the synaptic activation through the fiber.

Dr. Sotelo: You say, Dr. Caviness, that there is a correlation between the birthdays of the neurons and their location in the cortex. I believe this to be correct in the case of long-projecting neurons, but what about interneurons?

Dr. Caviness: The idea that there is a systematic relationship between the position of a neuron and its time of origin comes from studies based on autoradiographic labeling of cells, identifying their birthdays by tritiated thymidine. What we observe is the systematic inside-out relationship of cells with regard to their order of final division. This can easily be confirmed by other methods, such as the Golgi technique. In fact this ''inside-out'' observation goes back to Kinicku, who made the point that the younger cells are always the most superficial. There is one thing missing in this argument: He and every other student of the Golgi method has referred specifically to the long-projection neurons and in particular to the pyramidal cells. Interneurons have not been well visualized by the Golgi method for some reason, particularly the stellate neurons, so we do not have this independent correlation. One has to infer that they are taking their position in this inside-out sequence from their appearance in Nissil preparations, though there has been no independent confirmation with specific cell morphology studies.

Dr. Sotelo: It has been done, here in Madrid at the Cajal Institute, using acetyl-carboxylase (a good interneuron marker) and double labeling techniques. There is a convincing correlation between age and the position in the cortex of long-projecting neurons but not of interneurons. These appear relatively late in the mouse, in a burst over 2 to 3 days in all layers almost simultaneously.

Dr. Barbin: You mentioned during your talk, Dr. Caviness, that the migration of neurons occurred along RGFs. Would you consider the possibility of other mechanisms for neuron migration? The examples you have given concern laminated structures where there is an inside-out migration, but what about nucleated structures? Don't you think it possible that in such structures there could be neurono-neuronal interactions which could lead to the migration of some neuronal subset?

Dr. Caviness: Yes, I think this is an important qualification of the general phenomenon. We know from studies of the behavior of dissociated cells *in vitro* that they are motile organisms which can move around in tissue culture outside their original habitat. We also know that they have preferred substrates for movement. The glial substrate appears to be the preferred one for granular cells derived from cerebellar tissue. However, if this substrate is lacking, or if it is modified in some way that the cells find disagreeable, they will accept other substrates for movement. I think that the matter of cells moving along RGFs is consistent with the body of evidence about the formation of the cerebral cortex, at least for major periods of migration. On the other hand there is no reason to view this as the universal panacea for neuronal or axonal migration.

Dr. Evrard: I should like to add that we have recently had the opportunity, working with Dr. Gadisseux, to use the new glycogen-labeling technique which stains all RGCs easily at ultrastructural level. From our most recent data we find that all migrating neurons labeled by autoradiography at E16 or E17 in the mouse are constantly in contact with glial cells stained by the technique which I showed in my talk. This does not mean that there are no other mechanisms, but it does mean that there are additional arguments for the importance of glial cells at this stage of migration at least.

Dr. Barbin: I recall some recent work by Moody which showed that the migration of a given neuronal population was very much dependent on the presence of another afferent neuronal population. Has anyone seen these types of relationships in the migration of neurons? In Moody's experiments, the removal of a critical neuronal afferent results in failure of other types of neurons to migrate to their definitive targets.

Dr. Mariani: Do you think that factors such as plasminogen activators can play a role in cell migration?

Dr. Caviness: This is beginning to look below the surface of the individual cell to the molecular mechanisms, which I suspect is going to be very important because of their relation to the function of cytoskeletal elements, and particularly the microfilaments that invent the inner aspect of the cell surface. These may well be pivotal in the capacity of the cell to move.

Dr. Dubowitz: I should like to ask Dr. Caviness whether the destruction of the norepinephrinergic projections, which you say is associated with a terminal delay in pruning of the synapses, can be accelerated in stressed animals.

Dr. Caviness: This is an important and as yet unanswered question. There is work relating to the developmental history of organisms where the mother has been stressed. From my imperfect understanding of this literature, it has much to do with the sexual identity of the organism. Where stress has been great there has been an aberration of the hormonal milieu of cellular development and a shift from male to female mode of operation. I do not recall whether this has been examined particularly from the point of view of synaptogenesis but I suspect there would be a rich future in looking into it with this in mind.

Dr. Minkowski: I should like to ask Dr. Evrard a question. I think the disappearance of the famous subpial layer is rather a strange phenomenon since it appears to cause malformations. Is there anything more that you can add to throw light on what it represents? You also mentioned perfusion failure as a cause of malformation, but I think proof of this is difficult until we have proper measurements. Finally, could you comment on the prognosis of prenatal hydrocephalus?

Dr. Evrard: We do not know the importance of the subpial Brun layer which I showed. It may simply be a descriptive point in the histogenic events of the second half of gestation. As to perfusion failure, I feel that in many cases we really do have proof of this from our ultrasound studies. Prenatal hydrocephalus raises important ethical problems. I do not agree at all with the view that prenatal hydrocephalus usually has a good prognosis and that as much as possible should be done for these fetuses. I think that prenatal hydrocephalus often has a severe prognosis, even when derived prenatally or during early postnatal life.

Dr. Caviness: Dr. Kretchmer brought up the question of the energetics of migration and there was mention of the fibrillar systems and the molecular mechanisms which are involved in their function. These are important aspects of cell migration and they touch on the biology of the individual cell, independent of the context in which migration occurs. I should like to introduce now a whole new conceptual area which, instead of looking at the individual cell, looks more at the modulation of the overall phenomenon of cell migration: its timing and rate, and the specific elements involved that have to do with molecular species distributed on cells which determine their affinities with interacting cells in the course of migration. These ideas and observations come from the work of Thiery and Edelman and their associates and form the most provocative current hypothesis. Unfortunately their work has been concerned with migratory behavior in the neural crest rather than the central nervous system, but in summary they observed a set of molecules which contributed to the adhesion of cells and substrate during the period of development of neural tissues, stabilizing relationships and interfering with "shear", that is, relative movement. They also found substances which appeared to facilitate shear, particularly fibronectin and neural cell adhesion molecule (NCAM). During the period of migration of neural crest elements, there is a reciprocal and complementary relationship in the expression of these two types of substance. The stable structure prior to and after migration is strongly invested with NCAM, a stabilizing substance preventing shear. During the period of migration NCAM drops precipitously and fibronectin increases, affording the hypothesis that these are mirror images of a regulatory phenomenon which implements migration. There are mutant animals in which neural crest migration is defective. For example, there is a recessive mutant gene that is lethal in mice, giving rise to a phenotype which is identical to Hirschsprung's disease in man, and in which the final phase of neural crest migration into the terminal colon is not only not completed but continues for an abnormally long time into the postnatal period.

This mutant may be an interesting test of the hypothesis and it will be important to see whether there is a defect in the reciprocal development of fibronectin/NCAM regulation that would be consistent with the hypothesis put forward by Thiery and Edelman.

Developmental Neurobiology, edited by
Philippe Evrard and Alexandre Minkowski.
Nestlé Nutrition Workshop Series, Vol. 12.
Nestec Ltd., Vevey/Raven Press, Ltd.,
New York © 1989.

Cellular Interactions During Neuronal Development

Gilles Barbin

*INSERM Unité 114 Collège de France, Chaire de Neuropharmacologie,
75231 Paris Cédex 05, France*

Synaptogenesis is one of the final events during neurogenesis and is preceded by a series of phenomena (both progressive and regressive) overlapping in time but yet distinguishable (see Caviness, *this volume*). This chapter briefly reviews some of these events, especially highlighting those which have received much attention during the past few years through the use of *in vitro* techniques.

Early in this century Cajal's observations demonstrated that neurons received signals from their environment, and subsequent *in vivo* studies have shown that there are cellular interactions during brain development. Tissue culture techniques simplified the experimental situation, allowing better control of the artificial environment and direct access to various probes. Cell-type-specific markers allow identification of the cells (1). Moreover, replacement of the serum-containing medium with chemically defined media (2) allows the establishment of highly enriched neuronal cultures with limited glial "contamination".

Once a given cell type is obtained and characterized in culture it is possible to mix it with another cell population in order to detect any cellular interaction resulting from the co-culture. Such a strategy has been fruitful in studying the peripheral nervous system (PNS) due to its relatively low heterogeneity. The task is much more complicated with the central nervous system (CNS), but several successful examples are already available.

Differentiation as well as early migration of cells during embryonic development of the CNS are beyond the scope of this chapter and have been discussed elsewhere (3). The following questions are of immediate relevance to the achievement of synapse formation:

How do axons arrive in the neighborhood of appropriate target areas?

How is the size of the innervation pool of a given neuronal subset matched to the size of the target population?

How does the target area affect the subsequent development of the afferent system via neuro-neuronal interactions?

How does the cellular environment dictate the morphology of the neurons, in particular via glia–neuron interactions?

Two experimental systems have been used in order to answer these questions.

TROPHIC AND NEURITE-PROMOTING FACTORS FOR THE CILIARY GANGLION

Neuronal Cell Death in the Chick Ciliary Ganglion

The chick ciliary ganglion is a parasympathetic ganglion composed of two neuronal populations (choroid and ciliary neurons) which are both cholinergic and cholinoceptive. Once inside the eye, choroid nerves provide a diffuse innervation through the choroid layer, whereas ciliary nerves reach the ciliary body and iris (Fig. 1). The ganglion, readily accessible and distant from its innervation territories, offers a convenient experimental system that can be manipulated.

Following the pioneering work of Hamburger and Levi Montalcini, Landmesser and Pilar studied naturally occurring neuronal cell death in detail (4). Descriptions

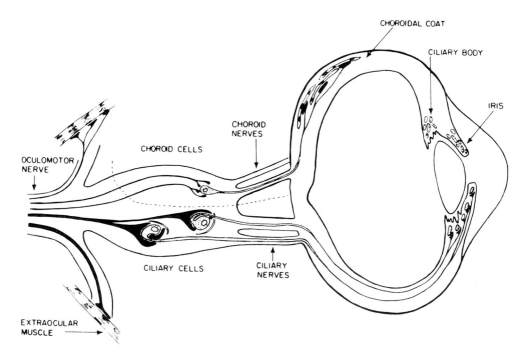

FIG. 1. Innervation of target territories within the eye by neurons from the chick ciliary ganglion.

of this phenomenon are based on data involving cell counts and can be summarized as follows: during the 8th and 14th day of embryonic life (E8 to E14) about 40-60% of the initial neuronal population of the ciliary ganglion degenerate. This process occurs when all the axons penetrate within the eye and is not due to an apparent lack of innervation. Prior to its onset, neurons appear to differentiate normally and their death occurs at the time of postganglionic synaptogenesis (Fig. 2). This implies that during normal development an excess of neurons is produced and that some of the cells degenerate owing to the inability of the periphery to support all of them. Indeed early removal of the eye primordium will exaggerate the neuronal loss, whereas the graft of a supernumerary eye primordium reduces the proportion of neurons, which subsequently die.

It was thus proposed that neurons from the ciliary ganglion compete within the target territories for limited amounts of one (or several) trophic factor(s); the latter might be taken up by the afferent axons and be retrogradely transported to the cell bodies in order to promote the survival of these neurons.

The Chick Eye Ciliary Neuronotrophic Factor

Ciliary ganglia can easily be dissected at E8, and then dissociated and grown in culture; neurons are distinguished from non-neuronal cells by their particular mor-

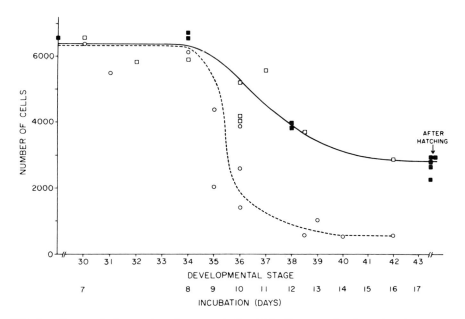

FIG. 2. Changes in the number of neurons in the chick ciliary ganglion through various stages of development. The solid line is based on data collected from normal unoperated animals; the broken line derives from those obtained after removal of the eye primordium (5).

phology. However when grown in a regular tissue culture medium without any supplement, all the neurons die within 24 hr. The addition of various exogenous sources, such as an extract of whole chick embryo (6), rescued the neurons under these artificial conditions. This activity can be quantified by a bioassay involving neuronal cell counts following serial dilutions of the active medium. Varon and his colleagues showed that within the embryo one third of the total activity is associated with the eye, the other two thirds being recovered in the carcass. Moreover subdissection of the eye reveals that all of the eye ciliary neuronotrophic factor (CNTF) activity resides in the iris, ciliary body, and choroid, that is, the innervation territories of the ciliary ganglion (7). During embryonic development there is a sharp increase in eye-CNTF activity between E11 and E15: within this period the specific activity, when expressed per unit of protein, doubles (8). In addition cultured ciliary ganglion neurons derived from younger (E5) as well as from older (E14) embryos will survive in the absence of added CNTF, whereas neurons taken between E7 and E11 show a marked dependence on its presence (9). This age dependence is not an artifact due to the dissociation procedure, since intact ciliary ganglia can be grown *in vitro* and shown to exhibit the same requirement for added CNTF in order to survive and continue their development (10). Taken together, these data show that the chick eye contains one (or several) neuronal survival factor(s) named CNTF, highly localized within the innervation territories of the ciliary ganglion and abundant at a time when neuronal cell death occurs *in vivo*.

The biochemical characterization and isolation of the CNTF has recently been achieved (11) using E15 chick embryos (at a time when specific activity is highest). Eye-derived tissues were dissected and homogenized, and an aqueous high speed supernatant was processed through various steps of biochemical fractionation (including ion-exchange chromatography, ultracentrifugation, and preparative gel electrophoresis). A protein, still retaining its biological activity (after removal of the detergent) and with an apparent molecular weight of 20,000 daltons and an isoelectric point around 5, could be eluted from the sodium dodecyl sulfate (SDS) gel. The CNTF molecule is different in its biochemical and biological properties from nerve growth factor, a trophic factor which is unable to promote the survival of ciliary ganglion neurons; the properties of CNTF are also distinct from the recently identified brain-derived growth factor (12). When sufficient amounts of purified CNTF can be generated, it will be possible to perform experimental manipulations to test its relevance during the *in vivo* development of the ciliary ganglion. The regulation of its production is also still unknown. Interestingly, Ebendal et al. (13) have reported that freezing and thawing rat irides releases a parasympathetic neuronotropic factor.

Neurite-Promoting Factors (NPF)

Besides the chick eye CNTF, other sources have been reported to support survival of ciliary ganglion neurons, such as muscle extracts or media collected from cultured muscle cells (conditioned media (6). Heart muscle cells in culture release two types of activities in the medium. These can be demonstrated when such a conditioned medium is transferred to culture dishes with dissociated ciliary ganglion neurons. The latter not only attach and survive but also exhibit a profuse neuritic extension which can be detected within a few hours following plating. This dual effect (survival and neurite outgrowth) is not shared by the eye-derived CNTF, which causes only survival and no outgrowth. The suspicion that two categories of molecules were involved in these phenomena was confirmed by Collins (14) and Adler and Varon (15) using the protocol schematically described in Fig. 3. Whereas the survival-promoting effect is shared by a soluble molecule, the neurite-promoting factor (NPF) is inactive unless it is properly reanchored to a tissue culture substratum (e.g., a polycationic surface such as polyornithine or polylysine) (Fig. 4). The NPF appears to exert a directive influence on neurite outgrowth (16).

Since the CNTF molecule is devoid of any neurite-promoting effect, what induces the neurons of the ciliary ganglion to send out processes? Adler and Varon (17), using intact ciliary ganglia plated on collagen as explants, noticed a correlation between the formation of an outgrowth of ganglionic non-neuronal cells and the timing and extent of neuritic development outside the ganglion. Neurites do not emerge from the explant until the onset of non-neuronal outgrowth, which occurs first. The growth cones move onto this preformed layer but never encompass it, indicating that the surface of non-neuronal cells bears signals competent for the elongation of neuritic processes.

NPF molecules present on the surface of non-neuronal cells and released into the medium are also produced by cultured glial cells from cell lines which include both PNS and CNS (18). The rat RN22 Schwannoma releases NPF in the culture medium and partial purification indicates that a large acidic glycoprotein is involved (19,20). Bovine corneal cells also secrete a substance with similar activity, associated with three or four proteins in a large complex containing a heparan sulfate proteoglycan (21).

Extracellular Matrix Components as NPF

The extracellular matrix is known to play an important role in cell interactions of various non-neuronal tissues (22). This material consists of a complex assembly of various molecules including collagen (of different types), several glycoproteins (laminin, fibronectin), and different proteoglycans (22). Laminin coated to a tissue culture dish is able to stimulate neuritic outgrowth in a manner similar to that observed for the various NPF sources described earlier (23). Indeed, Schwann cells or RN22 Schwannoma cells do produce laminin in their culture medium. However, antibodies directed against purified laminin are not able to block neuritic extension induced by the conditioned medium. To elucidate this apparent discrepancy Mattew and Patterson have recently been able to produce under particular conditions a monoclonal antibody that can block neurite outgrowth induced by one of these conditioned media (24). Preliminary experiments indicate that the elongation of neurites involves a macromolecular complex which includes laminin and heparan sulphate.

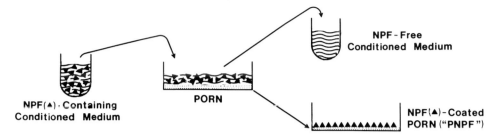

FIG. 3. Identification of the neurite-promoting factor (NPF) present in a conditioned medium derived from cultures of chick heart muscle cells. Although soluble, the NPF binds to polyornithine (PORN) in order to elicit neurite outgrowth.

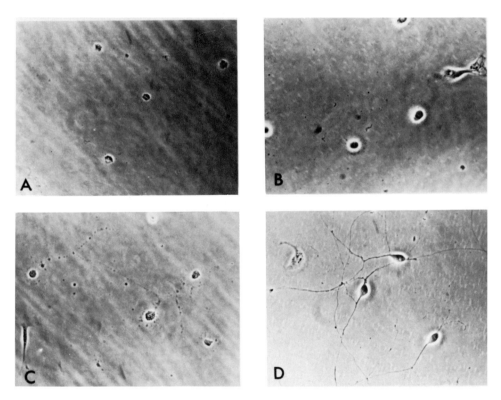

FIG. 4. Morphological aspect of chick ciliary ganglion neurons when grown for 24 hr under various conditions. **A:** In the absence of any supplement (basal medium), on polyornithine. **B:** In a NPF-free conditioned medium (prepared as described in Fig. 3, from heart muscle cells); neurons survive but do not extend neurites. **C:** In a basal medium using a polyornithine substratum previously coated with NPF (see Fig. 3); although they attach, neurons subsequently die due to lack of survival factor. **D:** In the presence of a complete conditioned medium (from heart muscle cells); neurons survive and send out processes. A similar picture is observed when combining conditions **B** and **C**.

The importance of laminin for neurite extension is puzzling since this molecule is known to be present around peripheral nerves but not along central axons of the adult brain (where it is only present around capillaries), although astrocytes can produce it under particular conditions (22).

CELLULAR INTERACTIONS DURING *IN VITRO* DEVELOPMENT OF DOPAMINERGIC NEURONS

In contrast to the results accumulated about the PNS, the information regarding specific growth factors directed to a given neuronal subset within the CNS is still preliminary (25–28). During the last few years A. Prochiantz's group (in J. Glowinski's laboratory) has addressed this topic using the dopaminergic (DA) nigrostriatal system in culture as an experimental model. In mice, postmitotic DA neurons are present at the level of the mesencephalic curvature as early as the 13th day of embryonic life. These can be visualized by DA-induced fluorescence (29); these perikarya begin to send out processes, particularly towards the striatum (Fig. 5). Innervation of this target territory is a progressive event which is achieved around the third postnatal week.

Influence of Striatal Target Cells

Using an embryonic mouse brain it is possible to dissect and dissociate a portion of the mesencephalon which includes the DA cell bodies. Cultures derived from this cell suspension exhibit a large heterogeneity with regard to the various neuronal phenotypes, among which the DA ones represent only a few percent. Fortunately the latter can easily be recognized either by fluorescence histochemistry or by immunocytochemistry with an antibody against tyrosine hydroxylase (the first enzyme

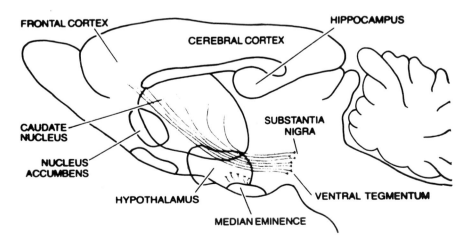

FIG. 5. Dopaminergic neuronal pathways in the rodent brain.

involved in DA biosynthesis) (30). Under appropriate conditions these cells are able to develop for a long period of time during which they extend processes. Their development is also assessed by their ability to synthesize the neurotransmitter from its tritiated precursor (L-tyrosine). Moreover they are capable of taking up exogenous tritiated dopamine (allowing their visualization by autoradiography) and to release this amine under depolarizing conditions (high potassium, veratridine) in a calcium-dependent manner (31).

When mesencephalic cells are grown in the presence of striatal target cells, the uptake of exogenous tritiated dopamine (^{3}H-DA) as well as its synthesis from ^{3}H-tyrosine by DA cells is increased at least twofold after 8 days or 2 weeks *in vitro* (32). Since the absolute number of DA neurons is not modified in the co-culture, this effect must reflect an enhanced maturation of DA cells in the presence of the striatal cells. However, the presence of both neuronal and glial cells in the culture (grown in the presence of serum) does not allow determination of which cell type is involved in this maturation effect. The relative contribution of glial cells to the total cellular population can be reduced to only a few percent when serum is omitted from a chemically defined medium (supplemented with hormones, proteins, and salts) (33). Under these conditions cultures of the striatum are highly enriched with neurons and are still able to stimulate ^{3}H-DA uptake, thereby reinforcing the hypothesis of a neuro-neuronal interaction (34). Such an interaction cannot be mimicked with a conditioned medium obtained from striatal cultures and thus favors the hypothesis of direct cellular interactions. Indeed, striatal membranes prepared from 2 to 3 week old animals stimulate ^{3}H-DA uptake by cultured DA neurons (35). This stimulation is not only age dependent (younger and older animals are incompetent) but also target specific (membranes issued from non-target tissues like cerebellum or hippocampus do not share the effect).

The enhanced uptake of ^{3}H-DA promoted by striatal neurons could result from an increase in length of DA processes. However under the co-culture conditions there is a significant reduction of the mean length of DA neurites; this reduction occurs when the neurites encounter the target neurons and is sometimes accompanied by a tendency to spread over and around the contacted cell (36). On the contrary, non-target cells (e.g., cerebellar neurons) are unable to retard DA neurite elongation. Thus it seems that the growth cones of DA neurons have a tendency to stop growing when they reach appropriate target cells, reflecting the ability for target areas to provide signals which limit further outgrowth.

Neuron–Glia Relationships

Besides neurons, glial cells can also affect the development of DA cells. When DA cells are cultured on confluent monolayers of glial cells from the mesencephalon or from the striatum they exhibit a different morphology (37). In both situations glial cultures are composed of astrocytes. On striatal glial cells DA neurons adopt an uncomplicated aspect and exhibit one long, very thin process with a few short ones around the cell body (Fig. 6); although a similar morphology is also observed

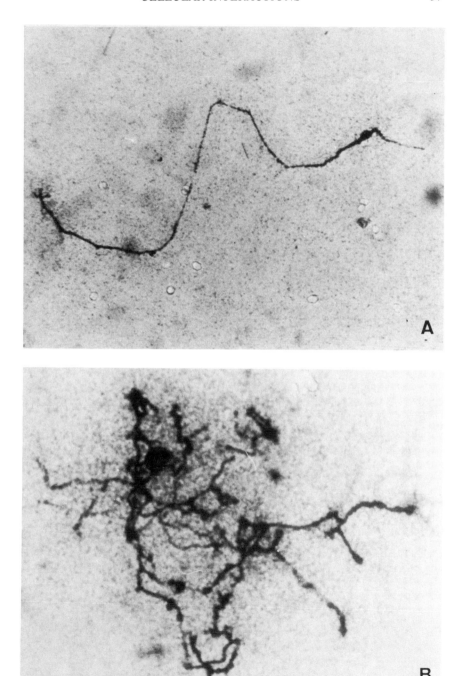

FIG. 6. Visualization of dopaminergic neurons after 2 days *in vitro* on monolayers of striatal **(A)** or mesencephalic **(B)** glial cells (37).

in the presence of mesencephalic glial cells, a larger proportion of the DA neurons develop several long and highly branched neurites with varicosities (Fig. 6). This morphological effect dictated by the origin of the glial monolayer does not result from the selection of a particular DA neuronal subpopulation: DA neurons grown on a given glial monolayer can be collected and replated on the other glial population, causing their morphology to change. Neither is this behavior influenced by any diffusible factor(s) released by the glial cells: When the two types of glial cells are present within the same dish, although physically separated, DA neurons adopt the shape dictated by the underlying glia. This phenomenon suggests direct cell-to-cell interaction. We infer that under the present experimental conditions the two types of glial cells (both astrocytes) exhibit different cell surface properties that we are presently characterizing with biochemical techniques. We have already found qualitative differences with respect to their glycoproteins.

The observed difference in morphology of DA neurons could be the *in vitro* counterpart of the axons and dendrites observed *in vivo*. Electron microscope studies performed by A. Autillo-Touati (*unpublished observations*) indicate that the processes of DA neurons grown on mesencephalic glia share some of the ultrastructural characteristics of dendrites (e.g., the presence of ribosomes).

To determine how DA neurons might modify their form under external influences we are looking at possible changes in the organization of cytoskeletal components, since a previous study has demonstrated the large heterogeneity of tubulin proteins within neuronal cells (38). Moreover it has recently been reported that a particular form of microtubules associated proteins, MAP_2, is preferentially if not exclusively localized in dendrites (39); processes of mesencephalic neurons were found to become heavily labeled with an antibody (kindly provided by A. Fellous, Paris, France) recognizing this protein, when astrocytes of the mesencephalon provided the underlying substratum.

CONCLUSIONS AND PERSPECTIVES

These two experimental systems have been chosen to illustrate some of the external influences that neurons receive from their immediate environment during embryonic development. These influences imply indirect (diffusible signals) or direct (cell-to-cell) interactions with other target neurons or tissues and glial partners (40). Alternatively, neurons can also influence their glial partners (e.g., by regulating glial cell proliferation). Target cells may deliver trophic factors essential for subsequent survival of the afferent input, thereby harmonizing the size of the neuronal population with that of the target area. Neuronal target cells can also bear specific signals allowing recognition by the appropriate growth cone (and future establishment of specific connections). Appropriate recognition will ensure subsequent maturation of the neuronal afference. Glial cells are well known to provide an adequate terrain for the adhesion of neurons and neurite outgrowth. Moreover it appears that these cells may exhibit a biochemical heterogeneity which could dictate the morphological appearance of the neurons. Only very recently have molecular clues been characterized for some of these interactions, though their mechanisms of action are at present unknown.

Undoubtedly future experiments will attempt to verify that such interactions, occurring *in vitro* and the involved molecular signals, are also relevant during *in vivo* development. Some of these factors appear to be very specific (e.g., those involved in cell–cell recognition) whereas others are rather ubiquitous and not restricted to the nervous system (e.g., extracellular matrix components). In this respect it is worth emphasizing the developmental regulation of these interactions. It is not yet known what triggers the expression of these signals at the appropriate time or what turns them off once their biological role has been achieved. Inhibitors might be involved to counteract their action. For instance, axonal growth inhibitors may be relevant to restrict outgrowth along preformed pathways or to stop the growth cone once the correct target cell has been reached.

The involvement of such critical interactions during development does not exclude their possible relevance in the adult nervous system, especially under pathological conditions. Preliminary experiments indicate, for instance, that the injured brain may produce some of these factors, which will be essential for neural repair (41).

ACKNOWLEDGMENTS

The author is most grateful to Ms. L. Belehradek for her efficient help in typing this chapter.

REFERENCES

1. Raff MC, Fields KL, Hakomori S-I, Mirsky R, Pruss R, Winter J. Cell-type specific markers for distinguishing and studying neurons and the major classes of glial cells in culture. *Brain Res* 1979;174:283–308.
2. Barnes D, Sato G. Methods for growth of cultured cells in serum-free medium. *Anal Biochem* 1980;102;255–70.
3. Jacobson M. *Developmental neurobiology*. New York: Plenum, 1978.
4. Landmesser L, Pilar G. Interactions between neurons and their targets during *in vivo* synaptogenesis. *Fed Proc* 1978;37:2016–22.
5. Landmesser L, Pilar G. Synapse formation during embryogenesis on ganglion cells lacking a periphery. *J Physiol (London)* 1974;241:715–36.
6. Berg DK. New neuronal growth factors. *Annu Rev Neurosci* 1984;7:149–70.
7. Adler R, Landa K B, Manthorpe M, Varon S. Cholinergic neuronotropic factors, II. Intracellular distribution of trophic activity for ciliary neurons. *Science* 1979;204:1434–6.
8. Landa K B, Adler R, Manthorpe M, Varon S. Cholinergic neuronotrophic factors. III. Developmental increase of trophic activity for chick embryo ciliary ganglion neurons in their intraocular target tissues. *Dev Biol* 1980;74:401–8.
9. Manthorpe M, Adler R, Varon S. Cholinergic neuronotrophic factors. VI. Age-dependent requirements by chick embryo ciliary ganglionic neurons. *Dev Biol* 1981;85:156–63.
10. Adler R, Varon S. Neuronal survival in intact ciliary ganglia *in vivo* and *in vitro:* ciliary neuronotrophic factor as a target surrogate. *Dev Biol* 1982;92:470–5.

11. Barbin G, Manthorpe M, Varon S. Purification of the chick eye ciliary neuronotrophic factor. *J Neurochem* 1984;43:1468–78.
12. Barde Y-A, Edgar D, Thoenen H. Purification of a new neurotrophic factor from mammalian brain. *EMBO J* 1982;1:549–53.
13. Ebendal T, Olson L, Seiger A, Hedlund KO. Nerve growth factors in the rat iris. *Nature* 1980;286:25–8.
14. Collins F. Induction of neurite outgrowth by a conditioned medium factor bound to culture substratum. *Proc Natl Acad Sci USA* 1978;75:5210–3.
15. Adler R, Varon S. Cholinergic neuronotrophic factors. V. Segregation of survival and neurite promoting activities in heart conditioned media. *Brain Res* 1980;188:437–48.
16. Collins F, Garrett JE. Elongating nerve fibres are guided by a pathway of material released from embryonic non-neuronal cells. *Proc Natl Acad Sci USA* 1980;77:6226–8.
17. Adler R, Varon S. Neuritic guidance by non-neuronal cells of ganglionic origin. *Dev Biol* 1981;86:69–80.
18. Adler R, Manthorpe M, Skaper S, Varon S. Polyornithine-bound neurite-promoting factors (PNPFs): culture sources and responsive neurons. *Brain Res* 1981;206:129–44.
19. Manthorpe M, Varon S, Adler R. Neurite promoting factor (NPF) in conditioned medium from RN22 Schwannoma cultures: bioassay, fractionation and other properties. *J Neurochem* 1981;37:759–67.
20. Adler R, Manthorpe M, Varon S. Lectin reactivity of PNPF, a polyornithine binding neurite promoting factor. *Dev Brain Res* 1983;6:69–75.
21. Lander AD, Fujii DK, Gospodarowicz D, Reichardt LF. Characterization of a factor that promotes neurite outgrowth; evidence linking activity to a heparan sulfate proteoglycan. *J Cell Biol* 1982;94:574–85.
22. Hay ED. *Cell biology of extracellular matrix.* New York: Plenum, 1982.
23. Carbonetto S. The extracellular matrix of the nervous system. *Trends Neurosci* 1984;7:382–7.
24. Mattew WD, Patterson PH. The production of a monoclonal antibody that blocks the action of a neurite outgrowth-promoting factor. *Cold Spring Harbor Symp Quant Biol* 1983;48:625–31.
25. Banker GA. Trophic interactions between astroglial cells and hippocampal neurons in culture. *Science* 1980;209:809–10.
26. Muller HW, Seifert W. A neurotrophic factor (NTF) released from primary glial cultures supports survival and fiber outgrowth of cultured hippocampal neurons. *J Neurosci Res* 1982;8:195–204.
27. Barbin G, Selak I, Manthorpe M, Varon S. Use of central neuronal cultures for the detection of neuronotrophic agents. *Neuroscience* 1984;12:33–44.
28. Hoffmann PC, Hemmendinger LM, Kotake C, Heller A. Enhanced dopamine cell survival in reaggregates containing telencephalic target cells. *Brain Res* 1983;274:275–81.
29. Golden GS. Postnatal development of the biogenic amine systems of the mouse brain. *Dev Biol* 1973;33:300–11.
30. Berger B, Di Porzio U, Daguet MC, et al. Long-term development of mesencephalic dopaminergic neurons of mouse embryos in dissociated primary cultures: morphological and histochemical characteristics. *Neuroscience* 1983;7:193–205.
31. Daguet MC, Di Porzio U, Prochiantz A, Kato A, Glowinski J. Release of dopamine from dissociated mesencephalic dopaminergic neurons in primary cultures in absence or presence of striatal target cells. *Brain Res* 1980;191:564–8.
32. Prochiantz A, Di Porzio U, Kato A, Glowinski J. *In Vitro* maturation of mesencephalic dopaminergic neurons from mouse embryos is enhanced in presence of their striatal target cells. *Proc Natl Acad Sci USA* 1979;76:5381–7.
33. Prochiantz A, Delacourte A, Daguet MC, Paulin D. Intermediate filament proteins in mouse brain cells cultured in the presence or absence of fetal calf serum. *Exp Cell Res* 1982;139:404–10.
34. Di Porzio U, Daguet MC, Glowinski J, Prochiantz A. Effect of striatal target cells on *in vitro* maturation of mesencephalic dopaminergic neurons grown in serum-free conditions. *Nature* 1980;288:370–3.
35. Prochiantz A, Daguet MC, Herbet A, Glowinski J. Specific stimulation of *in vitro* maturation of mesencephalic dopaminergic neurones by striatal membranes. *Nature* 1981;293:570–3.
36. Denis-Donini S, Glowinski J, Prochiantz A. Specific influence of striatal target neurons on the *in vitro* outgrowth of mesencephalic dopaminergic neurites: a morphological quantitative study. *J Neurosci* 1983;3:2292–9.

37. Denis-Donini S, Glowinski J, Prochiantz A. Glial heterogeneity may define the three-dimensional shape of mouse mesencephalic dopaminergic neurones. *Nature* 1984;307:641–3.
38. Moura Neto V, Mallat M, Jeantet C, Prochiantz A. microheterogeneity of tubulin proteins in neuronal and glial cells from the mouse brain in culture. *EMBO J* 1983;2:1243–8.
39. Huber G, Matus A. Differences in the cellular distributions of two microtubule-associated proteins, MAP1 and MAP2, in rat brain. *J Neurosci* 1984;4:151–60.
40. Varon S, Adler R. Trophic and specifying factors directed to neuronal cells. *Adv Cell Neurobiol* 1981;2:115–63.
41. Nieto-Sampedro M, Lewis ER, Cotman CW, et al. Brain injury causes a time-dependent increase in neuronotrophic activity at the lesion site. *Science* 1982;217:860–1.

DISCUSSION

Dr. Dubowitz: You briefly mentioned that an injury to the occipital cortex produced a cyst containing fluid with neuronotrophic properties. If this is so, is there any evidence that similar substances are present in infants with porencephalic cysts due to injury, perhaps identifiable in the CSF? If so, the removal of the fluid might have serious consequences.

Dr. Barbin: I cannot answer directly about the pathological situations to which you refer. We have been trying to detect and measure neuronotrophic activity in the CSF and have found evidence for it in some patients using tissue culture approach. The implications are uncertain.

Dr. Caviness: With regard to the different morphology of the striatal neurons maintained on glia derived from the striatum on the one hand and the mesencephalon on the other, is it your view that we are looking at different trophic effects, in other words the different degree to which these glia support the general growth properties of such cells, or are we seeing something more revolutionary: the view that the glial substrate in fact dictates a mode of growth?

Dr. Barbin: I do not think we are dealing with a trophic effect, at least judging from the cell morphology, though this does not exclude the possibility that glial cells contribute to trophic support. I think it is more likely that we are dealing with differences in surface properties and that there is, for instance, a difference in the adhesion of a growth cone which could be related to a constituent present on the surface of the glial cells. I have in mind that if you manipulate the surface of a cell by adding macromolecules such as heparin sulfate proteoglycan you can induce a very different morphology for some neuronal populations.

Dr. Sotelo: I think this is very important. I believe it is not a soluble factor we are seeing but something in the membrane of the astrocyte, of a specific astrocyte, which is important for the tridimensional disposition of the dendrites and axons in dopaminergic neurons. I do not know how general this phenomenon may turn out to be. It is certainly very difficult to investigate Purkinje cells, for example, because they are so hard to cultivate, but for these dopaminergic cells this is something very new and very important, indicating for the first time that there is local information contained in astrocyte membranes which is decisive in determining whether dopaminergic cells elongate or produce multiple neurites.

Dr. Minkowski: Is it known how nerve growth factor (NGF) acts?

Dr. Barbin: We still don't know this. There are several biological responses to NGF, some expressed very early, some expressed later. One of the early responses is to regulate the ion content of these nerve cells, so it is possible that it stimulates sodium-potassium-ATPase. This has to be confirmed but it does seem that NGF controls the equilibrium between the sodium and potassium content of the nerve cells.

Dr. Diamond: I was interested in the observation that adding glial cells promotes the dendritic branching of nerve cells in culture. I wonder whether this observation could be made with other kinds of cells, perhaps even non-neural cells, in that you are dealing with the surface properties of different layers. Or is this related specifically to a neuronal or glial membrane property of the added cells?

Dr. Barbin: I can only say that we have tried with fibroblasts in our glial experiments but have been unable to discriminate the two types of morphology.

Developmental Neurobiology, edited by
Philippe Evrard and Alexandre Minkowski.
Nestlé Nutrition Workshop Series, Vol. 12.
Nestec Ltd., Vevey/Raven Press, Ltd.,
New York © 1989.

Peroxisomes and Central Nervous System Dysgenesis and Dysfunction

Sidney L. Goldfischer

Department of Pathology, Albert Einstein College of Medicine,
The Bronx, New York 10461

Peroxisomes play a key role in a number of genetic diseases. These include disorders in which the activity of a peroxisomal enzyme is deficient and an extraordinary group of diseases in which the formation of the organelle itself is defective (1–3) (Table 1).

DISORDERS OF PEROXISOMAL BIOGENESIS

Zellweger's cerebrohepatorenal syndrome (CHRS) is the first disease in which defective formation of peroxisomes was described (4,5). Infants affected with this rare autosomal recessive disorder usually die within one year. Clinical features of the syndrome include a typical facial appearance, with hypertelorism, a high forehead, and pursed lips; minor skeletal abnormalities; renal cortical cysts; and severe hepatic fibrosis. Iron storage is frequently seen in the early stage of the disease. The most prominent findings are in the central nervous system and include profound hypotonia. Cerebral abnormalities include polymicrogyria, pachygyria, olivary dysplasia, and defective neuronal migration. Gliosis and accumulations of lipid in glia are associated with myelin breakdown, and the disease has been described as a sudanophilic leukodystrophy (6–9).

Hepatocellular peroxisomes have not been detected in children with this disease. This remarkable finding has been confirmed by many laboratories (10–13). It is particularly surprising in view of the fact that there are approximately 1,000 peroxisomes in a normal human hepatocyte (14). In hepatocytes and proximal renal tubules, where peroxisomes also appear to be absent, their diameter is approximately 0.5 microns and normally they are readily detectable. In addition to the peroxisomal defects, structural and chemical abnormalities in mitochondria have been described (4,5,10,13). The most common has been the report of diminished oxidation of succinate; further on in the respiratory pathway, electron transport is normal.

TABLE 1. *Peroxisomal diseases*

Defective peroxisomal biogenesis syndromes
  Zellweger's cerebrohepatorenal syndrome
  neonatal adrenoleukodystrophy
  infantile Refsum's disease
Deficiency of a peroxisomal enzymatic activity
  X-linked childhood adrenoleukodystrophy
  pseudo-Zellweger's syndrome (3-oxoacyl-coA thiolase deficiency)
  acatalasia
  cerebrotendinous xanthomatosis (?)

A variety of chemical abnormalities are seen in patients with CHRS, and many of these reflect the peroxisomal deficiency. These include markedly increased concentrations of pipecolic acid (15), very long chain fatty acids (VLCFA) in blood and tissues (16,17), and the presence of abnormal bile acid intermediates (18,19). The activity of a key peroxisomal membrane enzyme involved in the synthesis of plasmalogens, dihydroxyacetone phosphate acyltransferase (DHAP-AT), is reduced by approximately 90%, and tissue concentrations of plasmalogens are less than 10% of normal in cells and tissues from patients with CHRS (20–22). Assay of DHAP-AT has been utilized in the antenatal diagnosis of CHRS (23).

Neonatal adrenoleukodystrophy (NALD) is another disease in which the formation of hepatocellular peroxisomes is defective (24–26). Although not as severely affected as children with CHRS (affected individuals have survived for as long as 6 years), NALD patients also suffer from severe hypotonia and seizures. Plasma concentrations of VLCFA are increased six- to ninefold and cultured fibroblasts have a markedly diminished capacity to oxidize these fatty acids. Tissue deposits of VLCFA are widespread. We have examined the hepatocytes in two cases of NALD, and in both instances hepatocellular peroxisomes are markedly reduced in size and number (27). They are less than 0.2 μm in diameter, and one-tenth as numerous as in the normal hepatocyte. Indeed, they are so small and sparse that several reports have been published stating that they are absent in this disease (28). They can be identified unequivocally by incubation in a cytochemical medium that makes visible a marker peroxisomal enzyme, catalase. Other biochemical findings in this disease are similar to CHRS (27). These include elevated concentrations of pipecolic acid, the presence of abnormal bile acid intermediates, and reduced levels of DHAP-AT, a key enzyme in plasmalogen synthesis (Janna Collins *personal communication,* 1985).

The infantile variant of Refsum's disease is the third disorder in which formation of peroxisomes appears to be defective (29). Evidence for this comes from cytochemical and ultrastructural studies of the liver (30) and from biochemical studies of serum and fibroblasts (31,32). The classical form of Refsum's syndrome, which is an autosomal recessive disorder, manifests itself in the first or second decade of life and is characterized by retinitis pigmentosa, peripheral polyneuropathy, and cerebellar ataxia. Affected individuals have tissue stores of phytanic acid, a 20-carbon fatty acid derived from plant material. Because the stored material is exogenous in origin, a restricted diet is an effective therapy in this condition. The defect has been attributed to the failure in the first step of catabolism of phytanic acid, that is, the alpha oxidation of the terminal carboxyl group. Recently several cases have been described of young children with phytanic acid storage disease who manifested symptoms from birth. Electron microscopic studies by Dr. Frank Roels (30) have demonstrated that hepatocytes do not contain recognizable peroxisomes in this condition, and biochemical studies (31,32) have shown increased concentrations of the bile acid intermediate trihydroxycoprostanoic acid (THCA), as well as VLCFA. We are not aware of any studies in which the role of peroxisomes in the oxidation of phytanic acid has been analyzed. However, deficient oxidation of phytanic acid has been described in fibroblasts of such patients. We have recently found that serum phytanic acid is increased in CHRS and NALD, two diseases in which peroxisomes are deficient, but not in diseases associated with a more specific enzymatic defect, such as X-linked adrenoleukodystrophy (ALD) or a multiple peroxisomal oxidative activity deficiency syndrome (pseudo-Zellweger's disease) (33,34). This suggests that phytanic acid accumulation is secondary to a deficiency of peroxisomes, and that peroxisomal oxidative activity plays a critical role in the catabolism of phytanic acid. It is noteworthy that the number of peroxisomes is not diminished in fibroblasts from patients with the classical form of Refsum's disease (35).

It is unclear at the present time whether the CHRS, NALD, and infantile form of Refsum's disease are distinct entities or represent varying degrees of expression of a single disorder. It has recently been demonstrated that the absence of peroxisomes in CHRS is not absolute (36). Fibroblasts from four patients with CHRS or related diseases were examined. Two were classical Zellweger patients who died at the age of 6 months, and two others were longer-lived atypical patients (5 years, and alive at 3 years) who probably had NALD. Peroxisomes were detected, but reduced in number in all of these cell lines. Morphometric analysis demonstrated a reduction of approximately 90% in the first group of classical CHRS patients, and of 60% in the patients with longer survival. It will require much more extensive study to determine whether the severity of disease is a consistent reflection of the number of peroxisomes. The apparent inconsistency between hepatocytes and fibroblasts may reflect variations in the degree to which the deficiency manifests itself in different tissues. Intestinal peroxisomes do not appear to be reduced in NALD (27). It is noteworthy that in mice with testicular feminization syndrome there is a marked reduction in size and number of peroxisomes in the interstitial cells of the testes (37).

It is evident that there is considerable overlap between these syndromes (16). Even apparently distinctive pathologic phenomena, such as normal adrenals in CHRS and adrenal atrophy in NALD, may be a reflection of the shorter life span of these individuals. Recent studies have shown functional adrenal insufficiency in children with Zellweger's CHRS (38). Cerebellar heterotopia and olivary dysplasia occur both in classical CHRS and in NALD, but these phenomena have not been described in the infantile form of Refsum's disease. Other neurological findings, such as retinitis pigmentosa and demyelination, have been observed in all of these conditions, even though the degree of involvement may vary considerably. Comparison of conditions in which peroxisomal biogenesis is defective with several other disorders in which there appears to be defective activity of a single peroxisomal enzyme may be instructive in relating specific pathologic events to specific enzymatic activities. It must be stressed that there have been no studies of mitochondrial respiration in NALD and infantile Refsum's disease.

PEROXISOMAL DISORDERS AFFECTING SPECIFIC ENZYMATIC ACTIVITIES

A second group of peroxisomal disorders resemble the better known deficiency diseases. These are diseases in which the organelle is formed but a specific enzymatic activity is defective, analogous to the lysosomal storage diseases. It is not surprising that many of the manifestations of these conditions also appear in the syndromes in which the formation of the organelle and the functional activity of all its constituent enzymes are affected.

X-Linked Adrenoleukodystrophy (Schilder's Disease)

X-linked disease affects prepubertal boys who are normal until the age of 3 to 5 years. It is characterized by progressive destruction of the cerebral white matter and atrophy of the adrenals. Although neurological symptoms usually precede those of adrenal insufficiency, this is not always the case; their progression is usually relentless (39). These patients have markedly increased serum and tissue accumulations of VLCFA (C_{24}, C_{26}), visible in tissue sections as striated inclusions of acetone-insoluble lipid.

The presence of demyelination (or dysmyelination) as a common factor in CHRS and the adrenoleukodystrophies suggests that peroxisomal oxidation may be involved in the formation and maintenance of myelin (27,40). In the central nervous system, peroxisomes are present in oligodendroglia, the cells responsible for myelination (41). Enlarged hepatocellular peroxisomes with atypical inclusions have been described in a child with spongy degeneration of the CNS (van Bogaert and Bertrand type) in which dysmyelination is prominent (42).

Pseudo-CHRS or a Deficiency of Peroxisomal Thiolase

Peroxisomes were not reduced in number and were sometimes larger than normal in a liver biopsy from a 2 week old girl with an initial clinical diagnosis of CHRS. That diagnosis was based upon her characteristic facial appearance and severe hypotonia (34). Activity of two peroxisomal enzymes, DHAP-AT (measured biochemically) and catalase (demonstrated by cytochemistry), was normal. However, peroxisomal oxidative activities toward palmitoyl-CoA were reduced by about 90%. An abnormal bile acid intermediate, THCA, was increased in duodenal fluid and serum pipecolic acid concentrations were elevated. Death occurred at 11 months, and autopsy revealed adrenal atrophy, demyelination, gliosis, and neuronal heterotopia as well as storage of VLCFA. The underlying defect was a deficiency of 3-oxoacyl-coenzyme A thiolase (43). Plasmalogen concentrations were normal, indicating that these phospholipids are not implicated in the neuronal migration defect and dysmyelination that occur in these disorders.

Pipecolic Acidemia

Pipecolic acidemia has been described as a distinct entity; however, this metabolite is elevated in all of the disorders of peroxisomal biogenesis. Hepatocellular peroxisomes with normal morphology have also been reported in a male infant (one of two siblings) with hyperpipecolic acidemia (44).

Thus the situation with regard to pipecolic acid appears analogous to that which occurs with VLCFA and possibly phytanic acid; that is, increased concentrations of the metabolite occur in conditions in which either the formation of peroxisomes is inhibited or the activity of one or several of its constituent enzymes is diminished. Pipecolic acid is formed in a minor pathway of lysine catabolism; however, in the brain this is believed to be a principal product of lysine (45). Pipecolic acid is reported to compete for gamma amino butyric acid (GABA) receptors (46).

Cerebrotendinous Xanthomatosis

The principal features of cerebrotendinous xanthomatosis (CTX) are progressive dementia, cerebellar ataxia, demyelination, gliosis, and diminished bile acid formation associated with secretion of large amounts of bile alcohols. Cholesterol and cholestanol are deposited in brain, tendons, and elsewhere (47). The defect has been attributed to mitochondrial 26-hydroxylase deficiency (48). The likelihood that peroxisomes may have been present in the fraction that exhibits this activity was not considered. A peroxisomal 26-hydrolase has recently been described (49). Structural abnormalities in both mitochondria and peroxisomes have been demonstrated in CTX (50,51).

Acatalasemia

Human acatalasemia was first described by Takahara (52), an otolaryngologist who washed the gangrenous ulcers in the gums and jaw of a young girl with hydrogen peroxide, and noted that her blood turned brown-black and that few bubbles of oxygen were formed (see ref. 53 for review of this condition). Takahara attributed the color change to the formation of methemoglobin by H_2O_2 in the absence of catalase. The more general term acatalasia was proposed for this condition when the same phenomenon was detected in other tissues. Patients with different degrees of catalase deficiency have since been found in Europe, North Africa, and North America. Gangrenous oral lesions are not a common finding and have been attributed to a poor nutritional and hygienic status. No other functional or morphological abnormalities have been reported.

Mice with low or undetectable levels of blood and tissue catalase activity have been bred (54). Histochemical studies with the alkaline diaminobenzidine reaction for catalase (55) showed that peroxisomes in acatalasemic mice were more reactive than in normal mice. This paradoxical result was unexpected and was eventually explained by experiments which showed that the catalase in renal and hepatic peroxisomes of the "acatalasemic" mutant is present but altered so that its peroxidatic, rather than catalatic, activity is manifested (56,57). This is consistent with biochemical studies by Aebi et al. (58) who showed that catalase in these animals was labile and readily inactivated during the course of an assay at 37°C. Alkaline treatment and high temperature break catalase down into its four subunits, each of which functions as a peroxidase. Histochemical stains for catalase utilize fixation and incubation at pH 9–10, both conditions that inactivate the catalatic activity of catalase and favor its peroxidatic activity. In acatalasemia, catalase is readily degraded *in vivo* so that catalatic activity is lost while the peroxidase remains (57,59).

Caravaca et al. (60,61) demonstrated that there was a hypolipidemic and hypocholesterolemic response to the injection of hepatic catalase that had been degraded (presumably into peroxidase subunits) by highly alkaline treatment. Measurements of serum triglycerides and cholesterol indicated that acatalasemic mutant mice, apparently possessing an *in vivo* cataloperoxidase, had lower serum lipids than the wild strain. Cuadrado and Bricker (62) also showed that the synthesis of cholesterol was inhibited in the mutant mice.

PERSPECTIVES FOR FUTURE STUDY

Demyelination is not associated with defective neuronal migration in X-linked childhood ALD, a disease in which peroxisomes are synthesized but very long chain oxidase activity is diminished. Dysmyelination, demyelination, and a defect in neuronal migration are common features of CHRS and NALD, both diseases of peroxisomal biogenesis, and a newly described syndrome (pseudo-Zellweger's CHRS) in which peroxisomes are formed but ketothiolase is deficient. Included among the latter are oxidation of palmitoyl-CoA, VLCFA, and bile acids. Defects in the other enzymes involved in peroxisomal beta oxidation will undoubtedly be detected. Whether the defect in mitochondrial electron transport that has been described in CHRS is also present in NALD and infantile Refsum's is not known. Further studies of mitochondrial and peroxisomal metabolism in these disorders may provide new insights into the factors responsible for the defective development of the central nervous system.

REFERENCES

1. Goldfischer S. Peroxisomes in disease. *J Histochem Cytochem* 1979;27:1371–3.
2. Goldfischer S. The internal reticular apparatus of Camillo Golgi: a complex, heterogeneous organelle, enriched in acid, neutral and alkaline phosphatases, and involved in glycosylation, secretion, membrane flow, lysosome formation, and intracellular digestion. *J Histochem Cytochem* 1982;30:717–33.
3. Goldfischer S, Reddy JK. Peroxisomes (microbodies) in cell pathology. In: Richter GW, Epstein MA, eds. *International Review of Experimental Pathology,* vol 26. New York: Academic Press, 1984:43–84.
4. Goldfischer S, Johnson AB, Essner E, Moore C, Ritch RH. Peroxisomal abnormalities in metabolic diseases. *J Histochem Cytochem* 1973;21:972–7.
5. Goldfischer S, Moore CL, Johnson AB, et al. Peroxisomal and mitochondrial defects in the cerebro-hepato-renal syndrome. *Science* 1973;182:62–4.
6. Bowen P, Lee CSN, Zellweger H, Lindenberg R. A familial syndrome of multiple congenital defects. *Bull Johns Hopkins Hosp* 1964;114:402–14.
7. Passarge E, McAdams J. Cerebro-hepato-renal syndrome. A newly recognized hereditary disorder of multiple congenital defects including sudanophilic leukodystrophy, cirrhosis of the liver, and polycystic kidney. *J Pediatr* 1967;71:691–702.
8. Opitz JM, ZuRhein GM, Vitale L, et al. The Zellweger syndrome (cerebro-hepato-renal syndrome) birth defects. *Birth Defects* 1969;5:144–60.
9. Volpe JJ, Adams RD. Cerebro-hepato-renal syndrome of Zellweger. An inherited disorder of neuronal migration. *Acta Neuropathol (Berl)* 1972;20:175–98.
10. Versmold HT, Bremer HJ, Herzog V, et al. A metabolic disorder similar to Zellweger's syndrome with hepatic acatalasia and absence of peroxisomes, altered content and redox state of cytochromes, and infantile cirrhosis with hemosiderosis. *Eur J Pediatr* 1977;124:261–75.
11. Pfeifer U, Sandhage K. Licht-und elektronenmikroskopische leberbefunde beim cerbro-hepato-renalen syndrom nach Zellweger (peroxisomen-defizienz). *Virchows Arch [A]* 1979;384:269–84.
12. Müller-Höcker J, Bise K, Endres W, Hübner G. Zur morphologie und diagnostik des Zellweger syndroms. Ein beitrag zum kombiniert cytochemisch-feinstrukturellen nachweis der peroxisomen in autoptischem und tiefgefrorenem lebergewebe mit fallbericht. *Virchows Arch [A]* 1981;393:103–14.
13. Trijbels JMF, Berden JA, Monnens LAH, Willems JL, Janssen AJM, Schutgens RBH, van den Broek-van Essen M. Biochemical studies in the liver and muscle of patients with Zellweger syndrome. *Pediatr Res* 1983;17:514–17.
14. Rohr HP, Luthy I, Gudat F, et al. Stereology: a new supplement to the study of human liver biopsy specimens. In: Popper H, Schaffner F, eds. *Progress in liver diseases,* vol. V. New York: Grune and Stratton, 1976;24–34.
15. Danks DM, Tippett P, Adams C, Campbell P. Cerebro-hepato-renal syndrome of Zellweger. A report of eight cases with comments upon the incidence, the liver lesion, and a fault in pipecolic acid metabolism. *J Pediatr* 1975;86:382–7.
16. Brown FR III, McAdams AJ, Cummins JW, et al. Cerebro-hepato-renal (Zellweger) syndrome and neonatal adrenoleukodystrophy: similarities in phenotype and accumulations of very long chain fatty acids. *Johns Hopkins Med J* 1982;151:344–61.
17. Goldfischer S, Powers JM, Johnson AB, Axe S, Brown FR, Moser HW. Striated adrenocortical cells in cerebro-hepato-renal (Zellweger) syndrome. *Virchows Arch [A]* 1983;401:355–61.
18. Hanson RR, Szczepanik-Van Leeuwen P, Williams GC, Grabowski G, Sharp HL. Defects of bile acid synthesis in Zellweger's syndrome. *Science* 1979;283:1107–8.
19. Mathis RK, Watkins JB, Szczepanik-van Leeuwen P, Lott IT. Liver in the cerebro-hepato-renal syndrome: defective bile acid synthesis and abnormal mitochondria. *Gastroenterology,* 1980;79:1311–7.
20. Heymans HSA, Schutgens RBH, Tan R, van den Bosch H, Borst P. Severe plasmalogen deficiency in tissues of infants without peroxisomes (Zellweger syndrome). *Nature* 1983;306:69–70.
21. Schutgens RBH, Romeyn GJ, Wonders RJA, van den Bosch H, Schrakamp G, Heymans HSA. Deficiency of aryl-CoA:dihydroxyacetone phosphate aryl transferase in patients with Zellweger (cerebro-hepato-renal) syndrome. *Biochem Biophys Res Commun* 1984;120:179–84.
22. Datta NS, Wilson GN, Hajra AK. Deficiency of enzymes catalyzing the biosynthesis of glycerol-ether lipids in Zellweger syndrome. A new category of metabolic disease involving the absence of peroxisomes. *N Engl J Med* 1984;311:1080–3.

23. Hajra AK, Datta NS, Jackson LG, et al. Prenatal diagnosis of Zellweger cerebrohepatorenal syndrome. *N Engl J Med* 1985;312:445–6.
24. Ulrich J, Herschkowitz N, Heitz P, Sigrist T, Baerlocher P. Adrenoleukodystrophy: preliminary report of a neonatal case. Light and electron microscopical, immunocytochemical biochemical findings. *Acta Neuropathol (Berl)* 1978;43:77–83.
25. Haas JE, Johnson ES, Farrell DL. Neonatal-onset adrenoleukodystrophy in a girl. *Ann Neurol* 1982;12:449–59.
26. Jaffe R, Crumrine P, Hashida Y, Moser HW. Neonatal adrenoleukodystrophy. Clinical, pathological and biochemical delineation of a syndrome affecting both males and females. *Am J Pathol* 1982;108:100–11.
27. Goldfischer S, Collins J, Rapin I et al. Peroxisomal defects in neonatal-onset and x-linked adrenoleukodystrophies. *Science* 1985;227:67–70.
28. Partin JS, McAdams AJ. Absence of hepatic peroxisomes in neonatal onset adrenoleukodystrophy. *Pediatr Res* 1983;17:294A.
29. Scotto JM, Hadchovel M, Odievre M, et al. Infantile phytanic acid storage disease, a possible variant of Refsum's disease. Three cases, including ultrastructural studies of the liver. *J Inherited Metab Dis* 1982;5:83–90.
30. Ogier H, Roels F, Cornelis A, et al. Absence of hepatic peroxisomes in a case of infantile Refsum's disease. *Scand J Clin Lab Invest* 1985;45:767–68.
31. Poulos A, Pollard AC, Mitchell JA, Wise G, Mortimer G. Patterns of Refsum's disease. Phytanic acid oxidase deficiency. *Arch Dis Child* 1984;59:222–9.
32. Stokke O, Skride S, Ek J, Björkhem I. Refsum's disease, adrenoleukodystrophy, and the Zellweger syndrome. *Scand J Clin Lab Invest* 1984;44:463–4.
33. Collins JC, Rapin I, Van Hoof F, Goldfischer S. Pseudo-Zellweger's multiple peroxisomal oxidative deficiencies. *Pediatr Res* 1985; 19:246A, abstract 811.
34. Goldfischer SL, Collins J, Rapin I, et al. Pseudo-Zellweger syndrome: deficiencies in several peroxisomal oxidative activities. *J Pediatr* 1986;108:25–32.
35. Beard ME, Sapirstein V, Kolodny EM, Holtzman E. Peroxisomes in fibroblasts from skin of Refsum's disease patients. *J Histochem Cytochem* 1985;33:980–4.
36. Arias J, Moser AB, Goldfischer SL. Ultrastructural and cytochemical demonstration of peroxisomes in cultured fibroblasts from patients with peroxisomal deficiency disorders. *J Cell Biol* 1985;100:1789–92.
37. Reddy JK, Ohno S. Testicular feminization of the mouse. Paucity of peroxisomes in Leydig cells of the testis. *Am J Pathol* 1981;103:96–104.
38. Govaerts L, Monnens L, Melis T, Trijbels F. Disturbed adrenocortical function in cerebro-hepatorenal syndrome of Zellweger. *Eur J Pediatr* 1984; 143:10–2.
39. Powers JM, Schaumburg HH. The adrenal cortex in adrenoleukodystrophy. *Arch Pathol* 1973;96:305–10.
40. Holtzman E. Peroxisomes in nervous tissue. *Ann NY Acad Sci* 1982;386:523–5.
41. McKenna O, Arnold G, Holtzman E. Microperoxisome distribution in the central nervous system of the rat. *Brain Res* 1976;117:181–94.
42. Michaud J, Larbrisseau A. Enlarged peroxisomes in hepatocytes of a case of spongy degeneration of the central nervous system. *J Neuropathol Exp Neurol* 1984;43:295.
43. Schram AW, Goldfischer S, van Roermund CWT, et al. Human peroxisomal 3-oxoacyl-coenzyme A thiolase deficiency. *Proc Natl Acad Sci USA* 1987;84:2494–6.
44. Challa VR, Geisinger KR, Burton BK. Pathologic alterations in the brain and liver in hyperpipecolic acidemia. *J Neuropathol Exp Neurol* 1983;42:626–38.
45. Nishio H, Ortiz J, Giacobini E. Accumulation and metabolism of pipecolic acid in the brain and other organs of the mouse. *Neurochem Res* 1981;6:1241–52.
46. Takahama K, Miyata T, Hashimoto T, Okano Y, Hitoshi T, Kase Y. Pipecolic acid: a new type of α-amino acid possessing bicuculline-sensitive action in the mammalian brain. *Brain Res* 1982;239:294–8.
47. Salen G, Shefer S, Setouguchi T, Mosbach EH. Bile alcohol metabolism in man. Conversion of 5-cholestane-3,7,12,25-tetrol to cholic acid. *J Clin Invest* 1975;56:226–31.
48. Oftebro H, Björkhem I, Størmer FC, Pedersen JI. Cerebrotendinous xanthomatosis: defective liver mitochondrial hydroxylation of chenodeoxycholic acid precursors. *J Lipid Res* 1981;22:632–40.
49. Thompson SL, Krisans SK. Localization of 26-hydroxylase activity in rat liver peroxisomes. *Fed Proc* 1985;44:1155, abstract 4353.

50. Boehme DH, Sobel HS, Marguet E, Salen G. Liver in cerebrotendinosis xanthomatosis (CTX). A histochemical and EM study of four cases. *Pathol Res Pract* 1980;170:192–201.
51. Goldfischer S, Sobel HJ. Peroxisomes and bile acid synthesis. *Gastroenterology* 1981;81:196–7.
52. Takahara S, Hamilton HB, Neel JV, et al. Hypocatalasemia: a new genetic carrier state. *J Clin Invest* 1960;39:610–9.
53. Aebi H, Suter H. Acatalasemia. In: Harris H, Hirschara K eds. *Advances in human genetics,* vol. II. New York: Plenum Press, 1971;143–99.
54. Feinstein RN. Acatalasemia in the mouse and other species. *Biochem Genet* 1970;4:135–55.
55. Novikoff AB, Goldfischer S. Visualization of peroxisomes (microbodies) and mitochondria with diaminobenzidine. *J Histochem Cytochem* 1969;17:675–80.
56. Goldfischer S, Essner E. Further observations on the peroxidatic activities of microbodies (peroxisomes). *J Histochem Cytochem* 1969;17:681–5.
57. Goldfischer S, Essner E. Peroxidase activity in peroxisomes (microbodies) of acatalasemic mice. *J Histochem Cytochem* 1970;18:482–9.
58. Aebi H, Suter H, Feinstein RN. Activity and stability of catalase in blood and tissues of normal and acatalasemic mice. *Biochem Genet* 1968;2:245–51.
59. Feinstein RN, Savol R, Howard JB. Conversion of catalatic to peroxidatic activity in livers of normal and acatalasemic mice. *Enzymologia* 1971;41:345–58.
60. Caravaca J, Dimond EG, Sommers SC, Wenk R. Prevention of induced atherosclerosis by peroxidase. *Science* 1967;155:1284–7.
61. Caravaca J, May MD. The isolation and properties of an active peroxidase from hepatocatalase *Biochem Biophys Res Commun* 1964;16:528–34.
62. Cuadrado RR, Bricker LA. An abnormality of hepatic lipogenesis in a mutant strain of "acatalasemic" mice. *Biochim Biophys Acta* 1973;306:168–72.

DISCUSSION

Dr. Bourre: It is fascinating that this accumulation of long chain fatty acids is toxic for the cell when you consider how small the amount is in terms of a percentage of total fatty acids Does this mean that there are as yet unidentified molecules containing these very long chain fatty acids which disturb cell metabolism?

Dr. Goldfischer: It has been suggested that the accumulation of long chain fatty acids is toxic, but I do not know that anyone has actually shown this. It is equally possible that the cell is deprived of some important breakdown product of very long chain fatty acids and dies because of a deficiency. I have no idea of the metabolic consequences of this accumulation of substrate. There may be an analogy with the lysosomal diseases here; we know material accumulates because an enzyme is deficient but we do not know why the cell dies.

Dr. Bourre: In comparison with lysosomal diseases where the accumulation of sphingolipid is extremely high, the accumulation of very long chain fatty acids in the diseases you describe is relatively small. This could be related to the fact that the fatty acids which are not degraded come from the diet, as shown by Moser. These may have an extremely low turnover rate in myelin and a disproportionately large effect on cell machinery.

Dr. Goldfischer: Moser tried his patients on severely restricted diets with no very long chain fatty acids. This did not affect their serum lipids or their condition, so I think there must be an important degree of endogenous synthesis of these fatty acids.

Dr. Bourre: Plasmalogens are extremely important, especially in myelin membranes. If they are not synthesized in the peroxisomes, hypomyelination results. It is easy to understand how some sphingolipids and phospholipids may be synthesized in the microsomes, transferred to the Golgi apparatus and then to these transvesicles, which are in turn transferred to the plasma membrane, but how do you think plasmalogens are exported?

Dr. Goldfischer: It is easy to understand the endoplasmic reticulum-to-Golgi-to-vesicle pathway today because we have now accepted this as the principal method by which material from within the cell is transferred to the outside. But there are many other pathways. For example, no one knows how bile acids and the proteins in bile get from the liver cell into the bile, and there is no indication here of circular transport from the Golgi apparatus to the membrane. I think more pathways exist in the cell than we are aware of. Plasmalogens may be important for myelin synthesis, but the demyelination that occurs in X-linked adrenoleukodystrophy, which is very profound, occurs in children who have normal plasmalogen-synthesizing capacity. Furthermore, some children with this condition, or perhaps with less severe examples of Zellweger's syndrome, survive for relatively long periods instead of the usual 6 months to 1 year. In these children there are studies which have shown plasmalogen-synthesizing capacity reduced by 90% or so, which nevertheless seems to be compatible with relatively long-term survival. The problem is complex.

Dr. Guenet: Is there any possibility of detecting these abnormalities early enough to apply effective treatment?

Dr. Goldfischer: The defects can be detected during pregnancy using fibroblast or amniotic cell culture from amniotic fluid, and more recently chorionic villus biopsy. Originally the measurements involved very long chain fatty acid oxidating capacity, but now there are direct measurements of plasmalogen-synthesizing enzyme. The question of how to detect heterozygotes is an interesting one, and attempts have so far been unsuccessful. Very long chain fatty acids are normal in parents, and the limited studies of plasmalogen synthesizing enzyme in leukocytes have also been found to be normal. I think this lack of success is related to the fact that we do not know the exact nature of the underlying defect, that is, whether it is an enzyme defect or some other defect. The deficiency in affected children seems not to be in the ability to synthesize any of the known peroxisomal enzymes, whether membrane- or matrix-associated, but rather to be in some factor which is responsible for the assembly of the organelle.

Clofibrate and related compounds which stimulate proliferation of peroxisomes have been tried in some of these children with little effect. One other possible route to explore is pipecolic acid, which is elevated in blood more than in urine in these patients. The pathway from lysine to pipecolic acid is believed in general to be a minor metabolic pathway. However, there are studies which show that it may be a major pathway in the brain, competing with GABA. One study showed that injection of pipecolic acid produced profound hypotonia in animals.

There are many other possible explanations for these defects, but I cannot believe that there is both a mitochondrial and a peroxisomal problem. It could be that a toxic metabolite accumulating as a result of the peroxisomal deficiency blocks the mitochondria, or there could be some common factor that affects electron transport in the mitochondria and thus also affects peroxisomal assembly. Until we find the answer we shall not be able to identify heterozygotes.

Dr. Caviness: I understand that Professor van Hoof and associates have discovered that there are defects in amino acid oxidase in the kidney in the reeler mouse mutant; I also understand that this enzyme system is important in glial metabolism. It is interesting in this regard that one of the principal phenotypic characteristics of this mutant mouse is abnormal cell position due to failure of cell migration. I wonder if these various pieces of information go together.

The question I want to ask has to do with Zellweger's syndrome and the total absence of peroxisomes. Tell us something about the cell biology of the formation of these organelles.

Where might one look for a defect in their formation as a consequence of a single gene mutation?

Dr. Goldfischer: We were careful to say "absence of morphologically detectable peroxisomes"! We have recently looked at fibroblasts from four patients with Zellweger's syndrome. Two of these were classic cases and died within a year; the other two have since been called neonatal adrenoleukodystrophy, one having died at 6 years and the other still alive at 2 to 3 years. We were very surprised by the findings. In the Zellweger fibroblasts we found peroxisomes but there was a 90% reduction in their numbers, which is very consistent with the biochemical information about plasmalogen synthesis. In the two children with neonatal adrenoleukodystrophy there was a 60% reduction in peroxisomes. Whether this will prove to be a consistent finding remains to be seen, but there does not appear to be a total block in the formation of the organelle. There may also be a difference in numbers of peroxisomes from tissue to tissue. For example there is a mutant mouse with testicular feminization syndrome in which a marked deficiency of peroxisomes has been described in the interstitial cells of the testis. The liver of this mouse has not yet been examined for peroxisomes. We examined the intestine of a child with neonatal adrenoleukodystrophy and although we did not do morphometry, the microscopists had no trouble finding normal peroxisomes.

The most difficult part of the problem is the central nervous system. You cannot visualize peroxisomes by light microscopy, and although you can identify them in oligodendroglial cells (which are related to myelin formation) they are very tiny—not much larger than smooth endoplasmic reticulum—and also quite sparse. There may even be peroxisomes without catalase in the CNS so staining may not be possible. Thus any study on peroxisomes which relies on morphology is very difficult. We really know nothing about peroxisomes in the brains of these children.

Dr. Evrard: In one of our cases of neonatal adrenoleukodystrophy, clofibrate and barbiturates dramatically improved the clinical condition.

You spoke about demyelination and I agree with you to a certain extent. However, I have examined a lot of cases of Zellweger's syndrome myself and found that myelination was not bad in many of the structures in which myelin has normally developed by this age. Of course you do not expect to find much myelination in the neonatal cerebral hemispheres, but in certain parts of the brain stem it was not so bad.

Dr. Goldfischer: I am not a neuropathologist and I took that information from the literature. I have difficulty in separating demyelination from dysmyelination and have no opinion about current arguments on this subject.

Dr. Minkowski: I recently read that peroxisomes disappear as nervous tissue develops. They are seen in developing neurons but are rare in mature nervous tissue. Could you comment on this? The presence of peroxisomes in the developing nervous system could point to a role in the processes which control the immediate environment of neurons, perhaps filtering out components such as alcohol before they reach the neural surface.

Dr. Goldfischer: It is true that you cannot see peroxisomes in adult neurons. At least I have been unsuccessful in finding them, though I do not know whether they disappear or whether they lose their catalase activity and cease to stain. They are relatively more abundant in glial and supportive elements, which is not inconsistent with a role in myelinogenesis. Alcohol is a substrate for the peroxidasing activity of catalase, so it may well be a factor.

Developmental Neurobiology, edited by
Philippe Evrard and Alexandre Minkowski.
Nestlé Nutrition Workshop Series, Vol. 12.
Nestec Ltd., Vevey/Raven Press, Ltd.,
New York © 1989.

Peroxisomes and Brain Development: Search for an Animal Model

Joseph Vamecq, André M. Goffinet, Isabelle Labrique, Jean-Pierre Draye, and François Van Hoof

International Institute of Cellular and Molecular Pathology (ICP) and Department of Pediatric Neurology, Université Catholique de Louvain (UCL), B-1200 Brussels, Belgium

Until recently the assertion that mammalian peroxisomes play a role in the development of the central nervous system was received with incredulity by most investigators despite the demonstration by Goldfischer et al. (1) of the absence of recognizable peroxisomes in liver and kidney from patients with Zellweger's cerebrohepatorenal syndrome, together with the existence of neuronal heterotopias (2–4). There were several reasons for this. The idea that neuronal migration could depend on a metabolic process that takes place in a small subcellular organelle would have appeared revolutionary to neuroanatomists. A decade ago biochemists and cell biologists were still unaware of the multitude of physiological functions accomplished by peroxisomes. Furthermore, doubt existed concerning the peroxisomal nature of the tiny diaminobenzidine-reactive vesicles found in the brain, which are morphologically different from liver and kidney peroxisomes. The latter skepticism was overcome by the work of Gaunt and de Duve (5) who demonstrated that these tiny vesicles isolated from the cerebellum contain the bulk of sedimentable catalase and D-amino acid oxidase.

At the same time Lazarow and de Duve (6), by demonstrating that peroxisomes catalyze fatty acyl-CoA β-oxidation, considerably stimulated interest in this class of organelles. This interest was further increased by the discovery that the key steps in the anabolism of ether phospholipids, that is, those catalyzed by dihydroxyacetonephosphate acyltransferase (DHAP-AT) and by alkyl-dihydroxyacetonephosphate synthase, occur in hepatic and brain peroxisomes (7–9). Other established peroxisomal functions include the conversion of di- and trihydroxycoprostanoic acids to chenodeoxycholic and cholic acids, respectively, final steps of cholesterol catabolism (10–13), long chain dicarboxylyl-CoA oxidation (14–16), and a few other steps in intermediary metabolism, including glycolate oxidase (17–20), alanine-glyoxylate transaminase (21,22) and glutaryl-CoA oxidase (23,24). Furthermore, the accumulation in peroxisomal disorders of a C_{29} dicarboxylic acid, an unusual metabolite of bile acids, pipecolic acids, and phytanic acids (see S. Goldfischer, *this volume*), suggests the existence of still other enzyme activities in these subcellular organelles. Whatever the tissue considered, the biochemical recognition of peroxisomes should currently rest on the demonstration of sedimentable particles containing catalase (25–27), enzymes of very long chain fatty acid β oxidation (28,29), and those required for catalysis of the initial key steps of plasmalogen biosynthesis.

Plasmalogens are the end products of ether phospholipid biosynthesis and account for one fifth of all phospholipids of the human body (30). These ether lipids are abundant in the central nervous system and in myelin, where they may account for over 30% of the phospholipid content (30). In addition, it has been reported that the proportion of plasmalogens among the phospholipids greatly increases during brain embryogenesis (30). The mechanisms by which peroxisomal dysfunction interferes with brain development remain hypothetical. Two biochemical abnormalities have been reported in the brains of patients with peroxisomal disorders, and both could play a role in the occurrence of neuronal heterotopia. These are the decrease in plasmalogen content (31–33) and the accumulation of very long chain fatty acids, either free or in the form of cholesterol esters (34–37) (Fig. 1). It is conceivable that both these abnormalities, which can affect the composition of the plasma membrane, could interfere with neuronal migration. This effect might be direct or indirect, mediated by changes in the proteins which become integrated into glial and neuronal membranes. This chapter concerns the search for an animal model for the study of brain development disorders related to peroxisomal dysfunction. Cerebral lesions, morphological changes, biological and biochemical features, as well as the clinical

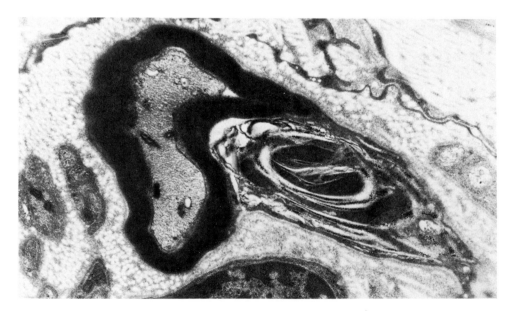

FIG. 1. Lipid deposition in a Schwann cell from a patient with peroxisomal dysfunction. Note the spicular inclusions not limited by a membrane. (Magnification × 13,500.) (Courtesy of J. Libert, Brussels.)

course in human patients with peroxisomal disorders are extensively documented by S. Goldfischer *(this volume)*.

PEROXISOMES IN THE REELER MOUSE

The reeler mutation is autosomal recessive. Affected mice are ataxic, and their cerebellums are atrophic and poor in granule cells. The fiber pattern and the cytoarchitecture of most of the brain structures are abnormal (Fig. 2) (38). This widespread disorganization attests to a defect of neuronal migration. In several aspects the cerebral abnormalities evoke those observed in the Zellweger patients (see S. Goldfischer, *this volume*) where an apparent arrest of neuronal migration has been suggested (3). It was therefore tempting to measure peroxisomal enzyme activities and to analyze the peroxisomal population in this strain of mouse. Preliminary investigations are presented here.

Ultrastructural analysis failed to reveal any abnormality in the number or size of liver and kidney peroxisomes. Biochemical assays performed as previously described (14,23) showed that the activity of peroxisomal oxidases on palmitoyl-CoA, glycolate, urate, and D-proline were normal in the liver and kidney cortex (Table 1). By contrast, the rate of D-proline oxidation was reduced by more than 65% in the

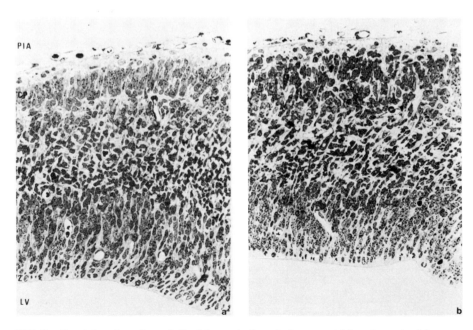

FIG. 2. Frontal sections through the telencephalic wall of a normal **(a)** and a reeler **(b)** mouse embryo at embryonic day 14. PIA, pial surface; CP, cortical plate; IZ, intermediate zone; VZ, ventricular zone; LV, lateral ventricle. The difference between both genotypes is apparent at the level of their cortical plate, well defined in the normal embryo, but more widespread and blunted in reeler embryos (semi-thin plastic section, × 180). (From ref. 38.)

TABLE 1. *Peroxisomal H_2O_2-generating oxidase activities in tissues from control (n = 12) and reeler (n = 10) mice[a]*

Substrate	Liver		Kidney cortex		Cerebellum	
	Control	Reeler	Control	Reeler	Control	Reeler
Palmitoyl-CoA	0.89	0.83	1.2	1.0	ND	ND
Glycolate	0.26	0.21	ND	ND	ND	ND
Urate	0.98	0.81	ND	ND	ND	ND
D-Proline	ND	ND	8.40	9.0	0.70	0.23

[a]Activities are expressed as μmol H_2O_2 produced per minute and per gram of tissue. ND, not detected.

cerebellum of these mutant mice. Protein concentration and enzyme activities in other subcellular organelles, including mitochondria (cytochrome c oxidase), endoplasmic reticulum (arylsulphatase C), and lysosomes (β-hexosaminidase), were in the normal range in both cerebellum and kidney cortex. The reduction of cerebellum D-proline oxidase activity thus appears to be specific. This abnormality is more likely to be accounted for by decreased amounts of enzyme than by structural modifications of the protein, since only the apparent V_m and not K_m is affected. Kinetic studies demonstrated that the apparent K_m of kidney cortex and cerebellum D-amino acid oxidases for various amino acids are similar, amounting to about 8.7 mM for D-proline. The difference between cerebellum D-amino acid oxidase activities in normal and reeler mice was not abolished by treating the animals with clofibric acid, a well-known peroxisomal proliferator (Table 2). The expected enhancement of both liver peroxisomal volume and capacity to oxidize the CoA esters of fatty acids was similarly induced in both strains of mice.

In reeler mice, the activity and distribution of catalase in the particular and sol-

TABLE 2. *Peroxisomal oxidase activities in tissues from control (n = 6) and reeler (n = 6) mice given a 0.5% clofibric acid-containing diet for 2 weeks[a]*

Substrate	Liver		Kidney cortex		Cerebellum	
	Control	Reeler	Control	Reeler	Control	Reeler
Palmitoyl-CoA	5.70	6.80	1.70	1.90	ND	ND
Glycolate	0.26	0.29	ND	ND	ND	ND
Urate	1.20	1.20	ND	ND	ND	ND
D-Proline	ND	ND	4.60	4.20	0.75	0.34

[a]Activities are expressed as μmol H_2O_2 produced per minute and per gram of tissue. ND, not detected.

TABLE 3. *Comparison between the activities of dihydroxyacetonephosphate acyltransferases in control and reeler mice tissues (nmol/min/g tissue)*

	Total	Peroxisomal	Extra-peroxisomal
Control kidney cortex (*n* = 17)	116.8	66.1	50.7
Reeler kidney cortex (*n* = 17)	120	56.4	64.3
Control cerebellum (*n* = 17)	13.3	6.2	7.1
Reeler cerebellum (*n* = 12)	13.8	5.8	8.0
Control liver (*n* = 5)	113.7	25.3	88.4
Reeler liver (*n* = 5)	126.6	25.6	101.0

uble fractions prepared from liver, kidney cortex, and cerebellar homogenates were unaffected. In the brain, the concentration and proportion of plasmalogens in phospholipids, as well as the activity and subcellular localization of DHAP-AT, were normal. As shown in Table 3, control values were obtained for the activities of both the extra- and intraperoxisomal DHAP-AT in tissues from the mutant animals.

Very long chain fatty acids did not apparently accumulate, as attested by the normal values obtained for the plasmatic cerotic acid (C_{26}).behenic acid (C_{22}) ratio. Bile acid precursors (di- and trihydroxycoprostanoic acids) could not be detected in plasma, where common bile acids were normally concentrated (Table 4).

With the exception of cerebellar D-amino acid oxidase activity it may be concluded that reeler mice apparently have normal peroxisomal functions.

TABLE 4. *Assay of bile acids in plasma from control and reeler mice*[a]

	Reeler mice	Control mice	Zellweger patient	NALD patient	Human controls
Common bile acids (cholic and chenodeoxycholic acids)	100	100	34	29	100
Bile acid precursors (di- and tri-hydroxycoprostanoic acids)	ND	ND	43	45	ND
C_{29}-dicarboxylic acid	ND	ND	23	26	ND

[a]Comparison is made with patients suffering from peroxisomal dysfunction (see S. Goldfischer, *this volume*). The concentrations of various bile acids are expressed as the percentage of the total bile acid content. ND, not detectable; NALD, neonatal adrenoleukodystrophy.

PEROXISOMAL ENZYMES IN NEWBORN MICE
GIVEN METHYLAZOXYMETHANOL

When injected intraperitoneally in normal newborn mice, methylazoxymethanol, an alkylating cytostatic agent, prevents the development of granule cells (39). These cells have intense mitotic activity shortly after birth, in contrast to other cells in brain and cerebellum. In the cerebellum of methylazoxymethanol-treated animals, the activity of D-amino acid oxidase on day 21 was markedly reduced when compared to the same enzyme activity in cerebellum from control mice (Fig. 3). By contrast, kidney D-amino acid oxidase was normally active. In both organs, the activities of the marker enzymes, including cytochrome c oxidase, arylsulphatase C, and β-hexosaminidase, were unaffected by the treatment. Other investigations on D-amino acid oxidase in normal mice included a study of the kinetics of the development of the activity of the enzyme in kidney and cerebellum from birth to adult age. Although the enzyme is already present in kidney cortex at birth, its activity could not be detected in the cerebellum at this time (Fig. 4). Cerebellar enzyme activity becomes detectable only around the end of the second week after birth. In both the kidney and cerebellum, the oxidase activity increases until adulthood is reached.

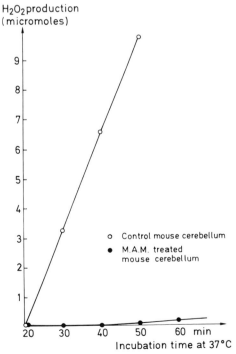

FIG. 3. D-Amino acid oxidase activity at postnatal day 21 in control and methylazoxymethanol (MAM)-treated mouse cerebellum. Same amounts of protein were used to assay the oxidase activity.

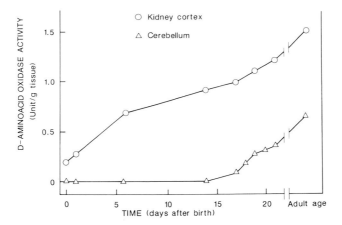

FIG. 4. Time course from birth to adulthood of D-amino acid oxidase activity assayed on 0.1M proline in kidney cortex and cerebellum from control mice. One unit is defined as the amount of enzyme which catalyzes the formation of 1 μmol H_2O_2 per minute.

BIOLOGICAL SIGNIFICANCE OF D-AMINO ACID OXIDASE ACTIVITY

D-Amino acid oxidase is a flavoprotein catalyzing the transhydrogenation depicted in Fig. 5, which results in the imine conversion of D-amino acids with the production of H_2O_2. A further spontaneous step then occurs, the hydrolysis of the imine to the corresponding α-ketoacid with the release of ammonia. However, this second step does not occur so readily for D-imino acids (*N*-alkyl-D-amino acids), in

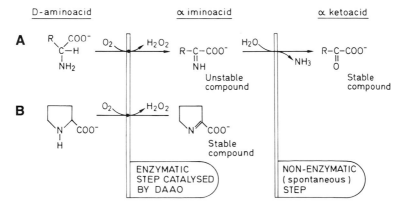

FIG. 5. Reactions catalyzed by D-amino acid oxidase (DAAO). **A:** D-α-amino acids. **B:** *N*-alkyl-D-α-amino acids. The molecular structure of D-proline is depicted.

which the imino configuration is more stable. Thus, D-proline and D-pipecolate oxidase reactions do not lead to ammonia production, unlike the oxidation of other D-amino acids, such as D-alanine, D-methionine, D-valine, or D-phenylalanine.

The physiological role of the peroxisomal flavoprotein is not obvious, as D-amino acids are neither produced by mammals nor incorporated into their proteins. However, Hamilton et al. (40) have demonstrated that thiazolidine-2-carboxylic acid, a cysteamine glyoxylate adduct, is a potential substrate for D-amino acid oxidase. This enzyme is also active on other unstable adducts formed nonenzymatically in solution from various molecules (see 41). Other metabolically important molecules could also be physiological substrates of D-amino acid oxidase.

Whereas the role of D-amino acid oxidase and its distribution in the different cerebellar cells remain poorly understood, the subcellular distribution of the enzyme activity in cytosol and in peroxisomal organelles of rodent tissues is well established. As both methylazoxymethanol-treated animals and reeler mice show atrophy of granule cells and reduced activity of D-amino acid oxidase, the suggestion that D-amino acid oxidase is localized in granule cells is certainly worth considering. However, the data do not rule out the possibility of secondary disappearance of D-amino acid oxidase-containing nongranular cells, following disorganization of the granule cell layer.

REELER MUTATION AND THE DEFICIENCY OF THE PRODUCTION OF CENTRAL NERVOUS SYSTEM D-AMINO ACIDS OR ANALOGS: AN ATTRACTIVE HYPOTHESIS

Convincing evidence to consider the reeler mutation as an appropriate model for the study of human peroxisomal disorders is lacking. Several hypotheses are discussed to explain the peroxisomal abnormality observed in reeler mice. One attractive hypothesis stems from the adaptive properties of D-amino acid oxidase activity.

First, it is unlikely that the reeler mutation affects the D-amino acid oxidase protein directly. As mentioned above, kinetic parameters argue against conformational changes in the structure of D-amino acid oxidase, at least in the domains of the enzyme which control its activity. A mutation affecting D-amino acid oxidase activity directly would also be likely to involve the kidney enzyme, which is not the case. Second, taking into account the reorganization in cerebellar anatomy, the decreased D-amino acid oxidase activity could be ascribed to a reduction of the peroxisome-rich cell population. The normal values and subcellular distribution of catalase and DHAP-AT activities in the cerebellum of reeler mice do not corroborate this assumption. The most striking finding is not the reduction of D-amino acid oxidase activity in the cerebellum of these mice but the fact that this deficiency, which is not related to direct mutation changes, occurs alone without abnormalities in the other peroxisomal functions studied. Intermixing experiments (combination of control and reeler mice cerebellum homogenates) have almost excluded the hypothesis of the existence of an inhibitor of reeler cerebellum D-amino acid oxidase.

Adaptative changes in kidney D-amino acid oxidase have been reported. This enzyme has been shown to be less active in germ-free mice, presumably as a consequence of the diminished production of D-amino acids of intestinal microfloral origin (42). In these animals, the administration of D-amino acids was shown to enhance the renal activity of the enzyme. By analogy, we suggest that the lower D-amino acid oxidase activity in the cerebellum from reeler mice results from a lesser exposure of the oxidase to D-amino acids or analog substrates. The normal activity of kidney D-amino acid oxidase precludes the involvement of general disturbances in D-amino acid production or resorption from the gut. Adaptation of cerebellar D-amino acid oxidase in response to modifications in brain substrates with structures analogous to those of D-amino acids should thus be considered.

Three structural analogs of glutamic acid, N-methyl-D, L-aspartate, kainic and quisqualic acids, are potent and specific agonists of receptors involved in synaptic transmission (43). The neuronal damage induced by these amino acids has been related to their neuroexcitatory action, kainic acid being by far the most neurotoxic agent (43). Some compounds with similar structure to D-amino acids (e.g., D-α-aminoadipic acid, D-glutamylglycine) can antagonize excitotoxic effects (43). For instance, D-glutamylglycine not only depresses the neuroexcitation by N-methyl-D,L-aspartate but also that induced by the potent neurotoxic kainic acid. Furthermore, the brain damage provoked by N-methyl-D,L-aspartate in the arcuate nucleus of the hypothalamus may be prevented by molecules such as D-α-aminoadipate. All these observations underline the fact that D-amino acid-like compounds may influence neuronal integrity and brain development. We suggest that the deficiency of cerebellar D-amino acid oxidase activity observed in reeler mice could reflect abnormal brain levels of such compounds.

PERSPECTIVES FOR FUTURE STUDY

Even if transplantation experiments (reeler cerebellum implanted in normal brain) would not correct the reeler phenotype, they would be expected to restore the mutant D-amino acid oxidase activity. A mutation directly affecting the structure of the oxidase with subsequent loss of the enzyme activity has been described in mice (44,45). These animals are clinically normal in contrast to reeler mice, supporting the idea that D-amino acid oxidase deficiency in the latter is a secondary consequence of a primary defect so far not elucidated. Besides inborn disorders, acquired pathology or dysfunction may alternatively be used to obtain animals with peroxisomal disturbances. The recent demonstration by Leighton et al. (46) that peroxisomal fatty acid oxidation can selectively be inhibited by phenothiazines is promising. The ability of many drugs (e.g., fibrates, nafenopin, tibric acid) to induce peroxisomal proliferation in rodents is extensively documented (47). Other peroxisomal proliferators such as phytol (48) or substrates for peroxisomal oxidases (e.g., glycolate, oleate) are also of interest. One might finally recall the inhibition of phospholipid biosynthesis by hypolipidemic agents (49).

ACKNOWLEDGMENTS

Professors Gilles Lyon and Philippe Evrard are gratefully acknowledged. The authors are indebted to Professor Hendrik Eyssen and Dr. Johan Van Eldere for the determination of plasmatic very long chain fatty acids and bile acids. This work was supported by grants of the Belgian Fonds National de la Recherche Scientifique (FNRS), by grant 84/90-74 of the Action de Recherche Concertée des Services du Premier Ministre, U.S. Public Health Services (Grant 2 R01 DK9235-21), and European Communities Twining Research Program. A.M. Goffinet is ''Chercheur Qualifié'' and J. Vamecq is ''Aspirant'' of the Belgian FNRS.

REFERENCES

1. Goldfischer S, Moore CL, Johnson AB, et al. Peroxisomal and mitochondrial defects in the cerebro-hepato-renal syndrome. *Science* 1973;182:62–4.
2. Volpe JJ, Adams RD. Cerebro-hepato-renal syndrome of Zellweger. An inherited disorder of neuronal migration. *Acta Neuropathol* 1972;20:175–98.
3. Evrard P, Caviness VS, Prats-Vinas J, Lyon G. The mechanism of arrest of neuronal migration in the Zellweger malformation: an hypothesis based upon cytoarchitectonic analysis. *Acta Neuropathol* 1978;41:109–17.
4. Della Giustina E, Goffinet AM, Landrieu P, Lyon G. A Golgi study of the brain malformation in Zellweger's cerebro-hepato-renal disease. *Acta Neuropathol* 1981;55:23–8.
5. Gaunt GL, de Duve C. Subcellular distribution of D-amino acid oxidase and catalase in rat brain. *J Neurochem* 1976;26:749–59.
6. Lazarow PB, de Duve C. A fatty acyl-CoA oxidizing system in rat brain peroxisomes, enhancement by clofibrate hypolipidemic drug. *Proc Natl Acad Sci USA* 1976;73:2043–6.
7. Hajra AK, Burke CL, Jones CL. Subcellular localization of acyl-coenzyme A: dihydroxyacetone phosphate acyltransferase in rat liver peroxisomes (microbodies). *J Biol Chem* 1979;254:10896–900.
8. Hajra AK, Bishop JE. Glycerolipid biosynthesis in peroxisomes via the acyl dihydroxyacetone phosphate pathway. *Ann NY Acad Sci* 1982;386:170–82.
9. Hajra, AK. Biosynthesis of O-alkylglycerol ether lipids: In: Mangold HK, Paultauf F, eds. *Ether lipids: biochemical and biomedical aspects.* New York: Academic Press, 1983:85–106.
10. Pedersen JI, Gustafsson J. Conversion of 3 alpha, 7 alpha, 12 alpha-trihydroxy-5 beta-cholestanoic acid into cholic acid by rat liver peroxisomes. *FEBS Lett* 1980;121:345–8.
11. Hagey LR, Krisans SK. Degradation of cholesterol to propionic acid by rat liver peroxisomes. *Biochem Biophys Res Commun* 1982;107:834–41.
12. Bjorkhem I, Kase BF, Pederson JI. Role of peroxisomes in the biosynthesis of bile acids. *Scand J Clin Lab Invest* 1985; 45 suppl 177:23–31.
13. Kase BF, Pedersen JI, Standvik G, Bjorkhem I. In vivo and in vitro studies on formation of bile acids in patients with Zellweger syndrome. Evidence that peroxisomes are of importance in the normal biosynthesis of both cholic and chenodeoxycholic acid. *J Clin Invest* 1985;76:2393–402.
14. Vamecq J, de Hoffmann E, Van Hoof F. The microsomal dicarboxylyl-CoA synthetase. *Biochem J* 1985;230:683–93.
15. Vamecq J. Peroxisomes and metabolism of dicarboxylic acids. In: Wirtz KWA, Tager, JM, eds. *Peroxisomes and their metabolites in cellular functions.* Zeist, The Netherlands: Joint UNESCO-IUB Workshop, August 22–24, 1985.
16. Vamecq J. Liver peroxisomal oxidizing activities in physiological and pathological conditions. In: Faihmi D, Sies H, eds. *Proceedings in life sciences. Peroxisomes in biology and medicine.* Heidelberg: Springer-Verlag, 1987:364–73.
17. Dohan JS. Glycolic acid oxidase. *J Biol Chem* 1940;135:795–6.

18. Kun E, Dechary JM, Pitot HC. The oxidation of glycolic acid by a liver enzyme. *J Biol Chem* 1954;210:269–89.
19. Schuman M, Massey V. Purification and characterization of glycolic acid oxidase from pig liver. *Biochem Biophys Acta* 1971;227:500–20.
20. Masters C, Holmes R. Peroxisomes: new aspects of cell physiology and biochemistry. *Physiol Rev* 1977;57:816–82.
21. Hsieh B, Tolbert NE. Glyoxylate aminotransferase in peroxisomes from rat liver and kidney. *J Biol Chem* 1976;251:4408–15.
22. Danpure CJ, Jennings PR. Deficiency of peroxisomal alanine: glyoxylate aminotransferase in primary hyperoxaluria Type I. *Eur J Cell Biol* 1986;41 Suppl 14:11.
23. Vamecq J, Van Hoof F. Implication of a peroxisomal enzyme in the catabolism of glutaryl-CoA. *Biochem J* 1984;221:203–11.
24. Vamecq J, de Hoffmann E, Van Hoof F. Mitochondrial and peroxisomal metabolism of glutaryl-CoA. *Eur J Biochem* 1985;146:663–9.
25. de Duve C. Functions of microbodies (peroxisomes). *J Cell Biol* 1965;27:25A–26A.
26. de Duve C, Baudhuin P. Peroxisomes (microbodies and related particles). *Physiol Rev* 1966; 46:323–57.
27. Baudhuin P. Liver peroxisomes, cytology and function. *Ann NY Acad Sci* 1969;168:214–28.
28. Kawamura N, Moser HW, Kishimoto Y. Very long chain fatty acid oxidation in the rat liver. *Biochem Biophys Res Commun* 1981;99:1216–25.
29. Singh I, Moser AE, Goldfischer S, Moser HW. Lignoceric acid is oxidized in the peroxisome: Implication for the Zellweger cerebro-hepato-renal syndrome and adrenoleukodystrophy. *Proc Natl Acad Sci* 1984;81:4203–7.
30. Horrocks LA, Sharma M. Plasmalogens and O-alkylglycerophospholipids. In: Hawthorne JN, Ansell GB, eds. *Phospholipids*. Oxford: Elsevier Biomedical Press, 1982:51–93.
31. Heymans HSA, Schutgens RBH, Tan R, van den Bosch H, Borst P. Severe plasmalogen deficiency in tissues of infants without peroxisomes (Zellweger syndrome). *Nature* 1983;306:69–70.
32. Heymans HSA, van den Bosch H, Schutgens RBH, et al. Deficiency of plasmalogens in the cerebro-hepato-renal (Zellweger) syndrome. *Eur J Pediatr* 1984;142:16–20.
33. Borst P. Animal peroxisomes (microbodies), lipid biosynthesis and the Zellweger syndrome. *Trends Biochem Sci* 1983;8:269–72.
34. Igarashi M, Schaumburg HH, Powers J, Kishimoto Y, Kolodni E, Suzuki K. Fatty acid abnormality in adrenoleukodystrophy. *J Neurochem* 1976;26:851–60.
35. Menkes JH, Corbo LM. Adrenoleukodystrophy: accumulation of cholesterol esters with very long chain fatty acids. *Neurology* 1977;27:928–32.
36. Powers JM, Schaumburg HH, Johnson AB, Raine CS. A correlative study of the adrenal cortex in adrenoleukodystrophy. Evidence for a fatal intoxication with very long chain saturated fatty acids. *Invest Cell Pathol* 1980;3:353–76.
37. Goldfischer S, Collins J, Rapin I, et al. Peroxisomal defects in neonatal-onset and X-linked adrenoleukodystrophies. *Science* 1985;227:67–70.
38. Goffinet AM. Events governing the organization of postmigratory neurons. *Brain Res* 1984; 7:261–96.
39. Slevin JT, Johnston NV, Biziere K, Coyle JT. Methylazoxymethanol acetate ablation of mouse cerebellar granule cells: effects on synaptic neurochemistry. *Dev Neurosci* 1982;5:3–12.
40. Hamilton GA, Buckthal DG, Mortensen RM, Zerby KW. Reactions of cysteamine and other amine metabolites with glyoxylate and oxygen catalysed by D-amino acid oxidase. *Proc Natl Acad Sci USA* 1979;76:2625–9.
41. Hamilton GA. Peroxisomal oxidases and suggestions for the mechanism of action of insulin and other hormones. *Adv Enzymol* 1985;57:85–178.
42. Lyle CR, Jutila JW. D-amino acid induction in the kidneys of germ free mice. *J Bacteriol* 1968;96:606–8.
43. Coyle JP, Bird SJ, Evans RH, et al. Excitatory amino acid neurotoxins: selectivity, specificity and mechanisms of action. *Neurosci Res Program Bull* 1981;19:355–427.
44. Konno R, Yasumura Y. Mouse mutant deficient in D-amino acid oxidase activity. *Genetics* 1983;103:277–85.
45. Konno R, Yasumura Y. Coat color genes of D-amino acid oxidase deficient ddY/DAO⁻ mice and nonlinkage of gene for D-amino acid oxidase to coat color genes. *Jpn J Genet* 1984;59:159–63.

46. Leighton F, Persico R, Nehcochea C. Peroxisomal fatty acid oxidation is selectively inhibited by phenothiazines in isolated hepatocytes. *Biochem Biophys Res Commun* 1984;120:505–11.
47. Reddy JK, Warren JR, Reddy MK, Lalwani ND. Hepatic and renal effects of peroxisome proliferators: biological implications. *Ann NY Acad Sci* 1982;386:81–108.
48. Van den Branden C, Vamecq J, Wybo I, Roels F. Phytol and peroxisome proliferation. *Pediatr Res* 1986;20:411–5.
49. Parthasarathy S, Kritchevsky D, Baumann WG. Hypolipidemic drugs are inhibitors of phosphatidylcholine synthesis. *Proc Natl Acad Sci* 1982;79:6890–3.

Developmental Neurobiology, edited by
Philippe Evrard and Alexandre Minkowski.
Nestlé Nutrition Workshop Series, Vol. 12.
Nestec Ltd., Vevey/Raven Press, Ltd.,
New York © 1989.

Gene Mapping Techniques

Jean-Louis Guénet

Institut Pasteur, 75724 Paris Cédex 15, France

Very accurate gene mapping is essential in both man and laboratory mammals (1–3). Several techniques have been used over the last 50 years to localize mammalian genes on the chromosomes of a given species. This chapter reviews these techniques, with special emphasis on the most recent ones that represent a true breakthrough in formal genetics.

CLASSICAL GENE MAPPING TECHNIQUES AND THEIR LIMITATIONS

When two genes are linked they have a tendency to cosegregate during successive generations. The closer the linkage, the more absolute is the cosegregation. This is the fundamental principle of gene mapping, which has been successfully applied to all species, including plants, over many years. In mammals such as humans and mice, the continued discovery of marker genes scattered throughout the genome has facilitated the mapping of new genes so that we now possess for these two species, particularly the mouse, linkage maps that are far more detailed than those existing for other mammals.

In the mouse, special matings can be set up, with appropriate stocks, to test for possible autosomal linkage after two successive reproductive rounds: In general, cross-back crosses are used, cross-intercrosses being reserved for studies in which the viability or the fertility of the homozygous mutant under study is impaired. In humans investigations concerning linkage are based on pedigree analysis.

In other words, for both species it is essential to define as a starting point a situation where two genes are heterozygous and either in repulsion $A + / + B$ or in coupling $AB/ + +$, then to look for changes in this configuration after a reproductive cycle (forms in coupling giving rise to forms in repulsion and vice versa), and finally to count the percentage or frequency of these recombination events. The smaller the frequency, the tighter is the linkage.

At the population level other approaches have been used to test for possible linkage. One such method used in human populations is the lod score, which assesses abnormally high frequencies of association between genes within populations having common ancestors. In the mouse the use of congenic strains, and especially recombinant inbred strains (RIS), has proved very useful. The use of RIS for the detection of linkage has been extensively reviewed by Taylor (4), who has considered each strain as the equivalent of an F2 individual with a unique reassociation of parental characters. Here, however, the new genotype is permanent since the strain is inbred.

Although such classic techniques have been very useful over the years they share several drawbacks and have in addition two intrinsic major limitations.

The drawbacks include their time-consuming nature, particularly in human studies; their expense, since several hundred mice may have to be bred to test for a hypothetical linkage or to ensure the necessary precision (since by definition as many recombinants as possible must be scored if tight linkage is to be detected or established with accuracy); and the fact that many mutant genes cause reductions in viability or are not fully expressed in all individuals bearing them. This is particularly likely to happen in the mouse and may prevent the determination of the true segregation ratio, and thus the proportion of recombinants in linkage crosses.

The two main limitations arise because: (a) The mapping methodology only allows for linkage detection with already known marker genes. By definition, linkage cannot be detected if the gene under investigation is "far away" from all other known genes. (b) The genes coding for invariant products, which by definition have no allelic forms, cannot be mapped using these methods.

It is mainly for these reasons that nonsexual techniques have been developed by mammalian geneticists over the last twenty years. These methods use somatic cells of different species grown *in vitro* and artificially hybridized. Although fundamentally different, these new techniques are complementary to the classic ones and should be considered as additions rather than alternatives to the classic mapping technologies.

GENE MAPPING WITH SOMATIC CELL HYBRIDS

Our knowledge of the mammalian genetic map (and especially the human map) has increased considerably during the past 15 to 20 years as a result of a number of very important advances in cell genetics. Among these were the discovery of human–rodent and rodent–rodent cell hybridization and the study of the segregation of different chromosomes occurring in such hybrids; the development of chromosome staining techniques (the so-called banding techniques) which permit unambiguous identification of all human, hamster, and mouse chromosomes at the metaphase stage; and the discovery of several hundreds of biochemical markers in the different species which can be identified and characterized as electrophoretic variants (the so-called electromorphs or allozymes, when the particular protein is an enzyme).

At present, every human chromosome and every mouse chromosome has at least one biochemical marker and often many more. These technical advances have permitted tremendous progress in mapping of both human (mostly) and mouse genes.

For rapid chromosomal assignment of human genes, a panel consisting of a collection of cloned human–rodent cell-hybrids containing specific combinations of human chromosomes can be used. The genes coding for proteins that are specific to the human species can be identified by their product, using special biochemical assays. In parallel, it is also possible to identify individual human chromosomes among the chromosomal set of the cell hybrids. Thus genes coding for unique human markers can be mapped to the individual human chromosome that matches its particular pattern in the hybrid panel. In some instances only one chromosome of a given species (humans in general) is present in addition to the normal complement of the partner species of the hybrid, so that a nonambiguous localization of the gene can be made almost immediately.

In order to increase such gene assignments, the following efforts have been made: (a) To characterize more gene products physically, chemically, and immunologically in order to distinguish clearly human from rodent products. Monoclonal antibodies, electrophoresis, and isoelectrofocalization techniques and study of thermal stability of proteins have been of cardinal importance in this field. (b) To devise methods for inducing gene activities which are not normally expressed in cell hybrids. (c) To construct additional hybrid panels containing new combinations of human, mouse, or chinese hamster chromosomes, either as intact chromosomes or partially rearranged with each other. (d) To develop sets of deletion hybrids each containing only one chromosome of a given species, with more or less extensive terminal deletion.

More than 100 genes have been localized using these somatic cell hybrid techniques, and about 40 new genes are mapped each year. It is, however, impossible with these techniques to localize genes coding for monomorphic gene products (those which exhibit no variation between the partners of the cell hybrids); they are also characterized by a certain lack of precision in gene localization due to the limited number of chromosomal breakages available. This results in most assignments being less precise than those obtained using the classic techniques.

Finally it must be pointed out that genes whose products are not expressed *in vitro* cannot be mapped using these techniques.

THE USE OF RECOMBINANT DNA PROBES IN GENE MAPPING

With the recent development of molecular DNA technology, new techniques have become available for mapping genes. Again, these new techniques are complementary to those already discussed. They involve the use of DNA probes.

A DNA probe consists of a small DNA segment, containing a specific sequence of the genome, which is used for hybridization at the molecular level with genomic DNA. To be easily kept and prepared in large quantities for hybridization, the DNA sequence of the probe is incorporated within an autoreplicative structure, either a bacteriophage or a plasmid, prior to hybridization. To be easily recognizable (the primary role of a probe) the DNA sequence is labeled, usually with a radioactive isotope.

Probes containing more or less extensive parts of specific genes are able to hybridize with the homologous segment of the chromosome carrying the particular gene if used under appropriate technical conditions. Thus if a radioactive probe is hybridized with a sample of DNA prepared from interspecific cell hybrids segregating for a given set of chromosomes it is possible to identify, at least roughly, where the locus coding for this gene is located by matching the pattern of positive hybridizations with the pattern of chromosome presence or absence in the panel (Fig. 1).

These techniques represent an important advance in formal genetics because they allow gene detection without requiring their expression. Mapping of the sequences of several important structural genes has been performed using heavily labeled cDNA probes and restricted (cut in small segments) genomic DNA from several sources: human–mouse hybrid cell lines have shown the localization of the α globin gene on human chromosome 16 and the assignment of the β globin gene complex to human chromosome 11; human–chinese hamster hybrid cell lines have allowed the assignment of the insulin gene to human chromosome 11 (5): mouse–chinese hamster hybrid cell lines have allowed the assignment of the cluster of genes coding for β interferon to mouse chromosome 4 (6).

In situ molecular hybridization constitutes another promising development in gene mapping. When DNA probes are labeled with ^3H with a high specific activity, rather than with ^{32}P, and hybridized to well spread mitotic metaphase preparations of somatic chromosomes, attachment of the probe to homologous regions on the chromosomes occurs (5). Again it is possible to determine where a given sequence is located on the chromosomes of a given species after autoradiography and computation of the grain count.

These hybridization techniques have proven very useful in formal mammalian genetics. However, they have a few disadvantages: a gene cannot be mapped unless a specific radioactive probe has been made available; in the genome of a species there are frequently sequences partially matching the probe (e.g., pseudogenes, genes coding for isoforms) which makes the recognition of a given sequence difficult; and

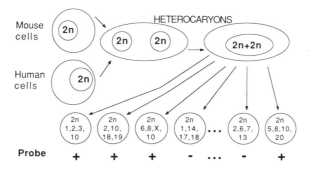

FIG. 1. Detection of syntenic relationships with cellular hybrids. The probe is localized on chromosome n°10.

since no use is made of sexual reproduction the process of meiotic recombination does not operate and thus no precise assignment is possible for a given gene.

DNA PROBES AS GENETIC MARKERS

With the increasing number of studies being carried out on the structure of genomic DNA it has become quite clear that polymorphism at the level of DNA is much more intense than it is at the level of transcribed and translated gene products. This can easily be explained by what geneticists call silent mutations, such as changes at the level of DNA resulting, for example, in the substitution of an ACA for an ACG codon, both coding for the amino acid phenylalanine. Moreover, most DNA polymorphism goes undetected simply because the DNA is not translated into proteins. According to a recent theoretical estimate no more than 1% to 3% of the genomic DNA is actually translated. If on the other hand one assumes (which is almost certainly true) that the coding sequences are randomly spread over the entire genome it is possible to use polymorphism at the DNA level as a source of markers.

This has been achieved by the use of so-called restriction endonucleases. These particular enzymes have the property of cutting the DNA in a nonrandom manner. They cut when a particular short sequence of 4 to 8 nucleotides is detected on the DNA strand; each restriction endonuclease recognizes a specific sequence of nucleotides. It is thus possible with a given enzyme to cut an entire genome into segments of various sizes (a few kilobase pairs in general); this dissection of the genomic DNA into small pieces can be made on different samples with two or more enzymes. If two individuals differ by just one base pair in a restriction site (a mutation) the size of the restriction fragment will be different. If these two individuals belong to two different species, such as mouse and man, the restriction fragment length will almost always be very different. This is the so-called restriction fragment length polymorphism (or RFLP).

After DNA restriction, the DNA fragments can be separated according to their size using gel electrophoresis. It is possible to recognize a particular segment of the genome hybridizing to a radiolabeled probe either directly on the electrophoretic gel or more frequently on a transfer replica of it. The tandem probe-restriction fragment can be considered as a marker which is normally unique for the genome since the probability of finding two sequences giving a restriction fragment of the same size and having a similar affinity for a given probe is very small indeed.

With the so-called restriction polymorphism it is possible to recognize an individual homozygous for a RFLP from another who is heterozygous. After electrophoresis of restricted DNA from a homozygous individual all fragments hybridizing with a radiolabeled probe will be of the same size, producing a single line. Two classes of labeled fragments will be recognized on DNA from a heterozygous animal, giving two lines.

Another advantage of RFLP is that the sequence which is used for the recognition of a particular fragment does not necessarily code for a protein. It is not even obligatory for the sequence to be expressed; any "anonymous" segment of DNA, provided that it is present in the genome under the form of a single copy, will do. About 1% of the recombinant phages in the human genomic library contain only unique sequences. Chromosomal localization of such unique sequences is then possible using the techniques already reported (e.g., hybrid cells, *in situ* chromosome hybridization). It is also possible using conventional markers in conjunction with normal sexual reproduction. Together with Robert and co-workers (7) we have mapped the gene coding for the light chain of myosin very close to the mouse *Idh-1* locus (chromosome 1) using sexual reproduction (and thus meiotic recombination) and two different mouse species: *Mus musculus domesticus* (the normal laboratory mouse) and *Mus spretus* (a line derived from a wild population of mice). These two lines, which have been separated for millions of years, have lost mutual sex appeal. They no longer interbreed and behave like two different species. In the laboratory, however, interbreeding is possible. This allows a tremendous amount of polymorphism to segregate since the genetic divergence has produced many translated or untranslated changes at the DNA level. What we did originally, using a known α actin probe, can now be generalized to any fragment, even an "anonymous" one. Once the DNA fragment contained in the probe has been mapped to a given chromosome the information is permanent and can, for instance, be used as a marker for other fragments. Data are cumulative and fresh information is now accumulating at an exponential rate. Avner and co-workers have used a similar approach for the study of a particular part of the genome. After preparing a DNA library from an almost pure preparation of mouse X chromosomes sorted by flow cytometry (8), X-chromosome-specific DNA probes have been localized using these probes at the molecular level in conjunction with studies on animal phenotype using classical marker genes for X chromosomes such as Tabby (Ta), jimpy (jp), α galactosidase (α gal), and hypoxanthine phosphoribosyl transferase (HPRT).

All these probes have been linearly arranged and can now be used to map further sequences. It is obvious that the system is autocatalytic. It can also be generalized to any chromosomes of a given species so that having a marker every milli-Morgan is now a reasonable perspective. These molecular approaches to the mapping of mammalian genes are universally applicable. For example, no understanding of the biochemical nature of a given inherited disease is required for mapping its genetic determinant. They open new and very promising perspectives in terms of genetic counseling, as most common genetic diseases will probably soon become detectable in carriers and pregnancies at risk identifiable. In the mouse, conventional mapping techniques, although still in use even in the more advanced laboratories, are going to be irreversibly transformed.

REFERENCES

1. Cooper DN, Schmidtke J. DNA restriction fragment length polymorphisms and heterozygosity in the human genome. *Hum Genet* 1984;66:1–16.
2. Green MC. Gene mapping. In: *The mouse in biomedical research*. New York: Academic Press, 1981:105–17.

3. Puck TT, Kao F-T. Somatic cell genetics and its application to medicine. *Annu Rev Genet* 1982; 16:225–71.
4. Taylor BA. Recombinant inbred strains: use in gene mapping. In: MORSE MC, III, ed. *Origins of inbred mice*. New York: Academic Press, 1978:423–38.
5. Malcolm S, Barton P, Murphy C, Ferguson-Smith MA. Chromosomal localization of a single copy gene by in situ hybridization—human beta globin genes on the short arm of chromosome 11. *Ann Hum Genet* 1981;45:135–41.
6. Naylor SL, Gray PW, Lalley PA. Mouse immune interferon (IFN-gamma) gene is on chromosome 10. *Somatic Cell Genet* 1984;10:531–4.
7. Robert B, Barton P, Minty Y, et al. Investigation of genetic linkage between myosin and actin genes using an interspecific mouse backcross. *Nature* 1985;314:181–3.
8. Baron B, Metezeau P, Kelly F, et al. Flow cytometry isolation and improved visualization of sorted mouse chromosomes. *Exp Cell Res* 1984;152:220–30.
9. Taylor X, Bailey X. *Proc Natl Acad Sci (USA)*.

DISCUSSION

Dr. Devilliers-Thiery: Do you have any idea how polymorphic genes are? In other words what is the percentage of homology in terms of nucleotide sequences between two strains of mice?

Dr. Guénet: Between two human beings one base per thousand per chain is different, so you probably have 1,000 bases that are different from your neighbors'.

Dr. Devilliers-Thiery: To be able to map a variant gene, you have to have polymorphism. Have you ever encountered a situation in which you had no polymorphism?

Dr. Guénet: No. There are so many restriction enzymes that the probability of not finding polymorphism within an interspecific cross is very close to zero. You must bear in mind that as well as the huge number of restriction enzymes you can use methylation, either independently or in addition, to change the restriction site. This gives you a tremendous advantage compared with formal genetics.

Dr. Devilliers-Thiery: How close is the genetic map of the mouse to that of the human? In other words, when you have mapped the mouse what are the chances that the human map will be the same in terms of linkage for invariant proteins? If you know that in the mouse genome gene A is next to gene B which is next to gene C, what are the chances that the same order will also be found in the human genome?

Dr. Guénet: Invariant proteins have a tremendous degree of homology. Thus a probe obtained from the mouse will have a very good chance of matching the homologous human gene. It is another matter for variant proteins, of course. As far as order is concerned, Taylor and Bailey (9) recently reported that there are sequential homologies between the mouse map and the human map. For example, chromosome 4 on the mouse map is almost a replicate of the branch q of human chromosome 1. So if you find your receptor to be in chromosome 4 in the mouse I would recommend that you look in branch q of human chromosome 1. There are exceptions of course, but there are a large number of homologies.

Dr. Campagnoni: Can you map genes within a chromosome by taking somatic cell hybrids that contain, for example, one human chromosome in a background of mouse chromosomes?

Dr. Guénet: Yes, this has been done. Attempts were made to map myosin with this technique, but the results were incorrect because several rearrangements caused confusion. When multiple rearrangements occur the segments of the human chromosome may become so small that they are no longer easy to identify.

Dr. Sotelo: You talk about hybridization *in situ*. If I understood you correctly, you have a cDNA probe and you use a single chromosome from one cell and try to find where the cDNAs hybridize. Is it necessary that the gene is expressed?

Dr. Guénet: No. The big advantage of *in situ* hybridization and of all nuclear techniques is that the gene does not have to be expressed. For example, the gene for phenylalanine hydroxylase is not expressed *in vitro* but, nevertheless, you can detect where this gene is located. This is not the problem with these techniques. The problem is the large amount of background "noise". You have to count the grains and make the map by a process of addition.

Developmental Neurobiology, edited by
Philippe Evrard and Alexandre Minkowski.
Nestlé Nutrition Workshop Series, Vol. 12.
Nestec Ltd., Vevey/Raven Press, Ltd.,
New York © 1989.

Expression of Myelin Basic Protein Genes in the Developing Mouse Brain

Anthony T. Campagnoni, H.J. Roth, M. Hunkeler, P.J. Pretorius, and C.W. Campagnoni

Department of Chemistry, University of Maryland, College Park, Maryland 20742

Myelination is a major biological event during the early postnatal development of the mouse brain, yet relatively little is known about the mechanism and regulation of myelin assembly. In view of the importance of the myelin sheath in the maintenance of a functionally normal brain, and because of the wide variety of neurological diseases and nutritional deficiencies that result in hypomyelination, studies into the mechanism by which the membrane is formed are particularly important.

Current understanding of the synthesis of myelin proteins and their assembly into the membrane is very incomplete, and research in this area is only at its earliest stages. The overall process by which proteins are synthesized and assembled into myelin may arbitrarily be divided into three rather broad stages: (a) the synthesis and processing of the mRNAs which code for the myelin proteins; (b) the translation of these mRNAs on ribosomes and subsequent posttranslational modification of the myelin proteins; and (c) the intracellular transport and assembly of these proteins into myelin.

MYELIN PROTEINS

The myelin basic protein (MBP) is one of the macromolecular constituents of myelin. It can be considered a peripheral membrane protein because of its particular topography within the myelin membrane and its solubility properties (1,2). It is a highly basic hydrophilic protein, in marked contrast to the other major myelin protein, the proteolipid protein, which is extremely hydrophobic. The MBP was first isolated from guinea pig brain (3), and its localization in the myelin sheath was subsequently established by a number of biochemical and immunocytochemical techniques. The protein has been isolated from a number of species and its complete primary sequence has been determined (4). The MBP from most species contains approximately 170 amino acid residues and has a molecular weight of 18,400. Table 1 summarizes some of the characteristics of the major myelin proteins.

TABLE 1. *Properties of the major myelin proteins*

	Type	Molecular weight	Primary sequence	Properties
Proteolipid protein	Integral	30 kdalton	known	Extremely hydropho-bic; contains 2%– 4% covalently bound fatty acid
Myelin basic protein(s)	Peripheral			Hydrophilic; pI greater
major forms		18.5 kdalton	known	than 10.8; highly en-
		14 kdalton	known	cephalitogenic
minor forms		21.5 kdalton	unknown	
		17 kdalton	unknown	

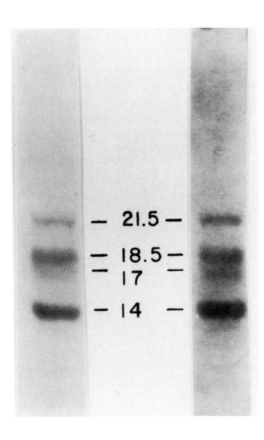

FIG. 1. Immunoblot of mouse my-elin showing the four myelin basic proteins (MBPs). Two preparations of myelin were separated by SDS-poly-acrylamide gel electrophoresis, trans-ferred to nitrocellulose, treated with anti-MBP; and the antibody-MBP complexes were visualized by immu-noperoxidase staining. The presence of the 17K and 21.5K minor forms of the MBP are evident in addition to the two major forms of the protein (14K and 18.5K).

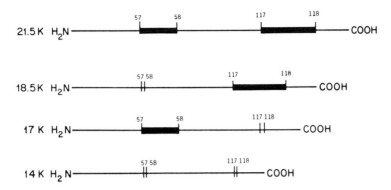

FIG. 2. Proposed structural relationship among the four mouse myelin basic proteins (MBPs) showing the positions of the two additional sequences in the N-terminal and C-terminal halves of the molecule. The 21.5K MBP contains both insertions. The 18.5K and 17K MBPs are each missing one of the two insertions. The 14K MBP is missing both insertions. The numbers refer to the residue numbers in the 14K MBP.

A number of species in the mammalian suborders *Myomorpha* and *Sciuromorpha* (which include the rat and mouse) contain two major MBPs which have been designated 18.5K and 14K, reflecting their apparent molecular weights (5). The rat 18.5K protein has been found similar in size, chromatographic properties, amino acid composition, and encephalitogenic activity to the single MBP found in other species, such as man and ox (6). The rat 14K protein has been isolated and sequenced, and it appears to be identical to the rat 18.5K protein except for a deletion within the interior of the molecule. The mouse 14K and 18.5K MBPs appear to bear the same structural relationship to each other, as do the rat proteins. In rats and mice the 14K MBP predominates over the 18.5K MBP by a ratio of 2–3:1 (7).

Two other low molecular weight MBPs can be detected in immunoblots of myelin (Fig. 1). These two MBPs, first described by Barbarese et al. (8), are immunologically related to the two major forms of the mouse basic proteins (i.e., 14K and 18.5K) and have apparent molecular weights of approximately 21,500 and 17,000. They appear to be structurally related to the 14K and 18.5K basic proteins, having an extra sequence of approximately 3,000 daltons in the N-terminal half of the molecule. Until recently, the exact position of this sequence was unclear; however, it has now been localized between residues 57 and 58 in sheep 21.5K MBP (9). Thus the four MBPs appear to be related through the 14K MBP primary sequence which is common to all four proteins, and they differ from each other by the presence or absence of one or two additional sequences inserted within the interior of the molecule (Fig. 2).

SYNTHESIS AND ASSEMBLY OF PROTEINS INTO MYELIN

In the developing mouse brain, expression of the two major forms of the MBP occurs synchronously and reaches a maximum at 18 days of age (10). Maximal ex-

TABLE 2. *Cell biological characteristics of myelin protein assembly*

	Myelin basic proteins	Proteolipid protein
Leader sequence	No	No
Site of synthesis	Free polysomes	Bound ribosomes
Transport mechanism	Unknown: possibly by ribosome movement, vesicles, or micro-tubules	Golgi involved
Order of assembly	14 and 18.5K MBPs before the proteolipid protein	

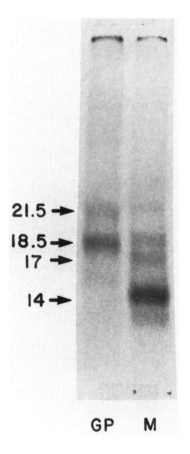

21.5 ➡

18.5➡

17 ➡

14 ➡

GP   M

FIG. 3. Autoradiogram of myelin basic proteins (MBPs) synthesized *in vitro* using mRNA isolated from either guinea pig (GP) or mouse (M) brain poly A(+) mRNA. Messenger RNA was isolated from either fetal guinea pig brain or 18 day old mouse brain and translated in reticulocyte lysates. Newly synthesized MBP labeled with ^{35}S-methionine was immunoprecipitated and analyzed by SDS-polyacrylamide gel electrophoresis. The autoradiogram shows that guinea pig brain synthesizes the two high molecular weight forms of the MBP (i.e., 18.5K and 21.5K) in contrast to the four forms synthesized by mouse brain.

pression of the other major myelin protein, the proteolipid protein, occurs several days later, suggesting that the "turning on" of the major myelin protein genes may be staggered (10).

Studies from our laboratory with isolated polyribosomes have shown that the predominant sites of synthesis of the MBPs are the free ribosomes in the oligodendrocyte (11). These studies have been confirmed elsewhere, and it has also been found that the proteolipid protein is synthesized on ribosomes bound to the endoplasmic reticulum (12). The proteolipid protein is synthesized without a leader sequence and it appears to be cotranslationally inserted into the endoplasmic reticulum (12–14). All the available biochemical and immunohistochemical data indicate that the basic proteins and proteolipid protein follow separate intracellular routes from their sites of synthesis to their assembly into the growing myelin membrane (15–19). Transport of the proteolipid protein probably involves the Golgi bodies, and transport of the basic proteins probably occurs through the cytosol by some other mechanism. Table 2 lists some of the cell biological characteristics of the major classes of myelin proteins.

When the 17K and 21.5K MBPs were first discovered there was a possibility that these proteins might be metabolic precursors of the quantitatively more important 14K and 18.5K MBPs. We undertook a study to determine whether or not this was the case, and it became apparent that the four MBPs were coded for by four separate mRNAs and that the four basic proteins were synthesized without leader sequences (20). The synthesis of all four mouse MBPs could be detected in mRNA-stimulated reticulocyte lysates which had been shown to contain no processing activity; and the kinetics of labeling of the four mouse MBPs did not support the concept of a precursor–product relationship among any of the MBPs. Figure 3 shows the anti-MBP immunoprecipitated products of a reticulocyte lysate stimulated with guinea pig and mouse polysomal mRNA. Note that the complete proteins are synthesized and that the guinea pig synthesizes only the two higher molecular weight forms of the MBP, whereas the mouse synthesizes all four forms.

CHARACTERIZATION OF THE MBP mRNA

Using two families of synthetic oligonucleotide probes corresponding to two regions of the MBP, Zeller et al. (21) were able to prepare and screen for a cDNA common to all four mouse MBP mRNAs. These two families of oligonucleotide probes corresponded to two different regions of the MBP. One family was used as a primer to prepare cDNAs which were cloned into pBR322, and both families were used to screen for cDNA clones containing an MBP insert. One clone, designated NZ111, contained 94 nucleotides and its sequence was found to correspond to residues 60 to 93 of the MBP. The clone was identified as an authentic MBP mRNA segment from its nucleotide sequence and from its ability to selectively hybridize to MBP mRNA using hybrid selection techniques.

This clone has been used to characterize the MBP mRNAs from mouse and

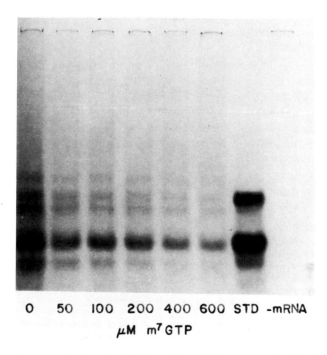

0   50   IOO   200   400   6OO   STD   -mRNA

μM m⁷GTP

FIG. 4. Autoradiogram showing the inhibition of the cell-free synthesis of the four mouse myelin basic proteins (MBPs) with increasing concentrations of the "cap" inhibitor, m7GTP. Reticulocyte lysates were programmed with 18 day old mouse brain poly A(+) mRNA, and MBPs were isolated by immunoprecipitation. The STD lane shows the migration of ^{125}I-labeled 14K and 18.5K mouse MBPs.

guinea pig brain (21,22). Northern blot analysis of 18 day old mouse poly A(+) mRNAs vary in size from approximately 2,100 to 2,400 nucleotides. Parallel Northern analysis of fetal guinea pig brain poly A(+) mRNA revealed a narrower band of MBP mRNA corresponding to the higher molecular weight half of the mouse MBP mRNA band. These data are consistent with the absence of the 14K and 17K MBPs in the guinea pig brain. Thus the mRNAs for the four mouse MBPs are of similar length and are encompassed within a range of 2,100 to 2,400 nucleotides. Since the coding region for the largest MBP (21.5K) would be approximately 600 nucleotides then, as has also been demonstrated from sequence data, there are large untranslated regions present in these mRNAs.

It has been known for some time that the MBP mRNAs are polyadenylated and it is now clear that they are very large. Another piece of information about mRNA structure that could have important regulatory implications is whether or not the mRNA contains a "cap" at its 5' end. Cap structures are 7-methyl guanosine residues linked from their 5' hydroxyl to the 5' hydroxyl group of the mRNA by a triphosphate bridge. One method commonly used to determine whether a mRNA is capped is to examine the ability of cap inhibitors, such as 7-methyl guanosine triphosphate, to inhibit the translation of that message. In cell-free translation experiments with brain mRNA-stimulated reticulocyte lysates the cap analog, m7GTP, significantly inhibited 35S-methionine incorporation in the four mouse MBPs. At the highest concentration examined, inhibition by 70% or more was observed (Fig. 4). The 14K mRNA appeared to be most inhibited by the cap analog and the 21.5K MBP mRNA least inhibited, but all four MBP mRNAs were substantially inhibited suggesting that all four MBP mRNAs are capped.

In summary, all the studies performed to date indicate that the various forms of the MBPs are coded for by separate mRNAs; that these mRNAs are polyadenylated at their 3' ends and capped at their 5' ends; that they are very large (2,100–2,400 nucleotides) considering the sizes of the proteins they code for; and that they contain substantial lengths of untranslated sequence. The rat 14K MBP mRNA has been cloned by Roach et al. (23) and its structure corresponds to that predicted by our results. It also supports the finding that the MBPs are the product of separate mRNAs.

EXPRESSION OF MBPs IN NORMAL AND MUTANT MICE

The mouse cDNA probe was also used in Northern and dot blot analyses to titrate the concentration of MBP mRNA in total polyribosomes isolated from the developing brains of normal and dysmyelinating mutant mice (22). Northern blots on mRNA isolated from 18 day old normal and mutant mice suggested that the three mutants, jimpy, quaking, and shiverer, contained greatly differing levels of MBP mRNA, although MBP mRNAs of apparently normal size were found to be associated with quaking and jimpy polyribosomes. Quaking polysomes contained much more MBP mRNA than jimpy, and virtually no MBP mRNA was detected in shiverer polysomes.

The concentrations of MBP mRNA were estimated by dot blot analysis (21,22) and maximal levels of MBP mRNA were observed to occur at 18 days in the normal developing mouse brain, in agreement with earlier *in vivo* synthesis studies (24). These studies were extended to the three hypomyelinating mutants, quaking *(qk/qk)*, jimpy *(jp/Y)*, and shiverer *(shi/shi)*, as well as heterozygote controls. A method was developed for quantifying the levels of MBP mRNA from dot blots which correlated well with estimates made from Northern blots (22). Figure 5 shows the levels of MBP mRNA present in C57BL/6J and mutant brains from 12 to 27 days postpartum. These studies were begun at 12 days, the earliest age at which clinical signs allowed definitive identification of the mutations. The data are presented relative to the levels of MBP mRNA present in 18 day old C57BL/6J control mice. Very low levels of MBP mRNAs were observed in *shi/shi* brain polyribosomes throughout early postnatal development, consistent with reports that there may be a deletion in the MBP gene in this mutant (22). Accumulation of MBP mRNAs in the brain polyribosomes of quaking homozygotes and heterozygotes (data not shown) was delayed by several days. In these animals, whereas MBP mRNA levels were below normal between 12 and 18 days, normal levels of message were found in polyribosomes

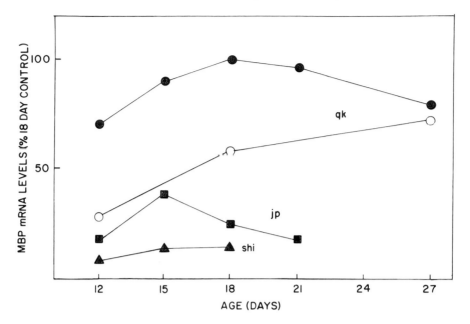

FIG. 5. Levels of myelin basic protein (MBP) mRNA in the developing brains of normal and mutant mice determined by dot blot analysis. *Closed circles,* normal C57BL/6J mice; *open circles,* quaking mice; *closed squares,* jimpy mice; *closed triangles,* shiverer mice. All results are presented as percent of 18 day old C57BL/6J MBP mRNA levels.

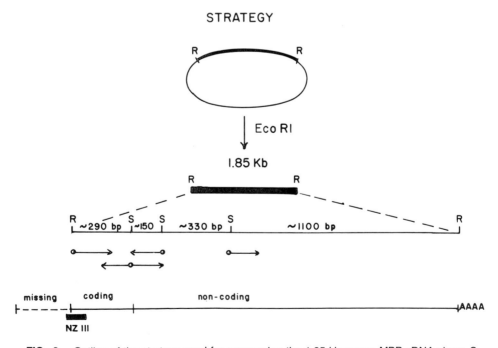

FIG. 6. Outline of the strategy used for sequencing the 1.85 kb mouse MBP cDNA clone. S and R refer to the Sau 3a and Eco RI restriction sites, respectively. *Arrows* indicate regions sequenced and in areas where *arrows overlap* both strands have been sequenced.

between 21 and 27 days. MBP mRNA levels remained well below control levels in *jp*/Y polyribosomes throughout early postnatal development. However, the levels did fluctuate slightly and peaked at 15 days in both *jp*/Y and *jp*/ + brains, three days earlier than in normal mice. Thus the expression of MBP is affected in all the mutants. In jimpy and quaking animals, the phenomenon is age dependent such that these mutants exhibit developmental patterns of MBP expression which are different from control mice as well as from each other. Thus the pattern of MBP gene expression in these mutants is more complicated than expected.

Although synthesis occurs in quaking mutants at all ages at a significant rate, very little of the newly synthesized MBP is incorporated into myelin (25–27), whereas in jimpy mutants not only is there reduced synthesis of the basic proteins, but there is also incomplete incorporation into myelin of those that are synthesized (22,27). Thus in these two mutants the expression of MBP is affected and in addition the assembly of the basic proteins into myelin appears to be blocked.

ISOLATION AND PARTIAL SEQUENCE OF A cDNA OF A MOUSE MBP mRNA

An examination of the expression of the multiple forms of MBP has generated a number of questions which are actively being explored in many laboratories. For example, what exactly is the structural relationship among the four mouse myelin basic proteins? How many genes code for the MBPs exist, and what, if any, MBP mRNAs are derived by differential splicing of a common primary transcript? One approach has been to attempt to clone all four mouse MBP mRNAs and determine their primary sequence. We have prepared an "expression" cDNA library in λgt11 which we have screened with both the mouse cDNA probe and with polyclonal antibodies directed against the MBP. The purpose of these studies has been to isolate and sequence the cDNAs corresponding to each of the four mouse MBPs in order to (a) establish the structure of the four MBP mRNAs, (b) unambiguously establish the structural relationships among the four mouse proteins, and (c) provide additional probes with which to study MBP mRNA metabolism in normal and mutant mice.

λgt11 libraries are prepared by inserting copies of cDNAs of mRNAs, in this case 18 day old mouse polysomal poly A(+) mRNA into λgt11 which contains the lac Z gene. This gene provides a promoter site such that when bacterial cells are infected with this phage a hybrid protein is made which consists of a portion of the lac Z gene product plus the protein of interest (28). The plaques containing a cDNA copy of this protein can then be detected by screening the library with an appropriate antibody.

Using the small NZ111 probe and this immunological approach we screened a λgt11 library and obtained a large number of clones varying in length from 0.44 to 3.7 Kb. We chose one of these clones (1.85 Kb) for further characterization and ascertained through a comparison of restriction maps and preliminary sequencing data that it probably was not a mRNA corresponding to the mouse 14K MBP. It was clear that the clone was not full length because of its size, and it appeared to begin (at its 5' end) within the NZ111 region of the coding region. Restriction maps indi-

```
Mouse 18.5K/21.5K  TAT GGC TCC CTG CCC CAG AAG TCG CAG CAC GGC
Rat 14K            TAC GGC TCC CTG CCC CAG AAG TCG CAG  -   -
NZ111              TAT GGC TCC CTG CCC CAG AAG TCG CAG CAC GGC

Mouse 18.5K/21.5K  CGG ACC CAA GAT GAA AAC CCA GTA GTC CAT TTC
Rat 14K            AGG ACC CAA GAT GAA AAC CCA GTA GTC CAC TTC
NZ111              CGG ACC CAA GAT GAA AAC CCA GTA GTC CAT TTC

Mouse 18.5K/21.5K  TTC AAG AAC ATT GTG ACA CCT CGA ACA CCA
Rat 14K            TTC AAG AAC ATT GTG ACA CCT CGT ACA CCC
NZ111              TTC AAG AA

Mouse 18.5K/21.5K  CCT CCA TCC CAA GGG AAG GGG AGA GGC CTG
Rat 14K            CCT CCA TCC CAA GGA AAG GGG AGA GGC CTG

Mouse 18.5K/21.5K  TCC CTC AGC AGA TTT AGC TGG GGG GCC GAG
Rat 14K            TCC CTC AGC AGA TTT AGC TGG  -   -   -

Mouse 18.5K/21.5K  GGG CAG AAG CCA GGA TTT GGC TAC GGA GGC
Rat 14K             -   -   -   -   -   -   -   -   -   -

Mouse 18.5K/21.5K  AGA GCT TCC GAC TAT AAA TCG GCT CAC AAG GGA
Rat 14K             -   -   -   -   -   -   -   -   -   -   -

Mouse 18.5K/21.5K  TTC AAG GGG GCC TAC GAC GCC CAG GGC ACG CTT
Rat 14K             -   -   -   -   -   -   -   -   -   -   -

Mouse 18.5K/21.5K  TCC AAA ATC TTT AAA CTG GGA GGA AGA GAC AGC
Rat 14K             -   -   -   -   -   -  GGA GGA AGA GAC AGC

Mouse 18.5K/21.5K  CGC TCT GGA TCT CCC ATG GCG AGA CGC TGA GAG
Rat 14K            CGC TCT GGA TCT CCC ATA GCA AGA CGC TGA GAG

Mouse 18.5K/21.5K  CCCTCCCCGCTCAGCCTTCCCGAATCCTGCCCTCGGCTTCTTAATATAACTGCC
Rat 14K            CC-TCCCTGCTCAGCCTTCCCGAATCCTGCCCTCGGCTTCTTAATATAACTGCC

Mouse 18.5K/21.5K  TTAAACTTTTAATTCTACTTGCACCGATTAGCTAGTTAGAGCAGACCCTCTCTT
Rat 14K            TTAAACGTTTAATTCTACTTGCACCAAATAGCTAGTTAGAGCAGACCCTCTCTT

Mouse 18.5K/21.5K  AATCCCGTGGAGCCGTGATC
Rat 14K            AATCCCGTGGGGCTGTGAAC
```

FIG. 7. A comparison of the mouse and rat MBP mRNA sequences. *Asterisks* refer to nucleotides that differ between the two species. The rat 14K sequence was obtained from Roach et al. (23) and the mouse NZ111 sequence was taken from Zeller et al. (21). The Sau 3a restriction sites in the mouse sequence have been *underlined*.

cated three Sau 3a sites, so the clone was digested with Sau 3a and the fragments were cloned into M13 for sequencing. One of the Sau 3a sites was just inside the coding region, as predicted from the rat 14K MBP sequence, but another site, unique to this mouse MBP mRNA, was found downstream from the coding region. Figure 6 illustrates the sequencing strategy. The arrows indicate the directions of sequencing and the regions where both strands were sequenced.

The sequence of this clone indicated that it was part of either the 18.5K or the 21.5K MBP mRNAs because it contained the extra sequence found in these two proteins. Approximately 450 bases were sequenced including all of the available coding region and part of the noncoding region. A comparison of the mouse sequence with the rat 14K MBP mRNA sequence (Fig. 7) indicated a high degree of homology with only 15 base substitutions and 7 deleted nucleotides within the 323 bases common to both mRNAs. There was a perfect correlation of the sequence of this clone with the smaller NZ111 sequence. The two Sau 3a sites are underlined in Fig. 7.

In Fig. 8 the sequence of the mouse MBP protein is compared to that of the rat 14K MBP obtained through its cDNA sequence (23) and to the bovine (29) and human (30) 18.5K MBPs obtained by conventional protein sequencing techniques. In the region sequenced, the mouse protein contains a His-Gly sequence at residues 78

```
Mouse 18.5K/21.5K   Tyr Gly Ser Leu Pro Gln Lys  Ser Gln His Gly  Arg Thr
Rat 14K             Tyr Gly Ser Leu Pro Gln Lys  Ser Gln  -   -   Arg Thr
Bovine              Tyr Gly Ser Leu Pro Gln Lys  Ala Gln Gly His  Arg Pro
Human               Tyr Gly Ser Leu Pro Gln Lys  Ala  -  His Gly  Arg Thr

Mouse 18.5K/21.5K   Gln Asp Glu Asn Pro Val Val His Phe Phe Lys Asn Ile Val
Rat 14K             Gln Asp Glu Asn Pro Val Val His Phe Phe Lys Asn Ile Val
Bovine              Gln Asp Glu Asn Pro Val Val His Phe Phe Lys Asn Ile Val
Human               Gln Asp Gln Asp Pro Val Val His Phe Phe Lys Asn Ile Val

Mouse 18.5K/21.5K   Thr Pro Arg Thr Pro Pro Pro Ser Gln Gly Lys Gly Arg Gly
Rat 14K             Thr Pro Arg Thr Pro Pro Pro Ser Gln Gly Lys Gly Arg Gly
Bovine              Thr Pro Arg Thr Pro Pro Pro Ser Gln Gly Lys Gly Arg Gly
Human               Thr Pro Arg Thr Pro Pro Pro Ser Gln Gly Lys Gly Arg Gly

Mouse 18.5K/21.5K   Leu Ser Leu Ser Arg Phe Ser Trp Gly Ala Glu Gly Gln  Lys
Rat 14K             Leu Ser Leu Ser Arg Phe Ser Trp  -   -   -   -   -    -
Bovine              Leu Ser Leu Ser Arg Phe Ser Trp Gly Ala Glu Gly Gln  Lys
Human               Leu Ser Leu Ser Arg Phe Ser Trp Gly Ala Glu Gly Gln  Arg

Mouse 18.5K/21.5K   Pro Gly Phe Gly Tyr Gly Gly Arg Ala Ser Asp Tyr Lys Ser
Rat 14K              -   -   -   -   -   -   -   -   -   -   -   -   -   -
Bovine              Pro Gly Phe Gly Tyr Gly Gly Arg Ala Ser Asp Tyr Lys Ser
Human               Pro Gly Phe Gly Tyr Gly Gly Arg Ala Ser Asp Tyr Lys Ser

Mouse 18.5K/21.5K   Ala His Lys Gly  Phe  Lys Gly  Ala Tyr  Asp Ala Gln Gly Thr
Rat 14K              -   -   -   -    -    -   -    -   -    -   -   -   -   -
Bovine              Ala His Lys Gly  Leu  Lys Gly  His  -   Asp Ala Gln Gly Thr
Human               Ala His Lys Gly  Phe  Lys Gly  Val  -   Asp Ala Gln Gly Thr

Mouse 18.5K/21.5K   Leu Ser Lys Ile Phe Lys Leu Gly Gly Arg Asp Ser Arg
Rat 14K              -   -   -   -   -   -   -  Gly Gly Arg Asp Ser Arg
Bovine              Leu Ser Lys Ile Phe Lys Leu Gly Gly Arg Asp Ser Arg
Human               Leu Ser Lys Ile Phe Lys Leu Gly Gly Arg Asp Ser Arg

Mouse 18.5K/21.5K   Ser Gly Ser Pro  Met  Ala Arg Arg STOP
Rat 14K             Ser Gly Ser Pro  Ile  Ala Arg Arg STOP
Bovine              Ser Gly Ser Pro  Met  Ala Arg Arg
Human               Ser Gly Ser Pro  Met  Ala Arg Arg
```

FIG. 8. A comparison of the protein sequence of the mouse 18.5K myelin basic protein (MBP), deduced from its nucleotide sequence, with the rat 14K MBP and the bovine and human 18.5K MBPs. The rat 14 K MBP sequence was deduced from its mRNA sequence (23), and the bovine (29) and human (30) sequences are those published using conventional protein sequencing techniques. The regions where the sequence of the mouse protein differs from the sequences of one or more of the other proteins have been blocked in.

to 79 which is missing in the rat 14K MBP, and a methionine in place of an isoleucine near the C-terminus of the molecule. Within the sequence which is missing from the rat 14K MBP the mouse protein has four substitutions which distinguish it from the bovine and human proteins. This cDNA has been used to analyze the other cDNA clones by Southern analysis and several of these others appear to represent different mRNAs.

Information about the structure of the MBP gene is itself now beginning to emerge. It appears to be very large (>30 Kb) and to contain a number of relatively small exons (perhaps 7–9) distributed among some very large introns (31–33). It is not yet clear how many MBP genes there are in the mouse or whether some of the exons may appear as sequences in mRNAs which code for proteins other than the MBPs in brain (34).

SUMMARY

In summary, studies on the expression of myelin proteins at the molecular biological level in normal brain are now beginning and it is possible to answer some fundamental molecular biological questions about the nature of the myelinogenesis defect in the dysmyelinating mutants for the first time since they were discovered. It seems clear that the mechanisms governing the expression of the MBPs will prove to be complex and that it is possible that an examination of this system may provide us with important insights into brain genetic regulatory mechanisms.

ACKNOWLEDGMENTS

The authors wish to thank Mr. J.E. Moskaitis for assisting with some of the *in vitro* translation experiments and Ms. Barbara Sorg for the immunoblot of mouse MBPs.

This work was supported, in part, by grants NS15469 and NS20971 from the National Institutes of Health (to A.T. Campagnoni) and by a grant from the South African Medical Research Council (to P.J. Pretorius).

REFERENCES

1. Braun PE. Molecular organization of myelin. In: Morell P, ed. *Myelin*. New York: Plenum Press, 1984:97–116.
2. Carnegie PR, Moore WJ. Myelin basic protein. In: Bradshaw RA, Schneider DM, eds. *Proteins of the nervous system*. New York: Raven Press, 1980:119–43.
3. Laatsch RH, Kies MW, Gordon S, Alvord EC Jr. The encephalitogenic activity of myelin isolated by ultracentrifugation. *J Exp Med* 1962;115:777–88.
4. Mendz GL, Moore WJ, Carnegie PR. N.M.R. studies of myelin basic protein. VI. Proton spectra in aqueous solutions of proteins from mammalian and avian species. *Aust J Chem* 1982;35:1979–2006.
5. Martenson RE, Deibler GE, Kies MW. The occurrence of two myelin basic proteins in the central nervous system of rodents in the suborders *Myomorpha* and *Sciuromorpha*. *J Neurochem* 1971;18:2427–33.

6. Kies MW, Martenson RE, Deibler GE. Myelin basic proteins. In: Davison AN, Mandel P, Morgan IG, eds. *Functional and structural proteins of the nervous system.* New York: Plenum Press, 1972:201–14.
7. Martenson RE. Myelin basic protein: what does it do? In: Kumar S, ed. *Biochemistry of the brain.* New York: Pergamon Press, 1980:49–79.
8. Barbarese E, Braun PE, Carson JH. Identification of prelarge and presmall basic proteins in mouse myelin and their structural relationship to large and small basic proteins. *Proc Natl Acad Sci USA* 1977;74:3360–4.
9. Carnegie PR, Dowse CA. Partial characterization of 21.5K myelin basic protein from sheep brain. *Science* 1984;223:936–8.
10. Campagnoni AT, Hunkeler MJ. Synthesis of the myelin proteolipid protein in the developing mouse brain. *J Neurobiol* 1980;11:355–64.
11. Campagnoni AT, Carey GD, Yu Y-T. *In vitro* synthesis of the myelin basic proteins: subcellular site of synthesis. *J Neurochem* 1980;34:677–86.
12. Colman DR, Kreibich G, Frey AB, Sabatini D. Synthesis and incorporation of myelin polypeptides into CNS myelin. *J Cell Biol* 1982;95:598–608.
13. Dautigny A, Alliel PM, Nussbaum JL, Jolles P. Cell-free synthesis of rat brain myelin proteolipids and their identification by immunoprecipitation. *Biochem Biophys Res Commun* 1983;110:432–7.
14. Sorg BJA, Agrawal D, Agrawal HC, Campagnoni AT. Expression of myelin proteolipid protein and basic protein in normal and dysmyelinating mutant mice. *J Neurochem* 1986;46:379–87.
15. Agrawal HC, Hartman BK. Proteolipid protein and other proteins of myelin. In: Bradshaw RA, Schneider DM, eds. *Proteins of the nervous system.* New York: Raven Press, 1980:145–69.
16. Sternberger NH, Itoyama Y, Kies NW, Webster HD. Immunocytochemical method to identify basic protein in myelin-forming oligodendrocytes of newborn rat CNS. *J Neurocytol* 1978;7:251–63.
17. Sternberger NH, Quarles RH, Itoyama Y, Webster HD. Myelin-associated glycoprotein demonstrated immunocytochemically in myelin and myelin-forming cells of developing rat. *Proc Natl Acad Sci USA* 1979;76:1510–4.
18. Benjamins JA. Protein metabolism of oligodendroglial cells *in vivo.* In: Norton WT, ed. *Oligodendroglia.* New York: Plenum Press, 1984:87–124.
19. Hartman BK, Agrawal HC, Agrawal D, Kalmbach S. Development and maturation of central nervous myelin: comparison of immunohistochemical localization of proteolipid protein and basic protein in myelin and oligodendrocytes. *Proc Natl Acad Sci USA* 1982;79.4217–20.
20. Yu Y-T, Campagnoni AT. *In vitro* synthesis of the four mouse myelin basic proteins: evidence for the lack of a metabolic relationship. *J Neurochem* 1982;39:1559–68.
21. Zeller NK, Hunkeler MJ, Campagnoni AT, Sprague J, Lazzarini RA. The characterization of mouse myelin basic protein specific messenger RNAs using a myelin basic protein cDNA clone. *Proc Natl Acad Sci USA* 1984;81:18–22.
22. Roth HJ, Hunkeler MJ, Campagnoni AT. Expression of myelin basic protein genes in several dysmyelinating mouse mutants during early postnatal brain development. *J Neurochem* 1985;45:572–80.
23. Roach A, Boylan K, Horvath S, Pruiner SB, Hood LE. Characterization of cloned cDNA representing myelin basic protein: absence of expression in brain of shiverer mutant mouse. *Cell* 1983;34:799–806.
24. Campagnoni CW, Carey GD, Campagnoni AT. Synthesis of myelin basic proteins in the developing mouse brain. *Arch Biochem Biophys* 1978;190:118–25.
25. Greenfield S, Brostoff S, Hogan E. Evidence for defective incorporation of proteins into myelin of the quaking mutant mouse. *Brain Res* 1977;120:507–15.
26. Brostoff SW, Greenfield S, Hogan EL. The differentiation of synthesis from incorporation of basic protein in quaking mutant mice myelin. *Brain Res* 1977;120:517–20.
27. Campagnoni AT, Campagnoni CW, Bourre JM, Jacque C, Baumann N. Cell-free synthesis of myelin basic proteins in normal and dysmyelinating mutant mice. *J Neurochem* 1984;42:733–9.
28. Young RA, Davis RW. Yeast RNA Polymerase II genes: isolation with antibody probes. *Science* 1983;222:778–82.
29. Eylar EH, Brostoff S, Hashim G, Caccam J, Burnett P. Basic A1 protein of the myelin membrane. The complete amino acid sequence. *J Biol Chem* 1971;246:5770–84.
30. Carnegie PR. Amino acid sequence of the encephalitogenic basic protein of human myelin. *Biochem J* 1971;123:57–67.
31. Campagnoni AT, Campagnoni CW. Synthesis and assembly of proteins into myelin. *Trans Am Soc Neurochem* 1984;15:83.

32. Prusiner SB, Roach AH, Takahashi N, Hood LE. Studies with cloned cDNAs encoding myelin basic protein. *Trans Am Soc Neurochem* 1984;15:252.
33. de Ferra F, Lazzarini RL. Structure and expression of the mouse myelin basic protein gene. *Trans Am Soc Neurochem* 1985;16:110.
34. Vaccarino F, Conti-Tronconi BM, Panula P, Guidotti A, Costa E. GABA-Modulin: a synaptosomal basic protein that differs from small myelin basic protein of rat brain. *J Neurochem* 1985;44:278–90.

DISCUSSION

Dr. Mariani: Are there genetic defects in the human that lead to abnormality in MBP? And is it possible to study such defects using molecular genetics, taking advantage of the homologous nature of the gene?

Dr. Campagnoni: To my knowledge there are no human diseases which involve the basic protein gene, but that does not mean we will not continue to look.

Dr. Caviness: Do you have any thoughts about why the MBP is not inserted in the myelin structure? Could this have to do with the posttranslational history of the MBP itself in relation to the mutation?

Dr. Campagnoni: That is one possibility. To start with, the mechanism by which the basic protein (which is synthesized on free ribosomes in the cytosol) is transported to the site of myelin assembly is simply unknown. It could possibly be related to posttranslational modifications such as methylation or phosphorylation. However, we have measured the activity of MBP-specific methylase in the brain and this appears perfectly normal in the quaking mutant where assembly is affected, though it is abnormal in the jimpy mouse. A more fundamental question is how the molecule is transported. Is the MBP inserted into small vesicles, or do the ribosomes move? There are two main theories so far. One is from Colman in Sabatini's laboratory who believes that the ribosomes actually move down the process and deposit the MBP in the region where myelin is assembled, after which it simply diffuses to the cytoplasmic surface of the plasma membrane which eventually becomes myelin. This is a testable hypothesis using *in situ* hybridization coupled with immunohistochemistry, and we are doing these experiments now. What you might expect if the ribosomes are moving is to see both the protein and the message moving together down the process. If the ribosomes do not move you would expect to see the protein move but the message stay behind in the cytosol of the oligodendrocyte. The second possibility that has been suggested is that there are vesicles which shuttle the protein back and forth, though I do not know of any other example where cytoplasmic protein is transported by a vesicular mechanism. One other possibility is that there is a specific transport molecule.

Dr. Guénet: Many countries continue to prepare rabies vaccine on baby mouse brain, though the basic protein may produce an immune encephalopathy. Do you think it would be a good idea to use a brain source such as shiverer or jimpy mutants?

Dr. Campagnoni: You do not really begin to see an accumulation of much MBP until about 8 to 10 days in the normal baby mouse. You can detect it immunocytochemically just after birth, but quantitatively it does not amount to very much; furthermore, mouse protein is not as encephalopathogenic as some other proteins, so on the whole I do not think it would be worthwhile to do as you suggest.

Dr. Sotelo: I should like to know whether the gene for MBP is the same in oligodendrocytes as it is in Schwann cells, since in many of these dysmyelinated mutant mice the peripheral nervous system seems to be totally normal.

Dr. Campagnoni: The same gene should be present in all cells and presumably there is a small amount of the basic protein made in peripheral nerve myelin. Whether the mechanisms which govern it and its expression in the Schwann cell and the oligodendrocyte are exactly the same I am not sure.

Dr. Caviness: Dr Sotelo's question is very interesting because is it not true that the shiverer mutant has normal myelination with MBP in the peripheral nervous system?

Dr. Campagnoni: It has a normal myelin-like structure but it has no MBP. The potential difference across the unit membrane is little different from normal, but there is no basic protein there.

Developmental Neurobiology, edited by
Philippe Evrard and Alexandre Minkowski.
Nestlé Nutrition Workshop Series, Vol. 12.
Nestec Ltd., Vevey/Raven Press, Ltd.,
New York © 1989.

Developmental Synthesis of Myelin Lipids: Origin of Fatty Acids—Specific Role of Nutrition

Jean-Marie Bourre

INSERM Unité 26, Hôpital Fernand Widal, 75475 Paris Cédex 10, France

Nerve cells and myelin require an adequate supply of nutrients, particularly lipids, for their formation and development. This chapter examines the role of nutrition in the synthesis of myelin lipids.

THE CELLS IN NEURAL TISSUE

The neural tissue in the brain is made up of three types of cells: neurons, astrocytes, and oligodendrocytes. Other cells such as the endothelial cells in the cerebral capillaries also play an important role. Each neuron communicates with other neurons by means of hundreds of thousands of synapses in order to transmit information. Oligodendrocytes ensure, among other things, the elaboration and the upkeep of the myelin sheath, a lipid-rich mantle which makes the high speed of nervous conduction possible. Astrocytes have an ill-defined role: among other things they multiply and produce a cicatricial tissue to fill spaces left vacant by dead neurons or oligodendrocytes since these two latter neural cell types do not further multiply after their histogenesis is finished, nor are they replaced if they die. Cerebral development is genetically programmed; if a stage is missing or upset, the possibilities of recovery are very small.

It is thus most important to ensure that in the course of their multiplication and differentiation the cells are adequately supplied with nutrients, particulary lipids. An anomaly in the lipid composition of the cell membranes can result in functional alterations. Cellular membranes ensure the individuality of the cells and serve as a support for a large number of specific physiological activities such as nerve transmission and interactions with other cells. The membrane can be schematized as a lipid double-layer, on and in which proteins are found. Each membrane in each organelle has an individual lipidic composition. Complex lipids are generally formed of fatty acids; these acids constitute the hydrophobic pole of the lipids and form the skeleton of the lipidic double-layer in biological membranes. The metabolism and

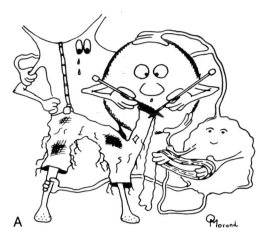

FIG. 1. A: Oligodendrocyte as a myelinating cell. **B:** The oligodendrocyte is extending long processes which are attached to and surround the axons. (Electron micrograph; rat spinal cord.) (Courtesy of Dr. Olivier Morand, INSERM U-154.)

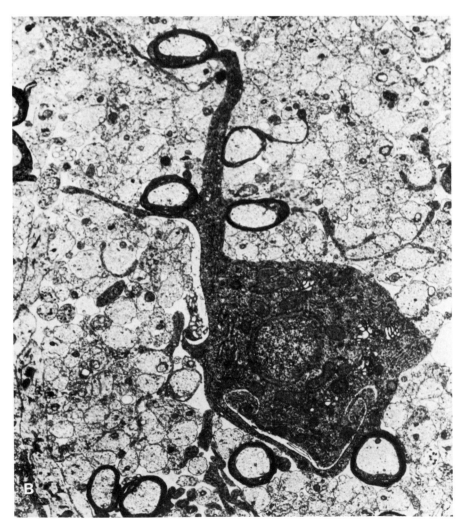

function of fatty acids in the brain have recently been reviewed (1). The fatty acid composition of phospholipids is specific to the membrane into which it is incorporated. This is particulary true for myelin.

MYELIN

Myelin, a multilamellar membrane surrounding nerve fibers of both the central and peripheral nervous systems, is derived from the plasma membrane of the oligodendrocyte (central nervous system) (Fig. 1) and Schwann cell (peripheral nervous system) (2). The metabolism of oligodendrocytes has now been largely unraveled (3). Dysmyelinating mutants have been used to study the myelination process (4,5) (Fig. 2). In the jimpy mutant, there is almost no myelination in the central nervous system, but the peripheral nervous system is normal. In the quaking mutant, myelination stops in a very early stage in the central nervous system and is quantitatively reduced in the peripheral nervous system (by 50%), but the composition of myelin is normal. The shiverer mutant and its allele mld present with a dramatic reduction of myelin with absence of the major dense line, as well as of basic protein; the peripheral nervous system is normal in these mutants, although devoid of basic protein. In the trembler mutant, dysmyelination affects the peripheral nervous system, the central nervous system being slightly hypermyelinated. Neurotoxicology provides a promising approach for the study of myelination processes.

The chemical composition of myelin differs markedly from that of its progenitor membrane. In addition, the chemical composition of myelin in the central nervous system differs from that in the peripheral nervous system. Myelin is relatively abundant in all parts of the nervous system. The appearance of the white matter is due to the high concentration of myelin in fiber tracts in the brain and spinal cord and in nerves. Myelin is biochemically unique and comprises 70% to 75% (dry weight) lipid and 25% to 30% protein (6). The high proportion of lipids gives the membrane a specific density. It can thus be isolated quite easily compared with other subcellular membranes.

The organization of myelin along axons permits the propagation of action potentials in a highly characteristic manner (saltatory conduction). The advantages of saltatory conduction over propagation in nonmyelinated fibers include a high velocity with increased economy in nerve size and energy consumption (1). The correspondence between myelin ultrastructure and its diffraction characteristics results from the precise ordering and regularity of the laminar structure.

Myelination is a major characteristic of late development in the nervous system. In the rat sciatic nerve, compaction of myelin lamellae begins at about 3 days of age (7), and the nerve is quite fully myelinated by 10 to 12 days of age. Lamellar compaction begins at about 10 days in the rat brain, and the rate of synthesis reaches a maximum at about 18 days. Between 15 and 30 days, there is a sixfold increase in myelin content (6), while brain weight increases by only 30% to 40%. At 20 days of age (6), each oligodendroglial cell produces daily more than three times its own

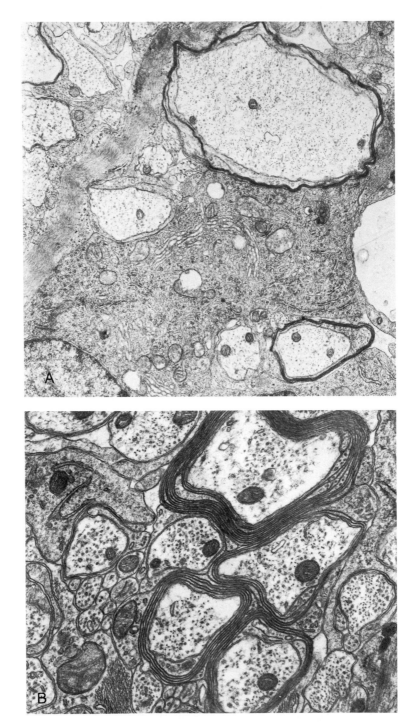

FIG. 2. Morphological aspects of myelin in neurological mutants. **A:** quaking (from Berger, ref. 188); **B:** shiverer (from Privat, ref. 189); **C:** trembler (courtesy of Dr. Herbert Koenig, from ref. 190). As shi and mld are alleles, mld would provide an aspect very similar to shiverer.

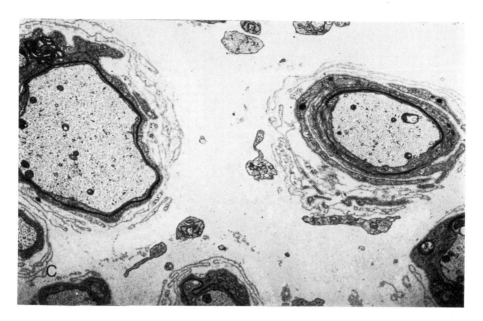

FIG. 2 (continued).

weight of myelin membrane. The final ratio of the myelin membrane surface area to the cell soma membrane surface is about 620:1 (8) (Figs. 3 and 4).

The development of myelin in the brain is subject to many nutritional and environmental influences, of which the most thoroughly analyzed are those associated with postnatal malnutrition, since myelination is largely a postnatal process for many species.

Because of the high metabolic activity associated with myelination, it is not surprising that nutritional disorders have various primary and secondary effects on myelin development (9). Furthermore, abnormalities of myelin development may occur in the absence of visible abnormalities affecting other organ systems. In contrast, teratogens acting early in fetal development typically cause gross abnormalities. The most vulnerable period of the myelination process is the one during which proliferation and development of the myelin-forming cells occur and the cellular mechanisms underlying myelin synthesis are initiated. As a result, nutritional deprivation during this period probably causes long-lasting reduction of myelin synthesis by oligodendroglia (10,11).

MYELIN LIPIDS

Structural Lipids

Only adipose tissue contains lipids in more abundance than the nervous system. These lipids are all structural; they are not oxidized for energy production.

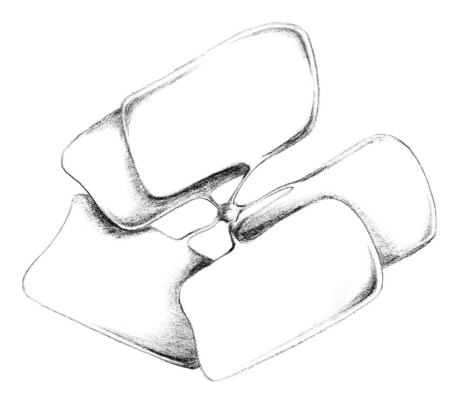

FIG. 3. Oligodendrocyte and unfolded myelin sheath. The oligodendrocyte perikaryon is in the center, and its attached myelin sheaths have been unfolded to demonstrate their extensive surface. In the optic nerve, for example, one oligodendrocyte synthesizes only a few sheaths, as shown here. In some parts of the central nervous system, one oligodendrocyte can synthesize many times more sheaths. Axons are not shown; the mechanism of formation of the myelin sheath is shown in Fig. 4.

They are essential for the functioning of cerebral cell membranes (Fig. 5), and their renewal rate is very slow.

All lipids which are found in other organs and even in plants, are present in the brain. Some are very abundant in the brain (e.g., sphingolipids) yet are minor components of other organs. Lipids from all organs are classified according to their complexity (Table 1).

The Elementary Lipids

Only minute quantities of free fatty acids and alcohols are found in nerve tissue, but they are structural components of simple and complex lipids. Alkanes are found in relatively important quantities in myelin, but free fatty acid formation occurs only under pathological conditions (12). Cholesterol is quantitatively a very important component of nerve membranes.

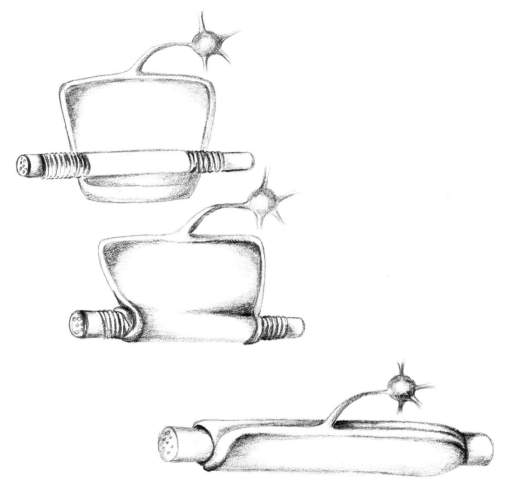

FIG. 4. Myelination of an axon by an oligodendroglial cell.

Single Lipids

The nervous system contains practically no glycerides; traces of cholesterol esters are transiently present in the course of normal brain development, but otherwise they are practically absent. However, they are found in large quantities during degenerative phenomena.

Complex Lipids

Myelin, like all membranes, is rich in phospholipids. Plasmalogens are found which have an alkenyl chain instead of an acyl chain at the 1 position. Mechanisms

TABLE 1. *Classification of lipids*

Elementary lipids
  Fatty acids
  Alcohols
    fatty alcohol
    sphingosine
    glycerol
    cholesterol
  Alkanes
Single lipids
  Glycerides
  Cholesterol esterol
Complex lipids
  Glycerophosphatides
    diacylphosphatides
      phosphatidylethanolamine
      phosphatidylserine
      phosphatidylcholine
      phosphatidylinositol
      phosphatidylinositol monophosphate
      phosphatidylinositol diphosphate
      phosphatidylglycerol
    cardiolipids
    plasmalogens
  Galactosyldiglycerides
  Sphingolipids
    ceramides
    cerebrosides
    sulfatides
    sphingomyelin
    gangliosides
    ceramides polyhexosides

---

of synthesis and degradation of phospholipids in the nervous tissue are similar to those found in other organs.

The galactosylglycerides, principally monogalactosyldiglycerides, are found in small quantities in myelin, ultimately as sulfate esters at the 6 positions of galactose.

Sphingolipids represent about 30% of the myelin lipids. Moreover, they are implicated in various hereditary neurological diseases in man (13) (Fig. 6). The two basic structural components of sphingolipids are fatty acids and sphingosine, which is an amino alcohol with a double bond. This diol is usually composed of 18 carbon atoms; the saturated molecule, dihydrosphingosine, is also present in small quantities.

Psychosine is a sphingosine with a galactose molecule bound to the primary alcohol at the 1 position (galactosylsphingosine). Although it is probably an important intermediary metabolite, only traces are detected in the nervous tissue and its presence in myelin is uncertain. In the ceramides the amino fraction of sphingosine is

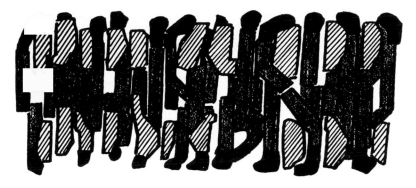

MYELIN

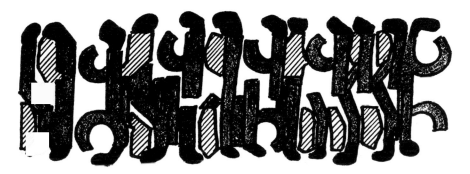

MITOCHONDRIA

FIG. 5. Molecular structure of the membrane lipid bilayer of myelin *(upper)* and mitochondria *(lower)*. The myelin membrane is a very compact structure. Polar groups in black, acyl groups gray, cholesterol dashed. From data of X. O'Brien.

acylated with a fatty acid whose chain length varies between 18 and 20 carbon atoms (*N*-acyl sphingosine). Sphingolipids are synthesized from ceramides.

The cerebrosides are synthesized from ceramides in the presence of UDP-galactose; the sulfatation of the cerebrosides by the 3'-phosphoadenosine 5'-phosphosulfate (PAPS) yields sulfatides. Conversely, the degradation of the sulfatides by a lysosomal enzyme (a sulfatase) produces cerebrosides; the activity of this enzyme is assayed *in vitro* as arylsulfatase. It is deficient in metachromatic leukodystrophy, thus provoking an accumulation of sulfatides. The galactocerebrosides are degraded by another lysosomal enzyme, galactosylcerebroside-β-galactosidase, which is deficient in Krabbe's disease (leukodystrophy with globoid cells). Finally, another lysosomal enzyme, ceramidase, degrades the ceramides; its activity is greatly reduced in Farber's disease.

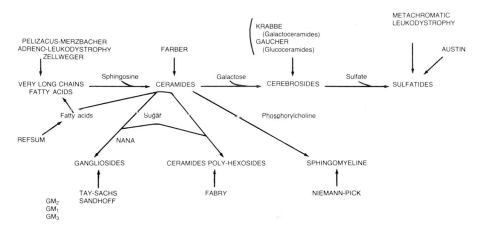

FIG. 6. Metabolic pathways of sphingolipids found in nervous tissues and related inborn errors.

Sphingomyelins are synthesized mainly from ceramides in the presence of cytidine diphosphate choline; their degradation takes place in the lysosome by means of a sphingomyelinase. The genetic deficiency of this enzyme causes an accumulation of sphingomyelin in Niemann-Pick disease.

The gangliosides are synthesized by the sequential addition of monosaccharides or of *N*-acetylneuraminic acid, catalyzed by specific, usually microsomal, glycosyl-transferases. The degradations are brought about in the lysosomes by glycosidases and neuraminidases; if one of these is deficient a lipidosis appears. The enzymatic activity can be measured in cultured amniotic fluid cells. Gangliosides are associated with myelin but account for less than 1% of the total lipid; GM_1 and GM_4 gangliosides represent 75% of the total ganglioside content. The fatty acid residues of myelin lipids vary considerably. The metabolism of myelin lipid has recently been reviewed (3).

Pure isolated myelin is not homogeneous. It is made up of a continuum of membranes having different densities. The differences in densities are due to variations in the proportion of lipids and proteins (Fig. 7).

Effects of Postnatal Undernutrition on Myelin Lipids

Brain Galactolipids: Sulfatides and Cerebrosides

Sulfatides are specifically associated with myelin, and the rate of sulfatide synthesis and its accretion in the brain closely reflect the metabolism of myelin (14); however, sulfatides are also constituents of other subcellular membranes such as mitochondria and microsomes (14,15). Consequently, large changes in sulfatide predominantly reflect changes in myelin; the rate of sulfatide synthesis in the brain

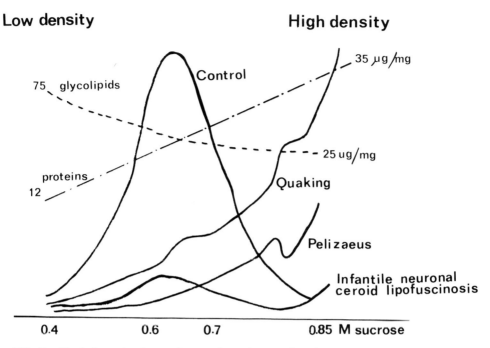

FIG. 7. Myelin is made of a continuum of membranes. Pure isolated myelin is not homogeneous; it is made of a continuum of membranes having different densities, owing to changes in the balance between lipids and proteins. The lightest fractions contain less protein and more sphingolipids (191,192). Different density profiles are obtained in various pathological conditions, such as dysmyelinating mutants in mice (193) and human neurological diseases. In Pelizaeus-Mersbacher disease myelin is primarily affected; in infantile neuronal ceroid lipofuscinosis hypomyelination is secondary to wallerian degeneration of the central nervous system (194). Intrauterine growth retardation also affects the myelin density profile (42).

of undernourished weanling rats of half normal body weight is depressed by 50% (15), comparable to the depression of myelin synthesis (11,16,17). Upon nutritional rehabilitation after weaning, there is no marked stimulation of either sulfatide or myelin synthesis (11). Nutritional deprivation at any time following birth produces a subsequent reduction in the rate of sulfatide synthesis between 15 and 30 days of age. The longer the deprivation, the more severe is the effect on sulfatide synthesis, at least during the first 14 days; no further effect is observed when starvation lasts for more than 20 days.

Cerebrosides are probably a more specific marker of myelin metabolism than sulfatides; however, their metabolism in undernourished rats is less well characterized than that of sulfatides. The specific depression of cerebroside concentration in the rat brain due to postnatal undernourishment is more marked than for cholesterol (18) and reflects more closely the severe depression characteristic in purified myelin membranes. Brain lipid deposition has been studied using different models of nutritional insufficiency. These data indicate that among the various classes of lipids, galactolipids are the most affected (19).

Cholesterol

The effect of undernutrition on overall brain cholesterol concentration differs from the effects on the cholesterol concentration in purified myelin membranes. Cholesterol is an important constituent of all cell membranes. Consequently, it lacks the myelin specificity of the galactolipids, and so the brain concentration of cholesterol is less depressed than sulfatide concentration (18,19). The cholesterol concentration in the brain of postnatally undernourished rats is slightly lower than in normal controls (20). Because of the close association between cholesterol and myelin metabolism (21), it has been suggested that postnatal undernourishment retards myelin formation. The effect of undernutrition on brain cholesterol has been found by many laboratories (22–25) and appears to have weighed heavily in the formulation of the hypothesis that myelination is a vulnerable period in brain development.

Other Brain Lipids

Proportions of other lipids such as the various phospholipids are also altered in case of postnatal nourishment. Additionally, the fatty acid composition of whole brain cerebrosides and phospholipids (26) is different in undernourished and normal rats. Various effects on whole brain gangliosides have been reported (12,14,27). Interpretation is equivocal; however, these data are probably more pertinent to neuronal maturation than to myelination (28).

Essential Fatty Acid Deficiency

Fatty acids of exogenous origin are essential for the synthesis of brain myelin and subcellular membranes. Essential fatty acid (EFA) deficiency during development results in numerous alterations in animals (29,30). For instance, myelin formation in developing rats deprived of essential fatty acids is severely disturbed. Histological analysis reveals a delay in the onset of myelination and a reduction in the level of myelin staining (31). There is qualitative evidence of recovery by 50 days of age. Similarly, the relatively specific myelin marker cerebroside is greatly reduced both in total amount and concentration (30), but this effect persists through adulthood. The lipoprotein of myelin is also severely reduced during the first 42 days in developing EFA-deficient rats (32). The cerebral concentrations of phospholipid and cholesterol, which are not particularly indicative of myelin metabolism, are nearly unaffected by EFA deprivation (30). Concentrations of DNA and total protein in brain are also only slightly affected, although brain weight as well as total amounts of these substances are reduced (30,33).

The activity of $2',3'$-cyclic nucleotide $3'$-phosphodiesterase (CNP), which is a marker of myelin synthesis, is affected by EFA deficiency. In mice, its activity is reduced from day 5 until day 11 after birth, whereas it is normal at later ages (32).

These results could indicate a delay in the early maturation of oligodendroglia, which precedes the formation of myelin in the third and fourth postnatal weeks.

EFA deficiency also produces various alterations in the acyl groups of different myelin lipids (34–38). Metabolic studies in deprived rats indicate that either the rate of turnover of myelin acyl groups is accelerated or the efficiency of acyl group reutilization is decreased (39).

In EFA deficiency, n-3 and n-6 polyunsaturated fatty acids in phospholipids are replaced by 20:3 n-9 (synthesized from oleic acid).

Effect of Prenatal Undernutrition (Intrauterine Growth Retardation) on Myelination

Prenatal undernutrition (40) is obtained by clamping a uterine artery; this operation is carried out in rats on the 17th day of gestation (E17). As a consequence, blood flow to the fetus is reduced, and the rat is born "small-for-date". The fetal blood supply per unit of body weight is also reduced; however, blood flow is preferentially directed towards the fetal brain rather than to the liver. The brain would therefore seem to be more particularly protected against dietary deficiency, though behavioral tests can be abnormal (41).

This type of prenatal malnutrition concerns a particular period in the development of the brain: The neurons are already formed from precursor neuroblasts; the glial cells are not yet in their definitive position and there is no myelin. Between the E17 and birth, brain weight doubles while considerable amounts of substances accumulate, corresponding to the growth of axons and dendrites, and to the organization of synaptic connections. Because the chronology of brain development is very closely programmed, a delay in maturation causing a deficit in the number of cells could prove irreversible.

In fact, the brain is also affected by hypotrophia; the weight of the brain in young adult hypotrophic rats is subnormal. This is not related to a noticeable variation in cell size but is the consequence of a decrease in the number of nerve cells, which could probably be attributed to slowing down of cell multiplication.

Although the brain is less affected than other organs in intrauterine growth retardation, forebrain weight and total lipids are reduced. The quantity of myelin is reduced by 27%, 17% and 9% at 15, 18, and 60 days after birth, respectively (42). Thus, even when postnatal nutritional intakes are adequate, intrauterine malnutrition affects myelination, a postnatal event. Prenatal growth retardation impairs brain maturation moderately but irreversibly, whereas the composition of myelin (density profile, amount of lipid and fatty acid pattern) during maturation is close to normal. Pre- and postnatal undernutrition affects myelination in different ways. In prenatal undernutrition, myelination is reduced, recovery is incomplete, and density profile and biochemical composition of myelin correspond to the age of the animal. In contrast, postnatal undernutrition delays myelination; myelin maturation seems to be delayed compared to the actual age of the animal, and a certain degree of recovery is possible.

Altered Myelination Due to Undernutrition in Humans

The development and biochemical composition of human myelin is similar to that of laboratory animals (6); however, very little is actually known about the neurochemical pathology of starved human infants. Lipoprotein concentration in white matter as well as cerebroside and plasmalogen concentrations were found to be reduced in brains of malnourished Puerto Rican infants compared with normal infants (43). Similarly, concentrations of cerebroside and sulfatide in the brain were below normal in Guatemalan infants who had died of malnutrition (44) and the cerebrum of undernourished children in Spain had a galactolipid concentration significantly below normal values (45). The lipid composition of isolated myelin was relatively normal (46) as in animal studies. DNA and total protein concentrations were normal. These data indicate that infant starvation specifically causes a relative reduction in the synthesis and accumulation of myelin membrane. Furthermore, brain cells are altered both in marasmus and kwashiorkor (47). Decreased nerve conduction velocity is observed in both conditions in children (48). Abnormal myelination would produce such neurophysiological effects (49).

IN SITU BIOSYNTHESIS OF FATTY ACIDS

Biosynthesis of Saturated and Monounsaturated Fatty Acids

These molecules (Fig. 8) are synthesized from acetyl-CoA and malonyl-CoA (50). The latter is obtained by carboxylation of acetyl-CoA. The regulation of the synthesis is different in brain and liver (51). Acetyl-CoA carboxylase in brain as well as in liver, adipose tissue, and mammary gland, is inhibited by excess malonyl-CoA and is strongly activated by citrate. Its activity is also lowered when ATP concentration is increased or decreased. But unlike the liver enzyme, the brain enzyme is not responsive to dietary changes and its K_m for acetyl-CoA is lower than that of the liver enzyme.

Besides acetate, ketone bodies are important precursors of fatty acids and lipids in the developing brain during the period of myelination (52,53).

De Novo Synthesis

In addition to obtaining fatty acids from the blood, the brain can synthesize fatty acids *de novo* (54) as efficiently as other organs such as the liver (55). The fatty acid synthetase of the soluble fraction obtained from cerebral tissue does not differ significantly from that of other tissues except in its regulation (56) and produces predominantly palmitic acid, which can be modified in microsomes or mitochondria. This fatty acid synthetase catalyzes the synthesis of medium chain fatty acids; acetyl-CoA and NADPH are required in the presence of malonyl-CoA. In the brain, this *de novo* synthesis occurs in three subcellular compartments: cytosol (57), mitochon-

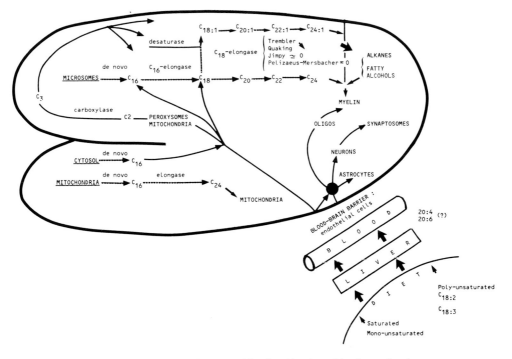

FIG. 8. Origin of brain fatty acids: diet, blood, and *in situ* synthesis.

dria (58), and microsomes (59,60). Palmitic acid (C16) is the main product, although small amounts of stearic acid (C18) and myristic acid (C14) are also produced. Synthesis in the three organelles is inhibited by long and very long chain acyl-CoA.

The microsomal system is different from the cytosolic(59) as it does not precipitate in the same way in the presence of ammonium sulfate. The optimum pH as well as the optimum concentrations for substrates are not identical.

The activity of the mitochondrial enzyme can be measured only after rupture of mitochondria (58); thus this system is fixed either on the inside of the external membrane of the organelle or on the inner membrane, or it is present in the matrix.

Activation of Fatty Acids (Fatty acyl-CoA Synthetase).

As *de novo* synthesis produces mainly fatty acids, these compounds have to be activated before elongation. The activated form is acyl-CoA.

Two enzymes are responsible for the synthesis and hydrolysis of acyl-CoA in microsomes: long chain fatty acyl-CoA ligase (61) and long chain fatty acyl-CoA hydrolase (62).

The specific activity of the ligase in the presence of either palmitic acid or stearic acid increases during development; the specific activity in the presence of arachidonic acid (C20:0) or behenic acid (C22:0) is considerably lower. The specific activities of palmitoyl-CoA hydrolase and of stearoyl-CoA hydrolase in the microsomal fraction decrease markedly (75%) between 6 and 20 days after birth; the corresponding specific activities in the soluble fraction show no decline. The specific activity of microsomal palmitoyl-CoA hydrolase and stearoyl-CoA hydrolase during the most active phase of myelogenesis declines sharply. This change in specific activity, together with the increase in the rate of fatty acid activation during development, will result in an increased availability of fatty acyl-CoA esters for phospholipid and sphingolipid biosynthesis. While stearoyl-CoA hydrolase is inhibited by bovine serum albumin the microsomal fatty acid chain elongation system is stimulated fourfold by albumin. Thus it is suggested that the decline in specific activity of the microsomal hydrolase and, to a lesser extent, the increase in the specific activity of the ligase is directly related to the increased demand for long chain acyl-CoA esters during myelogenesis as substrates in the biosynthesis of myelin lipids (61).

In the trembler dysmyelinating mutant, stearyl-CoA hydrolysis is increased in the peripheral nervous tissue (63) as well as the synthesis of acyl-CoA (64) when an ATP generating system is present. If not, acyl-CoA synthesis is reduced in total tissue as well as in Schwann cell cultures (65).

Microsomal Elongating Complex

Saturated fatty acids

Cytosolic and microsomal *de novo* synthesis produces mainly palmitic acid and little stearic acid. These two acids have approximately the same turnover in the brain. Stearic acid metabolism is normal in the quaking mutant (a mutant which has dramatically reduced amounts of myelin). Thus very long chain fatty acids (above C18) and stearic acid are not synthesized by the same enzyme complex.

Two elongating complexes are present in brain microsomes: a C16-elongase which uses palmityl-CoA as primer and produces stearic acid; and a C18-elongase which uses stearyl-CoA and produces very long chain fatty acids (up to C24 and C26) (65,66). These two systems have been partially purified by ammonium sulfate precipitation (11,12) and their specificity has been demonstrated with regard to cofactors, cosubstrates, ionic strength, optimal pH, and temperature. The elongating factor is malonyl-CoA (65,67).

The first elongating complex produces mainly stearic acid in both normal and quaking animals. However, the activity of the second elongating system is disturbed in mutants. It is nearly absent in the jimpy and largely decreased in the quaking mutant (60,68); it is probably altered in Pelizaeus-Merzbacker disease (69,70), a human leukodystrophy. This is a genetic disease in which the enzyme deficit concerns an anabolic process, but it is not equivalent to quaking or jimpy mutants.

The second elongating complex normally produces C20-C26 fatty acids and works with either stearyl-CoA, arachidyl-CoA (C20) or behenyl-CoA (C22) (71).

The existence of a third elongating system has previously been postulated (72) but could not be demonstrated.

The elongation of behenyl-CoA (the direct precursor of lignoceric acid) has been extensively studied. This acyl-CoA is elongated by malonyl-CoA in the presence of NADPH into lignoceric acid (24:0); small quantities of cerotic acid (C26) are also detected. The ratio of total radioactivity to radioactivity in the carboxyl carbon of the fatty acid synthesized is 1.05:1. Adding increasing amounts of behenyl-CoA inhibits the elongation of endogenous fatty acids and, at 17 μM (optimum yield), 90% of the radioactive malonyl-CoA used in fatty acid biosynthesis has elongated behenyl-CoA into longer chains. Free acid is not elongated (except in the presence of CoA, ATP, and Mg^{2+}, where the yield is much lower) and acetyl-CoA does not work at all. NADPH is the only effective nucleotide; adding NADH does not increase the synthesis (71).

Four percent of the added malonyl-CoA is found in lignoceric acid; 13% of the behenyl-CoA is elongated. This yield does not increase after addition of acceptors for the newly synthesized acids: increasing concentrations of α-glycerophospate, sphingosine, or psychosine have no effect. Adding diisopropylfluorophosphate, a thioesterase inhibitor (this enzyme is present in microsomes and rapidly splits acyl-CoA into nonreactive free fatty acids and CoA) has no effect; among various ions, Hg^{2+} and Cu^{2+} strongly inhibit the elongation, an effect which is possibly owing to alterations of the SH group in the enzyme complex (73).

Chain lengthening does occur in the peripheral nervous system. It is decreased in the trembler mutant (74).

Monounsaturated fatty acids

Three pathways have been proposed for the synthesis of monounsaturated fatty acids: (a) desaturation of the homologous saturated molecule; (b) elongation of dodecenoic acid (a pathway similar to the bacterial synthesis of palmitoleic acid from decenoic acid); and (c) elongation of oleyl-CoA.

The first hypothesis has been refuted; after direct injection of radioactive lignoceric acid into rat brain, no nervonic (24:1n-9) acid is detected (75). Moreover, very long chain acyl-CoA is not desaturated *in vitro* except for stearyl-CoA which is converted into oleyl-CoA in microsomes (76,77). The second proposed mechanism has been detected neither in microsomes nor in homogenate.

In homogenates of 10 day old rat brain, desaturation of stearyl-CoA requires O_2 and NADH or NAD, which is most likely first reduced to NADH. The monoene fraction produced by the desaturation of stearic acid contains mainly oleic acid (18:1n-9) (78,79) whereas palmitic acid yields some palmitoleic acid (16:1n-7) and *cis*-vaccenic acid (18:1n-7) in the monoene fraction. The desaturase activity of brain decreases with age to 10% of fetal values in the adult brain, whereas in liver the adult activity is 50-fold higher than the fetal activity (78,80). Fasting decreases desaturation only slightly in 10 day old and adult brains but markedly depresses desaturation in liver, especially in adults. Refeeding stimulates activity in adult livers but gives variable results with adult brains and 10 day old brains and livers.

Even though the specific activity of palmitoyl-CoA and stearoyl-CoA desaturases significantly decrease with development, the total activity for the whole brain remains nearly constant (76). Activity does not peak at the myelination period, in contrast with the activity of microsomal fatty acid synthesizing systems.

In mutants, the desaturase activity is not linked to myelination. This absence of correlation between the two processes is illustrated by the fact that in jimpy and quaking mice the decrease in desaturase activity is only 10%, whereas the activity of the myelin synthesizing enzymes decreases by about 60% (76).

Monounsaturated fatty acids are synthesized in brain microsomes by elongation of oleyl-CoA. Stearyl-CoA, behenyl-CoA, and erucyl-CoA are elongated in the same way (81). The chain length of the synthesized acids is the same for both saturated and monounsaturated acids; behenyl-CoA and erucyl-CoA are interchangeable. Adding increasing concentrations of one of these acyl-CoA derivatives in the presence of constant amounts of the others gives rise to identical curves. Results and kinetics are those obtained in the presence of only one acyl-CoA (81). This suggests that one enzyme complex elongates both saturated and monounsaturated fatty acids.

These results explain why the synthesis of both saturated and monounsaturated very long chain fatty acids is affected in the quaking mutant and corresponds to the n-9 structure of the very long monounsaturated myelin chains (since n-9 oleyl-CoA is the primer).

Activity of partial reactions

Partial reactions in the overall chain elongation of palmitoyl-CoA and stearoyl-CoA by mouse brain microsomes have been studied. The rate of the initial condensation reaction between palmitoyl-CoA and malonyl-CoA is more than five times faster than with stearoyl-CoA. Good agreement between condensation and overall chain elongation rates is observed (82).

By contrast, both β-hydroxyoctadecanoyl-CoA and β-hydroxyeicosanoyl-CoA are rapidly dehydrated by brain microsomes at comparable rates. Similar results are obtained with 2-*trans*-octadecanoyl-CoA and 2-*trans*-eicosanoyl-CoA; both substrates are rapidly reduced at nearly the same rate in the presence of NADPH. In all cases, intermediate reactions subsequent to condensation are much more rapid than overall chain elongation. These results suggest that the mechanism of malonyl-CoA-dependent fatty acid chain elongation in brain microsomes is similar to that observed in other tissues, and are consistent with an overall regulation of chain elongation mediated primarily by the initial condensation reaction (82).

Mitochondrial Elongating Systems

Contradictory results have been obtained in mitochondria of various organs. In brain, acyl-CoA is elongated by acetyl-CoA in the presence of NADH and NADPH (58,67,83,84). Palmityl-CoA and stearyl-CoA are elongated in the same way (84); in presence of NADH alone, more than 60% of the newly synthesized fatty acids are hydroxylated; NADPH alone does not provoke extensive synthesis. Adding both NADH and NADPH gives rise to saturated fatty acids. The synthesized fatty acids have two carbon atoms more than the primer. Lignoceric acid is synthesized from behenyl-CoA. This synthesis is altered in neither the quaking nor the jimpy mutant. As mitochondria contain small amounts of very long chain fatty acids (85) and *in vitro* synthesis is of the same order of magnitude as *in vivo* turnover, mitochondria seem to synthesize only their own fatty acids (68): only microsomes synthesize myelin fatty acids (86).

The difference between the requirements for acyl-CoA elongation in different organelles is striking (Table 2). In mitochondria, acetyl-CoA is the immediate precursor of the two carbon units; both NADH and NADPH are necessary for synthesis of saturated fatty acids. On the contrary, microsomal enzymes need only NADPH and malonyl-CoA. The physiological and genetic significance of these results is not yet known.

Fatty Acid Synthesis during Development

De novo synthesis

The activity of the cytosolic system is maximal about 6 days after birth (56,87,89); thus it precedes myelination. This however does not preclude a role in the deposition of myelin lipids. Nevertheless, this system seems more related to cell multiplication.

Microsomal and mitochondrial elongating systems

Ontogenic studies (68) confirm the existence of the three microsomal systems; they are directly related to myelination (87). Maximal *de novo* synthesis is at 10 to 12 days, the C16-elongase activity at 15 days, and the C18-elongase at 18 days. The evolution of the three microsomal systems from an ontogenic point of view is coherent; at 18 days, the age of most active myelination in mice, myelin deposition and maturation occur in two phases. Myelin contains sphingolipids first with medium chain fatty acids and later with very long chains (88).

Changes in the specific activity of malonyl-CoA-elongated behenyl-CoA in the

TABLE 2. *Requirements for acyl-CoA elongation in microsomes and mitochondria*

	Elongating complexes	Carbon atom donor	Reducing agent	Role in myelination	Alterations in mutants		Fate
					Quaking	Jimpy	
Microsomes	2	Malonyl-CoA	NADPH	+ + +	− 70%	− 97%	Myelin
Mitochondria	1	Acetyl-CoA	NADH + NADPH	0	− 0%	− 0%	Mitochondria

microsomal fraction of mouse brain from birth to maturity differ from changes in the specific activity of acetyl-CoA-elongated behenyl-CoA in mitochondria (68). The activity of the mitochondrial fatty acid elongating system is similar in normal and mutant animals; radioactive acetyl-CoA incorporation increases slightly but regularly during development. Age-dependent change in the activity of fatty acid biosynthesis in microsomes is quite different; there is a period of maximum activity by 15 to 18 days, when the specific activity is four times higher than in 4 day old or adult animals (though total synthesis of lignoceric acid for the whole brain is increased 11-fold). However, in the quaking mutant this increase is much less prominent, and it is absent in the jimpy. In controls, the specific activity of the microsomal elongating complex is five times (at 4 days) to seven times (at 15 to 20 days of age) higher than the specific activity of the enzyme in the mitochondrial fraction. But at adult age this activity is nearly the same in both organelles.

The specific activity in quaking mutants at 14 to 18 days is 50% of normal, but the mutant brain has only 75% of the normal amount of microsomes (71). Therefore the *in vitro* synthesis of lignoceric acid from behenyl-CoA is 30% of normal in quaking mice. These results agree with the data obtained from analysis of total brain lipids; in normal mice, lignoceric acid represents 1.9% of the total saturated fatty acids, but 0.6% in the quaking mutant. At adult age the synthesis of lignoceric acid is much less affected in the mutant, but myelination cannot occur normally any more at that time. The fate of lignoceric acid synthesized at adult age is unknown; it is probably incorporated in membranes other than myelin or it is involved in myelin turnover.

Changes with time of the elongating complex activity in the microsomal fraction indicate that this enzyme is implicated in myelin lipid formation: the period of maximum activity in the whole brain corresponds to the highest rate of lignoceric acid deposition. The rise of lignoceric acid synthesis, occurring coincidentally with myelination, is not found in the quaking mice brain.

Changes in cytosolic synthetase activity during brain development are related to changes in the enzyme content (84). One may thus speculate that the developmental change in the activity of very long chain synthesizing enzymes is the result of alterations in the rate of synthesis and degradation of enzyme complexes, possibly related to the differentiation of the oligodendrocyte through brain-specific regulatory mechanisms since enzymes in kidney follow different regulatory mechanisms (90).

Fatty Acid, Myelin, and Protein Synthesis and Oligodendrocyte Differentiation

Basic protein levels, level of glycolipids (which are major constituents of myelin), and enzymatic activities involved in their synthesis, including those responsible for the formation of basic components (e.g., ceramide from sphingosine) and those involved in completing complex molecules (e.g., cerebroside sulfotransferase), indicate that myelin is largely synthesized by active oligodendrocytes. All enzyme activities can be detected at about the same time in this cell (91). Correlation of these biochemical data with morphological findings indicates that maximal synthetic activity of all components of myelin occur in active oligodendrocytes (detected between 5 and 15 days after birth), and that these cells appear to be responsible for the initial synthesis of myelin. Both young and mature oligodendrocytes have limited capacity to synthesize these compounds. Furthermore, induction of the enzymes involved in the synthesis of myelin components appears to take place simultaneously, rather than sequentially (91).

Biosynthesis of Hydroxylated Fatty Acids

2-Hydroxy fatty acids are found in amide linkages in cerebrosides and cerebroside sulfates or as acyl moieties in 6'-acylcerebroside. Cerebronic acid (2-hydroxylignoceric acid, h 24:0) is the major hydroxy acid in the brain; h 22:0 and h 24:1 are second, and h 23:0, h 25:1 third highest in concentration. Fatty acids in the brain are dependent on chain elongation and α-oxidation reactions (92): 16:0→h 24:0→ 24:0→23:0→22:0. Cerebronic acid is formed by hydroxylation of lignoceric acid (93). Recent cell-free studies have demonstrated that the hydroxylating enzyme requires Mg^{2+}, molecular oxygen, and a reduced pyridine nucleotide; it is not inhibited by CO, which suggests that the enzyme is closely linked to the electron transfer system containing cytochrome b_5 rather than cytochrome p-450. The hydroxylation reaction in brain is stimulated by a heat-stable factor in the mitochondrial supernatant and by psychosine, which may act by accepting the cerebronic acid, a potent inhibitor of the hydroxylation reaction, to form cerebronyl-psychosine (94,95).

The precursor of sphingosine, L-serine, stimulates α-hydroxylation; α-hydroxylation is thus closely integrated with the synthesis of sphingosine, ceramide, and cerebroside. All hydroxycerebroside is made from hydroxyceramide. This synthesis is affected by nonphysiological compounds (95,96). The complex role of heat-stable and heat-labile factors in 2-hydroxylation and oxidation of lignoceric acid in the brain has recently been analyzed (97).

Comparisons of the conversion of lignoceric acid to cerebronic acid during development of normal mice and in quaking and jimpy mutants suggest that the synthesis of cerebronic acid is closely coupled with the synthesis of cerebrosides, a characteristic lipid class in myelin (94). The rate of hydroxylation peaks in normal mice during the period of maximum myelination, whereas the activity remains very low at all ages in the jimpy mice. In quaking mice, which exhibit less severe myelin deficiency than jimpy, the activity is higher than in the jimpy, although subnormal, and peaks during myelination.

Fate of the Fatty Acids

Mitochondria probably synthesize only their own fatty acids; microsomes synthesize plasma membrane fatty acids, including myelin fatty acids. The systems present in the brain are probably also operative in the peripheral nervous system (98). In microsomes stearyl-CoA enters the second elongating system leading to the synthesis of very long chain fatty acids; these acids are mainly incorporated into myelin sphingolipids, but are also found in nonesterified form (12). Newly synthesized fatty acids can be metabolized into fatty alcohols and alkanes.

Metabolism into Fatty Alcohols

Fatty acids are eventually reduced for the elaboration of alcohols (precursors of alkenyl bonds in plasmalogens) (99,100). Long chain alcohols, mainly hexadecanol, octadecanol, eicosanol, docosanol, and tetracosanol, are detected (101) in the developing rat brain at ages ranging from 5 to 40 days. Highest levels (0.02% of the total lipids) are found at the age of 10 days. The fact that substantial amounts of fatty alcohols having more than 20 carbon atoms are present in myelinating rat brain indicates a chain length specificity in their utilization for O-alkyl and O-ald-1-enyl glycerolipid biosynthesis.

In mouse brain microsomes, stearyl-CoA is reduced into stearyl-alcohol in the presence of NADPH (NADH is quite inactive). The presence of both NADPH and NADH does not increase the synthesis. Synthesis is reduced by 60% in presence of stearic acid + CoA + ATP + Mg^2 instead of stearyl-CoA, thus showing that stearic acid must be activated before reduction, stearyl-CoA being the substrate. Stearyl-alcohol synthesis increases during myelination and parallels plasmalogen deposition; this biosynthesis is reduced dramatically in jimpy and to 51% of normal in the quaking mouse brains (though at least 18% of this synthesis is used for plasmalogens found outside myelin) (99). The brain microsomes show maximal activity with stearic acid, the activities with palmitic or oleic acid being 65% and 38%, respectively, of that with stearic acid.

Metabolism into Alkanes

Fatty acids are eventually transformed into alkanes. This new class of neurolipids is found in normal mouse brains. They are concentrated in myelin. Their levels are reduced in the quaking mutant. The average content is 7.1 µg/mg in normal myelin, 2.2 µg/mg in quaking myelin. The distribution pattern of these alkanes has been determined by gas-liquid chromatography; it is different in normal and quaking myelin; the hydrocarbons consist mainly of *n*-alkanes ranging from C21 to C32 with even and odd aliphatic chains (102).

Only trace amounts of alkanes are found in other subcellular particles: 0.5 µg/mg in microsomes, 0.4 µg/g in mitochondria, and 0.13 µg/g in synaptosomes (102). The alkane content in normal myelin is at least three times higher than in quaking myelin. Since the quaking mouse has a much lower level of very long chain fatty acids, this suggests a close relationship between very long chain fatty acids and alkanes, as these molecular classes are reduced to the same degree in the mutant (102).

Alkanes are also found in the peripheral nervous system and the quantities as well as the chain length are affected in various neurological mutants, including trembler mutants (103).

The very long chain fatty acids synthesized by elongation of stearate by malonyl-CoA are partly transformed into alkanes (mainly odd chains); all molecular lengths, from C19 to C33, are formed. As acids have mainly even chains, it is proposed that alkanes could be synthesized by decarboxylation in microsomes of even very long chain fatty acids (104).

EXOGENOUS ORIGIN OF FATTY ACIDS

Very little information is available regarding the mechanisms of transport of lipids and fatty acids through the blood–brain barrier. The blood–brain barrier is made of endothelial cells which operate in a very specific manner. The presence of tight interendothelial junctions, in contrast with all endothelial cells from other organs, impedes diffusion between cells, and the paucity of pinocytotic vesicles in the endothelium as well as the absence of fenestrations are suggestive of the existence of very specific carrier mechanisms (105–107).

Nonessential Fatty Acids

Injection of Labeled Compounds

Cholesterol and fatty acids are rapidly synthesized from acetate in the adult rat brain, and the fatty acids are incorporated into complex lipids, as can be shown by ^{14}C acetate injection into the carotid artery (108). Carbon-14 palmitate is also incorporated into phospholipids at a rate comparable to ^{14}C acetate (109). The rapid synthesis observed in these experiments was unexpected, since the turnover of cholesterol and other lipids in brain is on the whole very slow. The existence of separate compartments, one with a very rapid turnover, and the other with a very slow turnover, has been proposed to account for these observations (109). These studies demonstrate that the adult brain is capable of very rapid uptake and assimilation of free fatty acids and fatty acid precursors from the blood. Furthermore, weanling rats synthesize lipids much more actively than adults. The blood–brain barrier definitely plays a role in the uptake and transport of fatty acids into the brain and in the myelination process. The uptake and metabolism of linolenic acid by the brain has also been studied (110).

Transport of stearic acid across the blood–brain barrier is studied by subcutaneous injection, since feeding also involves metabolism in the digestive tract, and direct injection into brain bypasses the blood–brain barrier (111).

Blood fatty acids are an important parameter in myelin membrane synthesis, an exogenous stearic acid is needed; labeled stearic acid, after subcutaneous injection into 18 day old mice, is transported into the brain and incorporated into myelin lipids (112). However, the acid is partly metabolized in the brain by elongation (providing very long chain fatty acids, mainly lignoceric acid) or by degradation to acetate units (utilized for synthesis of medium chain fatty acids such as palmitic acid or other lipids such as cholesterol) (113). These metabolites are subsequently incorporated into myelin lipids (112).

Myelin lipid radioactivity increases for up to 3 days; high activity is found in phospholipids, in which saturated as well as polyunsaturated fatty acids are labeled. But sphingolipids, especially cerebrosides, also contain large amounts of radioactivity (mainly found in very long chain fatty acids, principally in lignoceric acid). The presence of unesterified fatty acids needs to be mentioned. These molecules, unlike other lipids, are found only in minute amounts (112).

Subcutaneously injected acids are taken up by the brain and incorporated into synaptosomal lipids as well as into other brain compartments (113). Phospholipids (choline-phosphatides, ethanolamine-phosphatides, serine-phosphatides) are potent acceptors. Moreover, high levels of radioactivity are found in nonesterified fatty acids. It is not known whether these acids are derived from exogenous stearic acid after processing in synaptosomes, or if they are metabolized in another compartment, such as neuronal perikaryon, and thereafter fixed in nerve endings (114). This hypothesis could be correlated with synaptic transmission since these acids have been found in cerebral cortex in association with proteolipids (including cholinergic receptors), and the neurotransmitter-modulated release of unesterified fatty acids may be part of the mechanism for controlling membrane permeability (115).

Exogenous stearic acid is also necessary for the synthesis of the membranes of neurons and astrocytes. Subcutaneously injected 1-^{14}C stearic acid is taken up and incorporated into lipids of both cell types, the specific radioactivity being higher in astrocytes than in neurons. Phospholipids contain high amounts of radioactivity; glycosphingolipids contain low quantities of label in the two cell types. The injected acid is partly metabolized in the cells by elongation and desaturation (thus providing saturated, monounsaturated, and polyunsaturated very long chains); it is also partly degraded into acetate units (utilized for synthesis of palmitic acid) (116).

After injection of labeled palmitic or stearic acid, the specific activity of these acids is one order of magnitude less in the brain than in blood, showing that the incorporated labeled acid is largely diluted in the brain by newly synthesized acid. In contrast, after injecting lignoceric acid, the specific activities are similar in neurons and astrocytes and in blood, suggesting that most of the lignoceric acid in these cells comes the blood and probably from the diet, as nonneural tissue synthesizes very minute amounts of lignoceric acid (117).

Uptake During Development

During development stearic acid is transported from blood into the brain at varying rates. Total radioactivity (cpm in total brain lipids) increases parallel to myelination and decreases thereafter (Fig. 9) (118). Stearic acid contains most of the radioactivity in the brain and no other labeled molecule is found in blood. The importance of exogenous saturated fatty acids for brain lipid biosynthesis is thus clearly demonstrated. These results indicate a variation in the blood–brain permeability for fatty acids during development. However, stearic acid incorporation expressed in relation to the amount of brain lipids (specific radioactivity, cpm/mg lipids) decreases as a function of age (Fig. 9). This curve indicates the importance of exogenous fatty acids during glial cell multiplication, occuring in the first week after birth. Thus exogenous stearic acid seems to be relatively more important during early multiplication of glial cells than during myelination. These results are not caused by increased catabolism *in situ* as β-oxidation is very low in the brain.

Nonphysiological Fatty Acids

Trans unsaturated fatty acids

Trans unsaturated fatty acids are formed during partial hydrogenation of unsaturated fatty acids by some rumen microorganisms or by commercial processing of vegetable oils. Thus trans unsaturated fatty isomers, geometric opposite of the natural cis isomer, may be found in the diet in significant amounts.

Trans fatty acids are found in very minute amounts in tissues from mammals, including the brain (119). Trans fatty acids are absorbed and incorporated into most tissues of experimental animals and humans, but they seem to be selectively excluded by the brain (120). Although the rate of fatty acid metabolism is lower in the brain than in other tissues, and nervous tissue is more selective in utilizing circulating fatty acids, intragastrically injected elaidic acid is incorporated and metabolized by the developing brain (121), corroborating the fact that intracerebrally injected elaidic acid is utilized by the brain (122,123).

A culture of peripheral nerve cells enriched in Schwann cells incorporates a nonphysiological trans fatty acid (elaidic acid) as well as the physiological cis isomer (oleic acid). Both acids are incorporated similarly in all lipids studied (phosphatidylcholine is a very potent acceptor); only cholesterol-ester formation from elaidic acid is slightly reduced. Both acids are partially degraded into subunits, which are in turn used for synthesis of new fatty acids. However, elaidic acid is less degraded by the cells, thus providing more C14:1, C16:1 fatty acids and less cholesterol. The presence of elaidic acid diminishes the elongation–desaturation of EFAs (124).

Branched chain fatty acid: phytanic acid

Refsum disease (heredopathia atactica polyneuritiformis) is an autosomal recessive inborn error of metabolism with the accumulation of 3,5,7,11-tetramethylhexadecanoic acid (phytanic acid) (125). The phytanic acid is of exogenous origin, since no endogenous synthesis takes place. Preformed phytanic acid in dairy products, meat, and fish oils seems to be the main source. In addition, experiments both in animals and in humans show that free phytol may be converted to phytanic acid in the

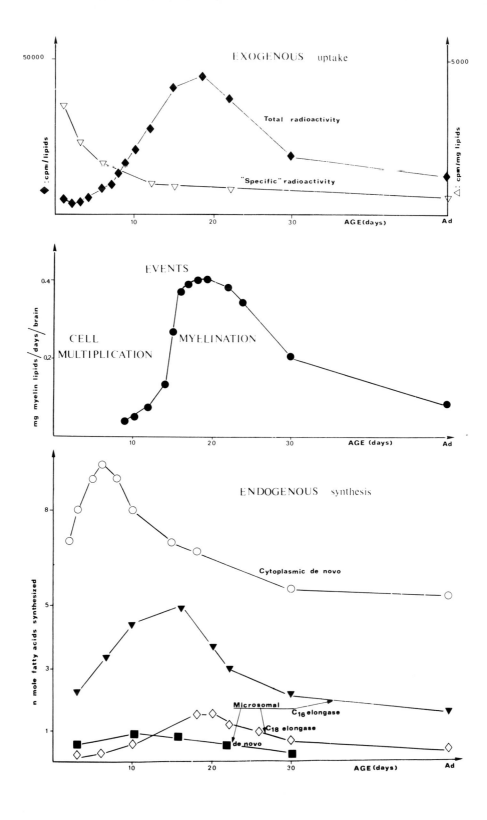

body, whereas phytol bound to the chlorophyll molecule is probably not absorbed in the intestine.

Phytanic acid cannot be degraded by ordinary β-oxidation since this is blocked by the methyl group in the β-position related to the carboxyl group. An alternative pathway was shown to be α-oxidation. Patients with heredopathia atactica polyneuritiformis have been shown to have a defect in the β-oxidation mechanism of β-methyl-substituted fatty acids (126–128). The enzyme defect has been identified in the very first step of phytanic acid oxidation, that is, the introduction of a hydroxyl group on the α-carbon of phytanic acid. The enzyme involved is phytanic acid α-hydroxylase. According to *in vitro* experiments, this enzyme is located in the mitochondria.

In cultures of skin fibroblasts from patients with phytanic acid storage disease, the rate of oxidation of phytanic acid was less than 5% of that found in fibroblasts from normal skin. Cells from parents of patients (clinically normal obligate heterozygotes) oxidized phytanic acid at about half the rate of normal subjects.

Refsum disease proves that a nonphysiological fatty acid can cross the blood–nerve barrier and the blood–brain barrier; this acid is incorporated in membranes and seriously disturbs their functioning, with consequent dramatic neurological problems presented by these patients (129).

Polyunsaturated Fatty Acids

The lipid composition of the brain is unique in a number of quantitative features, one of which is the high concentration of polyunsaturated fatty acids (PUFA) in the phospholipid fraction. This is true for the ethanolamine and serine phosphoglycerides and to some extent for the inositol phosphatides. Arachidonic(20:4n-6) and cervonic acids (docosahexaenoic acid) (22:6n-3) constitute over 30% of the total fatty acids of these fractions in human brain. Since ethanolamine phosphoglycerides and serine phosphoglycerides constitute about 45% of the brain phosphatide fraction, it is apparent that PUFA represent a considerable fraction of the total brain phospholipid fatty acids. Of the two major PUFA mentioned, 20:4 belongs to the n-6 series and 22:6 to the n-3 series of fatty acids. It has been shown *in vitro* and *in vivo* that no interconversion occurs between the two series. The fatty acids themselves, or a suitable precursor, must be provided for the deposition of these two polyenoic acids (130). The two major dietary precursors are linoleic acid for PUFA of the n-6 series and linolenic acid for those of the n-3 series.

The notion of essential and nonessential amino acids is familiar. There is a simi-

---

FIG. 9. Importance of exogenous essential fatty acids during brain development. **Top:** Total and specific radioactivity in animals injected with labeled stearic acid. (See text for more details.) **Middle:** Accumulation of lipids in brain myelin. The profile of stearic acid accumulation in myelin is similar to the profile of total radioactivity. **Bottom:** Synthesis of fatty acids during development. Only the microsomal C-16 elongase synthesizes stearic acid: *de novo* synthesis in cytosol and microsomes provides only very minute amounts of stearic acid. (From Bourre et al., ref. 118.)

larity between the amino acids and fatty acids, as animals can make some fatty acids but not others. In general, animal systems possess enzymes for both the degradation and synthesis of fatty acids. Mammalian systems can synthesize fatty acids and introduce at least one double bond between the carboxyl group and the 9 position in a C18 fatty acid. Plants can introduce double bonds beyond the 9 position. Two 18-carbon acids that occur in plants, linoleic and linolenic acids, have two and three double bonds, respectively, in position 9, 12 (and 15) numbered from the carboxyl group. These two PUFA are similar to the essential amino acids of proteins in that they cannot be made by animal systems but are found in structural lipids. PUFA occur in the β-position of phospholipids.

Biosynthesis of Polyunsaturated Fatty Acids

The synthesis of PUFA by successive desaturation and elongation of linoleic and linolenic precursors in the brain has scarcely been studied. However, one may presume that the mechanisms in the brain are related, if not similar, to those found in other organs, such as the liver (Table 3). Several different desaturases exist, each one introducing a double bond in a given position: $\triangle 6, \triangle 5$, or $\triangle 4$. $\triangle 8$ desaturase

TABLE 3. *Biosynthesis of polyunsaturated fatty acids*

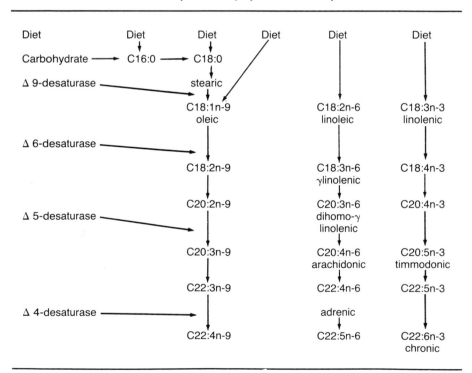

does not occur, thus preventing the formation of C20:3n-6 from C20:2n-6. Competition and limiting steps among these interconversions have been studied; elongation stages do not play an important role in their regulation.

In the brain, anabolism starts with the EFAs (C18:2n-6 and C18:3n-3), which, available in the diet, must be picked up by the brain before or after elongation and desaturation.

PUFAs are metabolized as acyl-CoA in microsomes (131). The process of elongation of PUFAs is presumed to be similar to that of the saturated chains, two-carbon units being provided by malonyl-CoA: there does not seem to be a specific enzymatic system for each series. However, condensation kinetics of malonyl-CoA are not similar: the possibility exists that elongations occurring in the n-3 and n-6 series are different. Moreover, the elongation of PUFAs in certain pathological cases is less affected than the elongation of their saturated homologs (81).

The quantitative importance of these elongation–desaturation mechanisms is debatable since they slow down rapidly after birth (131–133). Moreover, studies carried out on cell cultures (134) have shown that isolated nerve cells synthesize considerably smaller quantities of cervonic acid from linolenic acid (135–138).

Origin of Essential Fatty Acids in Brain

The brain contains only very small quantities of linoleic and linolenic acid. One could thus hypothesize that the truly essential fatty acids for nervous tissue are the longer chain derivatives obtained by elongation in the liver of linoleic and linolenic acid, as suggested by cell cultures in a chemically defined medium (without any fatty acid) contain only half as much PUFA as the original cells. They contain 20:3n-9, which proves that the medium lacks essential fatty acids. The decrease in PUFAs is balanced by an increase in monounsaturated fatty acids; saturated fatty acid levels remain unaffected. PUFAs introduced into the chemically defined medium are incorporated into phospholipids. The addition of acids from the n-6 series raises the level of arachidonic acid and moreover, induces an increase in acids from the n-3 series, which is probably owing to a better reutilization of the fatty acids contained in the original cells (139). The addition of linolenic acid to the culture medium inhibits the synthesis of acids of the n-6 series and proves to be toxic, even when greatly diluted.

After experimenting with various combinations of fatty acids, only the simultaneous addition of 20:4 and 22:6 to the chemically defined medium allows cultivation of cells whose fatty acid profile is similar to that of live tissue of the same age (139). Normal amounts of 22:5n-3 were only obtained when cells were incubated in the presence of 22:6n-3. Thus one metabolic function of 22:6 may be to serve as an intracellular storage pool for the formation of 20:5 through retroconversion. A similar hypothesis was derived from studies with retinoblastoma cells (140).

The addition of 20:4n-6 and 22:6n-3 stimulated the proliferation of small dense cells, probably oligodendrocytes. This is confirmed by the study of the fatty acids in these cells, very long saturated and monounsaturated chains of 24-carbon atoms being found, which are specific to the oligodendrocyte and to the membrane it synthesizes, myelin (139).

In addition, it appears that the addition of 20:4 and 22:6 into the culture medium of nerve cells allows better functioning of the neurons, evidenced by an increase in the stimulated liberation of neuropeptides (141), and by the multiplication and differentiation of the oligodendrocytes made possible by a normal composition of fatty acids in their membranes (139).

The likelihood that cervonic acid is essential for the brain is supported by results showing that when rats are compared on diets containing cervonic acid or linolenic acid, the former leads to the production of higher levels of cervonic acid in plasma and brain lipids than the latter (142). Moreover, preformed (dietary) cervonic acid seems to be incorporated into brain phospholipids much more rapidly than cervonic acid synthesized from linolenic acid (142,143).

Essential Fatty Acid Deficiency, Brain Development, and Myelination

Prenatal undernutrition (intrauterine growth retardation)

Oligodendrocytes in hypotrophic animals reveal two basic modifications: a deficit in monounsaturated fatty acids, balanced by an increase in the levels of saturated fatty acids and a sizeable imbalance between the n-6 and n-3 series, in favor of the n-6 series (144), in contrast with the imbalance in favor of the n-6 series observed in neurons (145). Since neurons are formed prenatally, it seems logical that there should be an alteration in the composition of their membranes. However, the changes in the composition of fatty acids of oligodendrocyte type during postnatal development remain unexplained. The quantity of PUFAs (n-6 + n-3) seems to be maintained and controlled by the nervous tissue, whereas the distribution between the two series is far more sensitive to external factors. The anomalies persist into adulthood, even though the animals are put on a normal diet; this is particularly true with regard to PUFAs.

Postnatal undernutrition

The development of brain myelin is subject to many nutritional and environmental influences, including postnatal undernourishment (28). Myelination is the neurogenic process most vulnerable to undernutrition in animals (146) and in humans (45). The deficit of myelin synthesis induced by nutritional deprivation is irreversible (16) and rehabilitation is difficult. Essential fatty acid deficiency which alters myelin formation and turnover, is one aspect of undernutrition.

The dietary treatment of female rats before mating and during gestation and lactation is important in producing EFA deficiency in the offspring. The newborn depends on the milk supply for all its nutrients and for the next 10 to 15 days the growth of the pup depends solely on an adequate milk supply. Lack of fat in the diet or low levels of linoleic acid in the diet does not seem to reduce the quantity of milk during lactation, but the linoleic acid content of milk is considerably reduced by the deficient diet (34,147). Thus the growing animal continues to receive very low amounts of linoleate during the important period of lactation in which myelin synthesis and deposition is proceeding at a rapid rate.

Most of the early work on EFA deficiency and the developing brain studied the effects of totally fat-free diets. Female rats, usually 1 or 2 weeks before mating, were started on a fat-free diet, and their progeny was examined at various intervals (148). The body and brain weights were severely reduced in all cases. The fatty acid analysis of the brain phospholipids indicated that n-6 fatty acids were decreased while 20:3n-9 fatty acids were detectable. The formation of 20:3n-9 (from 18:1n-9) (see Table 3) and its accumulation are considered an index of EFA deficiency (149). Fatty acid patterns of myelin lipids, in particular ethanolamine phosphoglyceride, were also affected indicating that the structure of the myelin may have been altered (150). Behavioral and performance tests were adversely affected by EFA deficiency (151). Essential fatty acid deficiency affects myelin metabolism, altering the turnover of phospholipids (152), and causes significant decreases of RNA and protein content in the brain and of protein in myelin (153).

Protein deficiency is thought to produce more permanent damage, whereas the effects of EFA deficiency seem to be reversible. However, this conclusion was drawn from the observation that lipid profiles in whole brain and subcellular fractions were restored in rats raised on an EFA-deficient diet up to one month or more after birth followed by an adequate diet during later adult life. Rats raised on a fat-free diet for the first 90 days followed by an adequate diet for an additional 90 days are able to completely restore lipid profiles. Upon introduction of an adequate diet, the level of n-6 fatty acids increased dramatically and the excess of n-9 fatty acids that had accumulated due to the deficient diet disappeared after rehabilitation (150).

Importance of n-3 Polyunsaturated Acids of Dietary Origin for the Nervous System

The position 2 of phospholipids is generally occupied by a PUFA, in most cases 20:4n-6, 22:5n-3 or 22:6n-3. There is a vast literature dealing with the influence of PUFAs on the structure and function of the brain (34,36,154–161). However, these authors have used diets that were deficient in fatty acids of the n-6 and n-3 series simultaneously, although the effects of a specific deficiency in fatty acids of the n-3 series (with a normal supply of n-6) are also interesting. A deficiency in EFAs will alter the course of brain development, during which the requirements for these EFAs are particularly high. Nerve tissue will partly make up for this deficit by synthesizing PUFAs of the n-9 series which will be incorporated into all membranes. If one single EFA is missing in the diet, the brain will maintain its PUFAs at a constant level by reciprocal interchange within the series (150), but the single deficit will inevitably cause a deficiency in long chains.

Animals put on a diet containing normal amounts of n-6 fatty acids but lacking fatty acids of the n-3 series (sunflower oil) were compared with animals put on a diet containing both types of acids (soya oil) (162,163). The level of total PUFAs in nerve cells and intracellular organelles remained normal, but a considerable deficit in cervonic acid (22:6n-3) was observed, which was eventually compensated for by an excess in 22:5n-6. The n-3:n-6 ratio is 20 times higher in a sunflower-oil-based diet than in a soya-oil-based diet; when animals are fed for 60 days on the former diet, the n-3:n-6 ratio in oligodendrocytes, myelin, neurons, synaptosomes, and astrocytes is 16, 12, 2, 6, and 3 times higher, respectively, than when they are fed the latter diet (Table 4) (162). The importance of fatty acids in the n-3 series (164,165) has also been shown by a specific study of phosphatidylethanolamine in animals put on a diet based on peanut oil or colza oil.

The rate of recovery after the transition from a sunflower-based diet to a soya-based diet is remarkably slow. It takes many months before the cells and brain organelles recover a normal quantity of cervonic acid (166). One could have predicted the recovery in myelin would be rather slow since its turnover is slow, but the low recovery rate in nerve endings was unexpected, since the renewal of the molecules which form their membranes is supposed to be rapid. The recovery depends perhaps either on hepatic production of chain ends (cervonic and arachidonic acids) or on the level of enzymatic desaturation and elongation activities which are known to be considerably weakened after birth (131–133).

Symptoms of deficiency in linolenic acid have been described in the monkey (167) and in humans (168). The deficiency in acids of the n-3 series is considered a syndrome of modern societies (169).

Insofar as PUFAs are concerned, the brain is undoubtedly an extremely well-protected organ which uses the nutritional fatty acids in a very selective manner. A restriction of very short duration of the n-3 fatty acids in the diets of animals which have been put on standardized diets causes few anomalies in the profile of PUFAs in the brain and its organelles, whereas other organs become rapidly deficient in these acids. A diet deficient in n-3 fatty acids does not cause anomalies in the brain unless it is prolonged over several generations; signs of deficiency will not become evident

TABLE 4. *The n-3/n-6 ratios in various cells and organelles of animals fed a soya-oil or a sunflower-oil-based diet, and in animals presenting with intrauterine growth retardation*

	Soya	Sunflower	Intrauterine growth retardation
Neurons	0.50	0.24	0.35
Oligodendrocytes	0.72	0.02	0.43
Astrocytes	0.76	0.25	0.62
Myelin	0.12	0.01	0.07
Synaptosomes	0.78	0.13	0.84
Microsomes	0.77	0.17	—
Mitochondria	0.74	0.11	—

in the brain unless the animals are the offspring of mothers who were already deficient before gestation. A deficiency in fatty acids of the n-3 series with a normal supply of fatty acids of the n-6 series causes disturbances in the animal's learning capacity (157) which can be correlated with the anomalies in the composition of fatty acids in the cerebral phospholipids (161). Moreover, this nutritional deficiency causes visual disturbances together with alterations in the electroretinogram (170,171). The n-3 PUFAs can control certain enzymatic activities, such as 5′-nucleotidase, a membrane enzyme, activity of which is reduced in the brains of animals deficient in PUFAs; only the addition of linolenic acid restores normal enzymatic activity (172). A linolenic acid-rich diet increases n-3 fatty acid levels in brain capillaries and alters their prostaglandin synthesis (173).

Adequate Nutritional Supplies for the Satisfactory Composition of Cerebral Membranes

The indispensable nature of PUFAs of the n-3 series has been questioned (174); this doubt is probably unwarranted. The brain clearly needs n-3 PUFAs, both for its structure and function. It is, therefore, particularly useful to determine the minimum supply required in order to obtain cerebral membranes of normal composition. Experiments were therefore performed with diets which were intermediary in their linolenic acid content (obtained by adding variable and increasing quantities of linolenic acid to the diet) (175). In all tissues examined (brain, liver, kidney, testicle), the increase in the supply of 18:3n-3 caused a global increase in the level of terminal fatty acids of the n-3 series and inversely a decrease in the level of fatty acids of the n-6 series. However, different fatty acids behave differently in the various tissues. In the brain, the level of 22:6n-3 increases linearly with increasing supplies of 18-3n-3, from 0.2 to 1.5% and then stabilizes (175). An inverse phenomenon is observed for 22:5n-3. On the other hand, variations at the hepatic level are continuous, which demonstrates the extreme sensitivity of the liver to exogenous supplies. The particular behavior of the brain can be explained on the one hand by the particular enzymatic patterns in brain tissue with regard to the n-3 and n-6 series and on the other hand by the selectivity of the uptake by the blood–brain barrier which seems to become dominant when the requirements for fatty acids of the n-3 series are met.

The study of the composition of PUFAs in lipoproteins has allowed us to demonstrate the importance of the intermediary intrahepatic metabolism for the supply of PUFAs to the brain; 18:2n-6 and 18:3n-3 precursors must be elongated and desaturated by the liver into longer chains, which are truly essential fatty acids for the brain, as has been demonstrated in cell cultures (139).

Disturbances in the profile of PUFAs can alter the functioning of membrane enzymes, disturb the interactions between receptor and ligand, disrupt intercellular interactions, and even upset the correct functioning of the organ (38,176,177). It could accelerate aging (178). For the rat, whose diet is composed of 10% lipids, the linolenic acid content should represent 1.5% of total fatty acids when the linoleic acid content is fixed at 25%. This quantity seems necessary and sufficient.

It has been suggested that it is important to maintain the linolenate/linoleate ratio in the diet at a level close to that found in the milk of mothers who are put on presumably normal diets. According to preliminary data, this ratio appears to be 6% in the rat, 8% in the rabbit, 16% in the guinea pig, and 30% in humans (179–181). Cervonic acid levels in human milk also depend on dietary intakes of the acid (182), whereas probably up to 50% of the ultimate mass of cervonic acid in the infant brain accumulates after birth. However, it must be taken into account that large quantities of linoleic acid (18:2n-6) in the diet could inhibit the transformation of linolenic acid into cervonic acid in the liver, thus causing suboptimal cervonic acid nutritional status.

FATTY ACIDS AND HUMAN PATHOLOGY

Various psychiatric (endogenous depression) (183) and neurological diseases (Friedrich's disease, multiple sclerosis) have been ascribed to anomalies of fatty acid metabolism. Treatment with PUFA has been proposed for multiple sclerosis (184), but its efficacy is questionable (185).Dietary phytanic acid is not catabolized in patients with Refsum's disease owing to a congenital enzymatic deficiency (128); the acid therefore replaces other fatty acids in phospholipids and seriously disturbs the functioning of membranes with resulting dramatic neurological defects. In adrenoleukodystrophy, fatty acids with very long saturated and monounsaturated chains cannot apparently be oxidized (186) and accumulate during the physiological renewal of membranes; although they are physiological molecules, they seem to cause toxic effects when present in excess. In adrenoleukodystrophy, as well as in the Zellweger cerebrohepatorenal syndrome, the peroxisomes are unable to oxidize the lignoceric myelinic acid (187). Very long chain fatty acids are probably not synthesized in Pelizaeus-Merzbacher's disease (69); as a result myelinic sphingolipids are not elaborated and myelin is not formed.

The structure as well as the function of membranes is altered in human PUFA deficiency (38,176). However, the specific role of each individual series (n-3 and n-6) has not been individualized and the best balance between the two series in the diet still needs to be determined. PUFAs represent only a few percent of total fatty acids in the diet; they do not play any specific role in energy metabolism, but their specific structural role, at least in nervous tissue, is extremely important. Hence the composition in terms of fatty acids both in enteral and parenteral nutrition, as well as in diets in developing countries, is important.

ACKNOWLEDGMENTS

This work was supported by INSERM. The author is most grateful to Mrs. Michelle Bonneil for her help in preparing the manuscript.

REFERENCES

1. Horrocks LA. Metabolism and function of fatty acid in brain. In: Horrocks LA, ed. *Phospholipids in the nervous system.* New York: John Wiley, 1985:173–99.
2. Morell P, ed. *Myelin,* 2nd ed. New York: Plenum Press, 1984.
3. Norton W. *Oligodendroglia.* New York: Plenum Press, 1984.
4. Baumann N. *Neurological mutants affecting myelination.* New York: Elsevier, 1980. (INSERM Symposium Series 4, no 14.)
5. Hogan EL, Greenfield S. Animal models of genetic disorders of myelin. In: Morell P, ed. *Myelin.* 2nd ed. New York: Plenum Press, 1984:489–534.
6. Norton WT. Formation, structure and biochemistry of myelin. In: Siegel GJ, Albers RW, Katzman R, Agranoff BW, eds. *Basic neurochemistry.* Boston: Little, Brown, 1976:74–102.
7. Webster H. The geometry of peripheral myelin sheaths during their formation and growth in rat sciatic nerves. *J Cell Biol* 1971;48:348–67.
8. Raine CS. Morphological aspects of myelin and myelination. In Morell P, ed. *Myelin.* New York, NY: Plenum, 1977:1–50.
9. Dobbing J. Vulnerable periods of brain development. In: *Lipids, malnutrition and the developing brain.* Amsterdam: Elsevier, 1972;9–23. (Ciba Foundation Symposium)
10. Wiggins RC, Fuller GN. Early postnatal starvation causes lasting brain hypomyelination. *J. Neurochem* 1978;30:1231–7.
11. Wiggins RC, Miller SL, Benjamins JA, Krigman MR, Morell P. Myelin synthesis during postnatal nutritional deprivation and subsequent rehabilitation. *Brain Res* 1976;107:257–73.
12. Bazan N, Aveldano M, Cascone G, Rodriguez E. *Neurochemical and clinical neurology.* In: Hashim G, Lajtha A, eds. New York: Alan R. Liss, 1980.
13. Suzuki K. Chemistry and metabolism of brain lipids. In: Siegel T, Alberts R, Katsman R, Agranoff B, eds. *Basic neurochemistry.* Boston: Little, Brown 1976;308–27.
14. Davison AN, Gregson NA. Metabolism of cellular membrane sulfolipids in the rat brain. *Biochem J* 1966;98:915–22.
15. Chase HP, Dorsey J, McKhann GM. The effect of malnutrition on the synthesis of a myelin lipid. *Pediatrics* 1967;40:551–9.
16. Wiggins RC, Benjamins JA, Krigman MR, Morell P. Synthesis of myelin proteins during starvation. *Brain Res* 1974;80:345–9.
17. Wiggins RC, Fuller GN. Relative synthesis of myelin in different brain regions of postnatally undernourished rats. *Brain Res* 1979;162:103–12.
18. Culley WJ, Mertz ET. Effect of restricted food intake on growth and composition of preweanling rat brain. *Proc Soc Exp Biol Med* 1965;118:233–5.
19. Crnic LS, Chase HP. Models of infantile undernutrition in rats: effects on brain lipids. *Dev Neurosci* 1980;3:49–58.
20. Dobbing J. The influence of early nutrition on the development and myelination of the brain. *Proc R Soc Lond (Biol)* 1964;159:503–9.
21. Davison AN, Dobbing J, Morgan RS, Payling Wright C. Metabolism of myelin: the persistence of (4-^{14}C) cholesterol in the mammalian central nervous system. *Lancet* 1959;1:658–60.
22. Ahmad G, Rahman MA. Effect of undernutrition and protein malnutrition on brain chemistry of rats. *J Nutr* 1975;105:1090–103.
23. Culley WJ, Lineberger RO. Effect of undernutrition on the size and composition of the rat brain. *J Nutr* 1968;96:375–81.
24. Howard E, Granoff DM. Effect of neonatal food restriction in mice on brain growth, DNA and cholesterol, and on adult delayed response learning. *J Nutr* 1968;95:111–21.
25. Nakhasi HL, Toews AD, Horrocks LA. Effects of postnatal protein deficiency on the content and composition of myelin from brains of weanling rats. *Brain Res* 1975;83:176–9.
26. Rao PS. Fatty acid composition of cerebrosides and phospholipids in brain of undernourished rats. *Nutr Metab* 1979;23:221–40.
27. Reddy PV, Sastry PS. Effects of undernutrition on the metabolism of phospholipids and gangliosides in developing rat brain. *Br J Nutr* 1978;40:403–11.
28. Wiggins RC. Myelin development and nutritional insufficiency. *Brain Res Rev* 1982;4:151–75.
29. Alling C, Bruce A, Karlsson I, Sapia O, Svennerholm L. Effect of maternal essential fatty acid

supply on fatty acid composition of brain, liver, muscle and serum in 21-day-old rats. *J Nutr* 1971;102:773–82.

30. Karlsson I, Svennerholm L. Biochemical development of rat forebrain in severe protein and essential fatty acid deficiencies. *J Neurochem* 1978;31:657–62.
31. Gozzo S, D'Udine B. Diet deprived in essential fatty acids affects brain myelination. *Neurosci Lett* 1977;7:267–75.
32. McKeena M, Campagnoni AT. Effect of pre- and postnatal essential fatty acid deficiency on brain development. *J Nutr* 1979;109:1195–204.
33. Balazs R, Patel AJ. Factors affecting the biochemical maturation of the brain. Effect of undernutrition during early life. *Prog Brain Res* 1973;110:115–28.
34. Galli C,Treciak H, Paoletti R. Effects of essential fatty acid deficiency on myelin and various subcellular structures in rat brain. *J Neurochem* 1972;19:1863–7.
35. Sun GY. Effects of a fatty acid deficiency on lipids of whole brain, microsomes and myelin in the rat. *J Lipid Res* 1972;13:56–62.
36. Sun GY, Sun AY. Induction of essential fatty acid deficiency in mouse brain: effects of fat deficient diet upon acyl group composition of myelin and synaptosome-rich fractions during development and maturation. *Lipids* 1974;9:450–4.
37. Trapp BD, Bernsohn J. Essential fatty acid deficiency and CNS myelin. *J Neurol Sci* 1978;37:249–66.
38. Brenner RR. Effect of unsaturated acids on membrane structure and enzyme kinetics. *Prog Lipid Res* 1984;23:69–96.
39. Winniczek H, Go J, Sheng SL. Essential fatty acid deficiency: metabolism of 20:3ω9 and 22:3ω9 of major phosphoglycerides in subcellular fractions of developing and mature mouse brain. *Lipids* 1975;7:365–73.
40. Minkowski A, Roux J, Tordet-Caridroit C. Pathophysiologic changes in intrauterine malnutrition. In: Winick M, ed. *Nutrition and fetal development,* vol 2. New York: John Wiley, 1974:45–78.
41. Matthieu JM, Leathwood P, Chanez C, Bourre JM. Influence of nutrition on animal brain development: a biochemical and behavioural approach. In: Aebi H, Whitehead R, eds. *Maternal nutrition during pregnancy and lactation.* Bern: Hans Huber, 1980:49–65. (Nestlé Foundation publication series; vol 1.)
42. Bourre JM, Morand O, Chanez C, Dumont O, Flexor M. Influence of intrauterine malnutrition on brain development: alteration of myelination. *Biol Neonat* 1981;39:96–9.
43. Fishman MA, Prensky AL, Dodge PR. Low content of cerebral lipids in infants suffering from malnutrition. *Nature* 1969;221:552–3.
44. Chase HP, Canosa CA, Dabiere CS, Welch NN, O'Brien D. Postnatal undernutrition and human brain development. *J Ment Defic Res* 1974;18:355–66.
45. Martinez M. Myelin lipids in the developing cerebrum, cerebellum, and brain stem of normal and undernourished children. *J Neurochem* 1982;41:1684–92.
46. Fox JH, Fishman MA, Dodge PR, Prensky AL. The effect of malnutrition on human central nervous system myelin. *Neurology* 1972;19:1863–7.
47. Winnick M, Rosso P, Waterlow J. Cellular growth of cerebrum, cerebellum, and brain stem in normal and marasmic children. *Exp Neurol* 1970;26:393–400.
48. Kumar A, Ghai OP, Singh H, Singh R. Delayed nerve conduction velocities in children with protein-calorie malnutrition. *J Pediatr* 1976;90:149–53.
49. Shah SN, Bhargava UK, Johnson RC, McKean CM. Latency changes in brain stem auditory evoked potentials associated with impaired myelination. *Exp Neurol* 1978;58:111–8.
50. Wakil SJ. Mechanism of fatty acid synthesis. *J Lipid Res* 1961;1:1–2.
51. Volpe JJ, Vagelos PR. Saturated fatty acid biosynthesis and its regulation. *Annu Rev Biochem* 1973;42:21–60.
52. Yeh YY, Streuli VL, Zee P. Ketone bodies serve as important precursors of brain lipids in the developing rat. *Lipids* 1977;12:957–64.
53. Koper J, Zeinstra E, Lopes-Cardozo M, Vangolde L. Aceto-acetate and glucose as substrates for lipid synthesis by rat brain oligodendrocyte and astrocyte in serum free culture. *Biochim Biophys Acta* 1984;796:20–6.
54. Lynen F. Biosynthesis of saturated fatty acids. *Fed Proc* 1961;20:941–51.
55. Brady RO. Biosynthesis of fatty acids. II. Studies with enzymes obtained from brain. *J Biol Chem* 1960;235:3099–4005.

56. Volpe JJ, Kishimoto Y. Fatty acid synthetase of brain. Development, influence of nutritional and hormonal factors and comparison with liver enzyme. *J Neurochem* 1972;19:737–41.
57. Pollet S, Bourre JM, Baumann N. Etude de la biosynthèse de novo des acides gras dans le cerveau de souris normale, Quaking et hétérozygotes pour le caractère Quaking. *CR Séances Acad Sci Paris* 1969;268:2146–9.
58. Paturneau-Jouas M, Baumann N, Bourre JM. Biosynthèse des acids gras dans les mitochondries de cerveau de souris en présence de malonyl-CoA ou d'acétyl-CoA. *Biochimie* 1976;58:341–9.
59. Pollet S, Bourre JM, Chaix G, Daudu O, Baumann N. Biosynthèse des acides gras dans les microsomes de cerveau de souris. *Biochimie* 1973;55:333–41.
60. Bourre JM, Pollet S, Chaix G, Daudu O, Baumann N. Etude "in vitro" des acides gras synthétisés dans les microsomes de cerveau de souris normales et Quaking. *Biochimie* 1973;55:1473–9.
61. Brophy PJ, Vance VE. The synthesis and hydrolysis of long-chain fatty acyl-coenzyme A thioesters by solubles and microsomal fractions from the brain of the developing rat. *Biochem J* 1976;160:247–51.
62. Kurook AS, Hokoki K, Yoshimura Y. Some properties of long fatty acyl-coenzyme. A thioesterase in rat organs. *J Biochem (Tokyo)* 1972;71:625–34.
63. Boiron F, Cassagne C, Darriet D, Bourre JM. Evidence of an abnormal stearoyl-CoA hydrolysis in a membrane pellet from Trembler sciatic nerves. *Neurosci Lett* 1982;33:91–6.
64. Boiron F, Heape MA, Cassagne C. Assay of stearoyl-CoA synthesis in microsomes from normal and Trembler mouse sciatic nerves. *Neurosci Lett* 1984;48:7–12.
65. Bourre, JM, Pollet S, Dubois G, Baumann N. Biosynthèse des acides gras à longue chaine dans les microsomes de cerveau de souris. *CR Séances Acad Sci Paris* 1970;271:1221–3.
66. Murad S, Kishimoto Y. Chain elongation of fatty acid in brain: a comparison of mitochondrial and microsomal enzymes activities. *Arch Biochem Biophys* 1978;30:300–6.
67. Aeberhard E, Menkes J. Biosynthesis of long chain fatty acids by subcellular particles of mature brain. *J Biol Chem* 1967;243:3834–40.
68. Bourre JM, Paturneau-Jouas M, Daudu O, Baumann N. Lignoceric acid biosynthesis in the developing brain. Activities of mitochondrial acetyl-CoA dependent synthesis and microsomal malonyl-CoA chain elongating system in relation to myelination. Comparison between normal mouse and dysmyelinating mutants (Quaking and Jimpy). *Eur J Biochem* 1977;72:41–7.
69. Bourre JM, Bornhofen JH, Araoz C, Daudu O, Baumann N. Pelizaeus-Merzbacher disease: brain lipid and fatty acid composition. *J Neurochem* 1978;30:719–27.
70. Bourre JM, Jacque C, Nguyen-Legros J, et al. Pelizaeus-Merzbacher disease: biochemical analysis of isolated myelin (electron microscopy; protein, lipid and unsubstituted fatty acids analysis). *Eur Neurol* 1978;17:317–26.
71. Bourre JM, Daudu O, Baumann N. Biosynthesis of lignoceric acid from behenyl-CoA in mouse brain microsomes. Comparison between normal and Quaking mutant. *Biochem Biophys Res Commun* 1975;63:1027–34.
72. Goldberg I, Schechter I, Block K. Fatty acyl-CoA elongation in brain of normal and quaking. *Science* 1973;182:497–99.
73. Bourre JM, Dumont O. Changes in fatty acid elongation in mouse developing brain by mercury; comparison with other metals. *Toxicol Lett* 1985;25:19–23.
74. Boiron F, Darriet D, Bourre JM, Cassagne C. Decreased biosynthesis of saturated C20-C24 fatty acids by the Trembler mouse sciatic nerve. *Neurochem Int* 1984;6:109–16.
75. Seidel D, Nowoczek G, Jatzkewitz H. In vivo studies on the metabolism of lignoceric acid in adult rat brain. *J Neurochem* 1975;25:619–22.
76. Carreau JP, Daudu O, Mazliak P, Bourre JM. Palmityl-CoA and stearyl-CoA desaturase in mouse brain microsomes during development in normal and neurological mutants (Quaking and Jimpy). *J Neurochem* 1979;32:659–60.
77. Horrocks LA, Harper LW. Fatty acids and cholesterol. In: Lajtha A, ed. *Handbook of neurochemistry,* vol 3. New York: Plenum Press, 1983:1–16.
78. Cook HW, Spence M. Formation of non enoic fatty acids by rat brain homogenate. Effects of age, fasting and refeeding and comparison with liver enzyme. *J Biol Chem* 1973;248:1793–6.
79. Seng A, Derbuch M, Strosznader A. Stearate desaturase in rat brain and liver. *J Neurochem* 1976;27:825–6.
80. Cook M, Spence M. Biosynthesis of fatty acids in vitro by homogenate of developing rat brain: desaturation and chain elongation. *Biochem Biophys Acta* 1974;369:129–41.

81. Bourre JM, Daudu O, Baumann N. Nervonic acid biosynthesis by erucyl-CoA elongation in normal and Quaking mouse brain microsomes. Elongation of other unsaturated fatty acyl-CoA (mono and poly-unsaturated). *Biochim Biophys Acta* 1976;424:1–7.
82. Bernert JT, Bourre JM, Baumann N, Sprecher H. Fatty acid biosynthesis in mouse brain microsomes: the activity of partial reactions in the chain elongation of palmitoyl-CoA and stearyl-CoA by mouse brain microsomes. *J Neurochem* 1979;32:85–90.
83. Boone S, Wakil S. In vitro synthesis of lignoceric acid and nervonic acid in mammalian liver and brain. *Biochemistry* 1970;9:1470–9.
84. Paturneau-Jouas M, Baumann N, Bourre JM. Elongation of palmitoyl-CoA in mouse brain mitochondria: comparison with stearyl-CoA. *Biochem Biophys Res Commun* 1976;71:1326–34.
85. Bourre JM, Paturneau-Jouas M, Daudu O, Baumann N. Biosynthèse de l'acide lignocérique dans deux organelles (mitochondries et microsomes) au cours du développement cérébral de la souris, normal et pathologique (Quaking et Jimpy). *CR Séances Acad Sci Paris* 1976;283:409–12.
86. Bourre JM, Pollet S, Daudu O, Baumann N. Evolution in brain mice microsomes of lipids and their constituents during myelination. *Brain Res* 1973;51:225–39.
87. Bourre JM, Daudu O, Baumann N. Ontogénèse des trois systèmes de biosynthèse des acides gras dans les microsomes cérébraux: relation avec la myélinisation. *Biochimie* 1976;58:1277–9.
88. Volpe JJ, Lyles TO, Roncari DA, Vagelos PR. Fatty acid synthetase of developing brain and liver. Content, synthesis, and degradation during development. *J Biol Chem* 1973;248:2502–13.
89. Baumann N, Bourre JM, Jacque C, Harpin ML. Lipid composition of Quaking mouse myelin; comparison with normal mouse myelin in the adult and during development. *J Neurochem* 1973;20:753–9.
90. Bourre JM, Daudu O, Baumann N. Fatty acid biosynthesis in mice brain and kidney microsomes; comparison between Quaking mutant and control. *J Neurochem* 1975;24:1095–7.
91. Tennekoon GI, Kishimoto Y, Singh I, Nonaka G, Bourre JM. The differentiation of oligodendrocytes in the rat optic nerve. *Dev Biol* 1980;79:149–58.
92. Fulco AJ, Mead JF. The biosynthesis of lignoceric, cerebronic and nervonic acids. *J Biol Chem* 1961;236:2416–21.
93. Hajra A, Radin NS. In vivo conversion of labelled fatty acids to their sphingolipid fatty acid in rat brain. *J Lipid Res* 1963;4:448–53.
94. Murad S, Kishimoto Y. Hydroxylation of lignoceric acid to cerebronic acid during brain development. Diminished hydroxylase activity in myelin deficient mouse mutants. *J Biol Chem* 1975;250:5841–6.
95. Singh I, Kishimoto Y, Vunnam RR, Rodin NS. Conversion by rat brain preparation of lignoceric acid in ceramides and cerebrosides containing both α-hydroxy and nonhydroxy fatty acids. Effects of compounds which affect sphingolipid metabolism. *J Biol Chem* 1979;254:3840–4.
96. Singh I, Kishimoto Y. α-Hydroxylation of lignoceric acid in brain. Subcellular localization of hydroxylation and the requirement for heat-stable and heat-labile factors and sphingosine. *J Biol Chem* 1979;254:7698–704.
97. Shimeno H, Wali A, Kishimoto Y. α-Hydroxylation and oxidation of lignoceric acid in brain: the role of heat-stable and heat-labile factors. *Neurochem Res* 1984;9:181–94.
98. Cassagne C, Darriet D, Bourre JM. Biosynthesis of very long chain fatty acids by the sciatic nerve of the rabbit. *FEBS Lett* 1978;90:336–40.
99. Bourre JM, Daudu O. Stearyl-alcohol biosynthesis from stearyl-CoA in mouse brain microsomes in normal and dysmyelinating mutants (Quaking and Jimpy). *Neurosci Lett* 1978;7:225–30.
100. Natarajan V, Schmid HHO. Biosynthesis and utilization of long-chain alcohols in rat brain: aspects of chain length specificity. *Arch Biochem Biophys* 1978;187:215–22.
101. Natarajan V, Schmid HHO. Docosanol and other long chain primary alcohols in developing rat brain. *Lipids* 1977;12:128–30.
102. Bourre JM, Cassagne C, Larrouquere-Regnier S, Darriet D. Occurence of alkanes in brain myelin. Comparison between normal and Quaking mouse. *J Neurochem* 1977;29:645–8.
103. Darriet D, Cassagne C, Bourre JM. Sciatic nerve contains alkanes. Comparison between normal mice and neurological mutants: Jimpy, Quaking and Trembler. *J Neurochem* 1978;31:1541–3.
104. Cassagne C, Darriet D, Bourre JM. Evidence of alkane synthesis by the sciatic nerve of the rabbit. *FEBS Lett* 1977;82:51–4.
105. Lefauconnier JM, Hauw JJ. Barrière hémato-encéphalique II: données physiologiques. *Rev Neurol (Paris)* 1984;140:3–13.

106. Lefauconnier JM, Hauw JJ. Barrière hémato-encéphalique II: données physiologiques. *Rev Neurol (Paris)* 1984;140:89–109.
107. Joo F. The blood-brain barrier in vitro: ten years of research on microvessels isolated from the brain. *Neurochem Internat* 1985;7:1–25.
108. Dhopeshwarkar GA, Subramanian C. Lipogenesis in the developing brain from intracranially administered carbon-14 acetate and uniformly labeled carbon-14. *Lipids* 1977;12:762–4.
109. Dhopeshwarkar GA. Uptake and transport of fatty acids into the brain and the role of the blood brain barrier system. *Adv Lipid Biochem* 1975;11:104–42.
110. Dhopeshwarkar GA, Subramanian C. Intracranial conversion of linoleic acid to arachidonic acid: evidence for lack of δ8 desaturase in the brain. *J Neurochem* 26:1175–9.
111. Gozlan-Devillierre N, Baumann N, Bourre JM. Incorporation of stearic acid into brain lipids in the developing brain: blood–brain relationships during development. *Dev Neurosci* 1978;1:153–8.
112. Gozlan-Devillierre N, Baumann N, Bourre JM. Distribution of radioactivity in myelin lipids following subcutaneous injection of (14C) stearate. *Biochim Biophys Acta* 1978;528:490–6.
113. Gozlan-Devillierre N, Baumann N, Bourre JM. Mouse brain uptake and metabolism of stearic acid. *Biochimie* 1976;58:1129–33.
114. Bourre JM, Gozlan-Devillierre N, Pollet S, Maurin Y, Baumann N. In vivo incorporation of exogenous stearic acid in synaptosomes: high occurence of nonesterified fatty acids. *Neurosci Lett* 1977;4:309–13.
115. Lunt GG, James JE. Unesterified fatty acids in rats cerebral cortex: their association with proteolipids. *J Neurochem* 1976;26:325–9.
116. Morand O, Baumann N, Bourre JM. In vivo incorporation of exogenous (1-14C) stearic acid into neurons and astrocytes. *Neurosci Lett* 1979;13:177–81.
117. Morand O, Masson M, Baumann N, Bourre JM. Exogenous (1-14C) lignoceric acid uptake by neurons, astrocytes and myelin, as compared to incorporation of (1-14C) palmitic and stearic acids. *Neurochem Int* 1981;3:329–34.
118. Bourre JM, Gozlan-Devillierre N, Daudu O, Baumann N. Is there a blood–brain relationship for saturated fatty acids during development? *Biol Neonate* 1978;34:182–6.
119. McBeath LS, Cook HW. Trans-octadecenoic fatty acids in human brain. *Clin Res* 1977;25:709A.
120. McConnell KP, Sinclair RG. Evidence of selection in the building up of brain lecithins and cephalins. *J Biol Chem* 1937;118:131–6.
121. Cook HW. Incorporation metabolism of the dietary trans-unsaturated fatty acid, elaidic acid, by developing rat brain. *J Neurochem* 1979;32:515–9.
122. Cook HW. Incorporation, metabolism and positional distribution of trans-unsaturated fatty acids in developing and mature brain: comparison of elaidate and oleate administered intracerebrally. *Biochim Biophys Acta* 1978;531:245–56.
123. Karney R, Dhopeshwarkar G. Trans fatty acids: positional specificity in brain lecithin. *Lipids* 1979;14:257–60.
124. Bourre JM, Boutry JM, Masson M, Hauw JJ. Peripheral nerve cells in culture rich in Schwann cells incorporate and metabolize trans-unsaturated fatty acid (elaidic acid) as well as physiological cis isomer (oleic acid). *Neurosci Lett* 1982;30:173–8.
125. Klenk E, Kahlke W. Uber das Vorkommen der 3,7,11,15-Tetramethyl-hexadecansaure (Phytansaure) in den cholesterinestern und anderen lipoidfraktionen der organe bei einem кrankheitsfall unbekannter genese (verdacht auf heredopathia atactica polyneuritiformis (Refsum-syndrome)). *Hoppe Seylers Z Physiol Chem* 1963;333:133–9.
126. Avigan J, Steinberg D, Gutman A, et al. α-Decarboxylation: an important pathway for degradation of phytanic acid in animals. *Biochem Biophys Res Commun* 1966;24:388–9.
127. Herndon JH, Steinberg D, Uhlendorf BW. Refsum's disease: defective oxidation of phytanic acid in tissue cultures derived from homozygotes and heterozygotes. *N Engl J Med* 1969;281:1034–8.
128. Steinberg D, Mize CE, Avigan J, et al. Studies on the metabolic error in Refsum's disease. *J Clin Invest* 1967;46:313–22.
129. Shorland FB, Hansen RP, Prior IAM. The effect of phytanic acid on the fatty acid composition of the lipids of the rat with further observations on its metabolism. In: *Proceedings of the seventh international congress on nutrition*, vol 5. Braunschweig, FRG: Vieweg & Sohn, 1966:399–405.
130. Mohrhauer H, Holman R. Alteration of the fatty acid composition of brain lipids by varying level of dietary essential fatty acids. *J Neurochem* 1963;10:523–30.
131. Cook HW. "In vitro" formation of polyunsaturated fatty acids by desaturation in rat brain: some

properties of the enzyme in developing brain and comparison with liver. *J Neurochem* 1978; 30:1327–34.
132. Strouve-Vallet C, Pascaud M. Désaturation de l'acide linoléique par les microsomes du foie et du cerveau du rat en développement. *Biochimie* 1971;53:699–703.
133. Purvis JM, Clandinin MT, Hacker RR. Chain elongation-desaturation of linoleic acid during the development of the pig. Implications for the supply of polyenoic fatty acids to the developing brain. *Comp Biochem Physiol [B]* 1983;75B:199–204.
134. Spector AA, Mathur SN, Kaduce TL, Hyman BT. Lipid nutrition and metabolism of cultured mammalian cells. *Prog Lipid Res* 1981;19:155–86.
135. Yavin E, Menkes JH. Incorporation and metabolism of fatty acids by cultured dissociated cells from rat cerebrum. *Lipids* 1974;9:248–53.
136. Yavin E, Yavin Z, Menkes JH. Polyunsaturated fatty acid metabolism in neuroblastoma cells in culture. *J Neurochem* 1975;24:71–7.
137. Robert J, Rebel G, Mandel P. Essential fatty acid metabolism in cultured astroblasts. *Biochimie* 1977;59:417–23.
138. Robert J, Rebel G, Mandel P. Utilization of polyunsaturated fatty acid supplements by cultured neuroblastoma cells. *J Neurochem* 1978;30:543–8.
139. Bourre JM, Faivre A, Dumont O, et al. Effect of polyunsaturated fatty acids on fetal mouse brain cells in culture in a chemically defined medium. *J Neurochem* 1983;41:1234–42.
140. Yorek MA, Bohnker RR, Dudley DT, Spector A. Comparative utilization of n-3 polyunsaturated fatty acids by cultured human Y-79 retinoblastoma cells. *Biochim Biophys Acta* 1984;795:277–85.
141. Loudes C, Faivre A, Barret A, Grouselle D, Puymirat J, Tixier-Viadal M. Release of immunoreactive TRH in serum free culture of mouse hypothalamic cells. *Dev Brain Res* 1983;9:231–4.
142. Sinclair AJ. Incorporation of radioactive polyunsaturated fatty acids into liver and brain of the developing rat. *Lipids* 1975;10:175–84.
143. Walker BL. Maternal diet and brain fatty acids in young rats. *Lipids* 1967;2:497–500.
144. Morand O, Chanez C, Masson M, et al. Intrauterine growth retardation (malnutrition by vascular ligation) induces modifications in fatty acid composition of neurons and oligodendrocytes. *J Neurochem* 1981;226:235–44.
145. Morand O, Chanez C, Masson M, et al. Alteration in fatty acid composition of neurons, astrocytes, oligodendrocytes, myelin and synaptosomes in intrauterine malnutrition in rat. *Ann Nutr Metab* 1982;26:111–20.
146. Krigman MR, Hogan EL. Undernutrition in the developing rat: effect upon myelination. *Brain Res* 1976;107:239–55.
147. Menon NK, Moore C, Dhopeshwarkar A. Effect of essential fatty acid deficiency on maternal, placenta and fetal rat tissues. *J Nutr* 1981;111:1602–10.
148. Paoletti R, Galli C. Effects of essential fatty acid deficiency on the central nervous system in the growing rat. In: *Lipids, malnutrition and the developing brain (Ciba Found Symp.)* Amsterdam: Elsevier, 1972;121–140.
149. Holman RT. Essential fatty acid deficiency. In: Holman RT, ed. *Progress in the chemistry of fats and other lipids*, vol 9, part 2. Oxford: Pergamon Press, 1968:279.
150. Galli C, Treciak H, Paoletti R. Effects of dietary fatty acids on the fatty acid composition of brain ethanolamine-phosphoglyceride: reciprocal replacement of n-6 and n-3 polyunsaturated fatty acids. *Biochim Biophys Acta* 1971;248:449–54.
151. Lampley M, Walker B. Learning behaviour and brain lipid composition in rats subjected to essential fatty acids deficiency during gestation, lactation and growth. *J Nutrition* 1978;108:358–67.
152. Miller S, Klurfeld D, Weinsweig D, Kritchevsky D. Effect of essential fatty acid deficiency on the synthesis and turnover of myelin lipids. *J Neurosci Res* 1981;6:203–10.
153. Miller S, Klurfeld D, Lotfus B, Kritchevsky D. Effect of essential fatty acid deficiency on myelin proteins. *Lipids* 1984;19:478–80.
154. Alling C, Bruce A, Karlsson I, Svennerholm L. The effects of different dietary levels of essential fatty acids on lipids of rat cerebrum during maturation. J Neurochem 1974;23:1263–70.
155. Crawford MA, Hassam AG, Stevens PA. Essential fatty acid requirements in pregnancy and lactation with special reference to brain development. *Prog Lipid Res* 1981;20:31–40.
156. Dhopeshwarkar GA, Mead JF. Uptake and transport of fatty acids into the brain and the role of the blood-brain barrier system. In: Paoletti R, Kritchevsky D, eds. *Advances in lipid research*, vol 11. New York: Academic Press, 1973:109–42.

157. Lampley M, Walker BK. A possible essential role for dietary linolenic acid in the development of the young rat. *J Nutr* 1976;106:86–93.
158. Sanders TAB, Naismith DJ. The metabolism of α-linolenic acid by the fetal rat. *Br J Nutr* 1980;44:205–8.
159. Sinclair AJ, Crawford MA. The accumulation of arachidonate and docosahexaenoate in the developing rat brain. *J Neurochem* 1972;19:1753–8.
160. Svennerholm L, Alling C, Bruce Å, Karlsson I, Sapia O. Effect on offspring of maternal malnutrition in the rat. In: *Lipids, malnutrition and the developing brain (Ciba Found Symp)*. Amsterdam: Elsevier, 1972;141–57.
161. Samulski M, Walker B. Maternal dietary fat and polyunsaturated fatty acids in the developing fetal rat brain. *J Neurochem* 1982;39:1163–8.
162. Bourre JM, Pascal G, Durand G, Masson M, Dumont O, Piciotti M. Alterations in the fatty acid composition of rat brain cells (neurons, astrocytes and oligodendrocytes) and of sub-cellular fractions (myelin and synaptosomes) induced by a diet devoid of n-3 fatty acids. *J Neurochem* 1984;43:342–8.
163. Foot M, Cruz TF, Clandinin MT. Influence of dietary fat on the lipid composition of rat brain synaptosomal and microsomal membranes. *Biochem J* 1982;208:631–40.
164. Nouvelot A, Bourre JM, Sezille G, Dewailly P, Jaillard J. Changes in the fatty acid patterns of brain phospholipids during development of rats fed peanut or rapeseed oil, taking into account differences between milk and maternal food. *Ann Nutr Metab* 1983;27:173–81.
165. Nouvelot A, Dedonder-Decoopman E, Sezille G, et al. Influence de la teneur en acide linolénique du régime maternel sur la composition en acides gras polyinsaturés des fractions subcellulaires au cours du développement cérébral chez le rat. *Ann Nutr Metab* 1983;27:233 41.
166. Youyou A, Durand G, Pascal G, Piciotti M, Dumont O, Bourre JM. Recovery of altered fatty acid composition induced by a diet devoid of n-3 fatty acids in myelin, synaptosomes, mitochondria and microsomes in developing rat brain. *J Neurochem* 1986;46:224–8.
167. Fiennes RN, Sinclair AJ, Crawford MA. Essential fatty acid studies in primates: linolenic acid requirements of capuchins. *J Med Primatol* 1973;2:155–69.
168. Holman RT, Johnson SB, Hatch TF. A case of human linolenic acid deficiency involving neurological abnormalities. *Am J Clin Nutr* 1982;35:617–23.
169. Rudin DO. The dominant diseases of modernized societies as omega-3 essential fatty acid deficiency syndrome: substrate beriberi. *Med Hypotheses* 1982;8:17–47
170. Neuringer M, Connor WE, Van Petten C, Barstad L. Dietary omega-3 fatty acid deficiency and visual loss in infant rhesus monkeys. *J Clin Invest* 1984;73:272–6.
171. Dedonder E, Nouvelot A, Dewailly P, Bourre JM. Influence du taux des acides gras de la série n-3 sur la composition et le fonctionnement de la rétine chez le rat. *Cah Nutr Diét* 1985;20:123–5.
172. Berhsohn J, Spitz FJ. Linoleic and linolenic acid dependency of some brain membrane-bound enzymes after lipid deprivation in rats. *Biochem Biophys Res Commun* 1974;57:293–8.
173. Brown ML, Marshall LA, Johnston PV. Alterations in cerebral and microvascular prostaglandin synthesis by manipulation of dietary essential fatty acids. *J Neurochem* 1984;43:1392–400.
174. Tinoco J, Babcock R, Hincenbergs I, Medwadowski B. Linolenic acid deficiency. *Lipids* 1979;14:166–73.
175. Nouvelot A, Delbart C, Bourre JM. Hepatic metabolism of dietary alpha-linolenic acid in suckling rats, and its possible importance in polyunsaturated fatty acid uptake by the brain. *Ann Nutr Metab* 1986;30:316–23.
176. Stubbs CD, Smith AD. The modification of mammalian membrane polyunsaturated fatty acid composition in relation to membrane fluidity and function. *Biochim Biophys Acta* 1971;248:449–54.
177. Clandinin M, Foot M, Robson L. Plasma membrane: can its structure and function be modulated by dietary fat? *Comp Biochem Physiol* 1983;76:335–9.
178. Horrobin DF. Loss of delta-6-desaturase activity as a key factor in aging. *Med Hypotheses* 1981;7:1211–20.
179. Smith S, Watts R, Dils R. Quantitative gas liquid chromatographic analysis of rodent milk triglycerides. *J Lipid Res* 1968;9:52–7.
180. Galli C, Spagnulo C, Agradi E, Paoletti R. Comparative effects of olive oil and other edible fats on brain structural lipids during development. In: Paoletti R, Porcellati G, Jacini G, eds. *Lipids, vol 1. Biochemistry*. New York: Raven Press, 1976:237–43.

181. Crawford MA, Sinclair AJ, Msuya PM, Munhambo A. Structural lipids and their polyenoic constituents in human milk. In: Galli C, Jacini G, Pecile A, eds. *Dietary lipids and postnatal development*. New York: Raven Press, 1973:41–56.
182. Harris WS, Connor WE, Lindsey S. Will dietary ω-3 fatty acids change the composition of human milk? *Am J Clin Nutr* 1984;40:780–5.
183. Ellis S, Sanders T. Long chain polyunsaturated fatty acid in endogenous depression. *J Neurol Neurosurg Psychiatry* 1977;40:168–9.
184. Horrobin DF. Multiple sclerosis: the rational basis for treatment with colchicin and evening primrose oil. *Med Hypotheses* 1979;5:365–78.
185. Bates D. Polyunsaturated fatty acid in treatment of acute remitting multiple sclerosis. *Br Med J* 1978;2:1390–1.
186. Singh I, Moser HW, Moser AB, Kishimoto Y. Adrenoleukodystrophy: impaired oxidation of long chain fatty acids in cultured skin fibroblasts and adrenal cortex. *Biochem Biophys Res Commun* 1981;102:1223–9.
187. Singh I, Moser AE, Goldfischer S, Moser HW. Lignoceric acid is oxidized in the peroxisome: implications for the Zellweger cerebro-hepato-renal syndrome and adrenoleukodystrophy. *Proc Natl Acad Sci USA* 1984;81:4203–7.
188. Berger B. Quelques aspects ultrastructuraux de la substance blanche chez la souris quaking. *Brain Res* 1971;25:35–53.
189. Privat A, Jacque C, Bourre JM, Dupouey P, Baumann N. Absence of the major dense line in myelin of the mutant mouse "shiverer". *Neurosci Lett* 1979;12:107–12.
190. Bourre JM, Boiron F, Boutry JM, et al. Biochemical aspects of the trembler mouse (dysmelinating mutant of the peripheral nervous system with onion bulb proliferation). In: Seatrice G, ed. *Neuromuscular diseases*. New York: Raven Press, 1984:237–46.
191. Bourre JM, Pollet S, Paturneau-Jouas M, Baumann N. Myelin consists of a continuum of particles of different density with varying lipid composition: major differences are found between normal mice and quaking mutant. *Biochimie* 1977;59:819–24.
192. Waehneldt TV, Lane JD. Dissociation of myelin from its enzyme markers during ontogeny. *J Neurochem* 1980;35:566–73.
193. Bourre JM, Jacque C, Delassalle A, et al. Density profile and basic protein measurements in the myelin range of particulate material from normal developing mouse brain and from neurological mutants (Jimpy, Quaking, Trembler, Shiverer and its MLD allele) obtained by zonal centrifugation. *J Neurochem* 1980;35:458–64.
194. Bourre JM, Haltia M, Daudu O, Monge M, Baumann N. Infantile form of so-called neuronal ceroid-lipofuscinosis: lipid biochemical studies, fatty acid analysis of cerebrosides, sulfatides and sphingomyelin; myelin density profile and lipid composition. *Eur Neurol* 1979;18:312–21.

DISCUSSION

Dr. Dubowitz: How do you know that when you ligate the uterine artery to produce delayed myelination the process is the same as in undernutrition? Ligation of the uterine artery could easily produce ischemia of the brain, as shown earlier by Dr. Evrard. Can you produce delayed myelination postnatally by ischemic lesions, and if so, what is the mechanism?

Dr. Bourre: These are good points. I do not know the answer, but I would accept that hypoxia or some other mechanism may be involved. However, the point is that when you interfere with intrauterine growth in this way in the rat you produce abnormal myelination without any recovery, whereas in postnatal malnutrition, although you also produce abnormal myelination, recovery can nevertheless occur. Remember that in the rat myelination is continuing throughout life, in contrast to the human, so if no recovery occurs in the rat the effect must be even more dramatic for a species in which myelination does not proceed throughout life.

Dr. Minkowski: Fetal and neonatal physiology texts state that reduction of uterine artery blood flow is one of the best ways to produce undernutrition, and there are many examples of its use. It is worth emphasizing that you get similar results in the fetus by uterine artery ligation as you do by maternal protein deprivation. There are many ways in which the effects of reducing blood flow to the fetus closely resemble the effects of undernutrition. It is true, however, that there is likely to be more sparing of the brain in undernutrition than in blood flow reduction, so the question remains open for discussion.

Dr. Martinez: When considering the two main families of fatty acids, do you think it is only the proportion that matters, or do the absolute amounts also have an influence? If so, what do you consider to be the optimal amounts? We studied a group of children receiving parenteral nutrition and although the proportions were right there was an extremely high concentration of linoleic acid, and the cianoic acid in the liver was reduced to half the normal.

Dr. Bourre: It is difficult to give an answer to this point. We need to know the minimum amount of dietary polyunsaturated fat that is compatible with normal brain membranes. We are currently trying to determine this in the rat, but nobody currently knows the minimum intake of polyunsaturates or the proportion between the two series necessary to get normal brain membranes.

Dr. Ballabriga: In humans it appears that the brain is very resistant to changes occurring because of fatty acid overload, for example, during parenteral nutrition. The study of phosphoglycerides in brain homogenates after prolonged parenteral nutrition shows only minor alterations in the choline phosphoglyceride:ethanolamine phosphoglyceride ratio, in contrast to major changes occurring in aorta, red cells, or liver. It seems that the brain is resistant to change in this respect, either as the result of fatty acid deficiency or of overload.

Dr. Bourre: The brain is heavily protected, but it has to be taken into account that the turnover of phospholipids in, for example, the myelin sheath is extremely low. It takes months for changes to be registered; thus the fatty acids acquired by phospholipids during brain development will be retained over a long period of time, and these fatty acids will be reutilized to synthesize other phospholipids. This means that, although there is considerable resistance to dietary aberrations, there is also extremely slow recovery if a defect has occurred; for example, it takes months for the brain of an animal to recover after a period of feeding with a diet deficient in linolenic acid.

Dr. Ballabriga: I think that the turnover is likely to change with age. For instance, when you change the diet of a neonate by introducing large quantities of linoleic acid the composition of subcutaneous fat changes in about 10 days, whereas in an adult it may take 3 months.

Dr. Campagnoni: Why is it only regarded as important if these lipid ratios change rapidly and by a large amount? Perhaps a small change in ratios in the brain may have an important effect on its function. We keep hearing that the brain is protected. Please explain to me how it is protected!

Dr. Ballabriga: I personally believe that there may not be any correlation between brain function and the sort of chemical change we have been discussing. We have observed gross biochemical changes in marasmic infants, with reduction in both galactolipids and plasmalogens, but normal myelin composition. It is difficult to determine in what way a particular biochemical alteration is reflected in particular clinical features. In malnutrition there are always factors other than dietary change and it is hard to determine the individual effect of each one of these factors.

Dr. Guesry: You say that what is important for myelination is not so much linoleic acid (C18) but more particularly the longer chain fatty acids C20 and C22. Can this finding be applied to the human infant? As you know human milk contains large amounts of linoleic and linolenic acids but only traces of arachidonic acid and no C22 at all. Is rat milk rich in C22, and could this account for species differences?

Dr. Bourre: I do not know the answer to this. However, I did not say that n-chain fatty acids were essential for the human, I said they were essential for the *brain*. Provided that you have an adequate intake of linoleic and linolenic acids, these are known to be transformed in the liver in young animals. What happens during aging, when the enzymatic machinery is drastically reduced both in liver and brain, is much less clear.

Dr. Martinez: In my experience human milk has more C22 than cow's milk. The amounts are small (about 0.5% C22 vs 1% C20), but C22 is nevertheless much higher than in cow's milk, which could have interesting implications.

Developmental Neurobiology, edited by
Philippe Evrard and Alexandre Minkowski.
Nestlé Nutrition Workshop Series, Vol. 12.
Nestec Ltd., Vevey/Raven Press, Ltd.,
New York © 1989.

Formation of Cerebellar Projection Maps: Development of Olivo- and Spinocerebellar Projections

Constantino Sotelo

INSERM Unité 106, Histologie Normale et Pathologique du Système Nerveux, Hôpital de la Salpêtrière, 75651 Paris Cédex 13, France

In spite of the apparent homogeneity of the cerebellar cortex, which is composed throughout of the same neuronal populations and the same types of afferent and efferent systems, the anatomical work of Voogd (1) and the electrophysiological studies of Oscarsson (2) have shown that the cerebellum has a longitudinal-zonal organization determined by the successive apposition of structurally and functionally distinct longitudinal strips. The specificity of each of these cerebellar compartments results from the precise pattern of its afferent and efferent connections, which constitute the cerebellar projection maps.

The study of the formation of cerebellar projection maps should provide some insight into the mechanisms underlying the acquisition of the longitudinal-zonal organization. This is the aim of a research program started a few years ago in our laboratory and carried out with ML Arsenio-Nunes, F. Bourrat, and M. Wassef. A summary of this research will be presented here, in relation to the following topics: (a) the establishment of the olivocerebellar projection; (b) the formation of spinocerebellar topography; and (c) the arrangement of Purkinje cells during their migration and subsequent segregation.

The rat was chosen as the experimental animal since most of the electrophysiological information concerning the development of olivocerebellar (3–5) and spinocerebellar systems (6,7) has been obtained from this species. Analysis of the immature organization of projections was based on tracing systems using autoradiography and peroxidase techniques. Purkinje cell compartmentalization was studied by means of immunohistochemical techniques with antibodies that specifically stain all cells belonging to this neuronal population in the adult cerebellum.

TOPOGRAPHIC ORGANIZATION OF THE IMMATURE OLIVOCEREBELLAR PROJECTION

The electrophysiological study carried out in Paris by Crépel, Mariani, and Delhaye-Bouchaud (4) indicates that synaptogenesis between climbing fibers (the nerve endings of all olivocerebellar projections) and Purkinje cells occurs postnatally in the rat, since the first functional synapses to be identified were observed in 3 day old animals (P3). Although of longer duration, these climbing fiber responses are already very similar to adult ones. However, they are not all-or-none in nature, as in the adult cerebellum (8), but are graded in parallel with increasing intensity of stimulus. By P15, the responses acquire their all-or-none adult character. The grading of early responses has been considered as demonstrating that during a transient period Purkinje cells have multiple innervation from climbing fibers. The analysis of intracellular recordings as these synapses mature (9,10) has allowed the determination of the evolution of multiple innervation. The peak of multiple innervation is reached at P5, from P7 to P10 an abrupt decrease occurs, followed by a slight decrease between P10 and P15. At this age, all Purkinje cells are monoinnervated.

In order to evaluate the presumptive influences of both synaptogenesis and regression (theoretically more important; see ref. 11) of the multiple innervation on the establishment of the olivocerebellar topography, we analyzed their organization in newborn rats (PO) before the onset of synaptogenesis, and up to 5 days (P5) when multiple innervation is maximal (12).

Before reporting the results, a brief description of the broad organization of the olivocerebellar system in adult rats will be given. As in the cat (13), this projection is organized in such a way that neurons in restricted sectors of the olivary complex innervate corresponding sagittally aligned strips of cerebellar cortex (14). First, the entire projection crosses the interolivary commissure; then the olivary axons ascend in the lateral aspect of the brain stem and enter the cerebellum mainly through the inferior peduncle. The caudal half of the medial accessory olive (MAO) projects almost exclusively to the vermis, whereas its rostral half projects to the flocculus, the paraflocculus, and a restricted portion of the paravermal zone (intermediate cortex). The ventral and dorsal lamellae of the principal olivary nucleus (PON) mainly supply innervation to the hemispheric cortex. The lateral portion of the dorsal accessory olive (DAO) projects to the paravermal zone (intermediate cortex) of the anterior lobe, and its medial portion innervates the intermediate cortex of the posterior lobe.

The results obtained from an experimental study using anterograde and retrograde transport techniques led to the following conclusions: Olivocerebellar fibers reach the cerebellum during intrauterine life, since these fibers are already present in the cerebellum at birth. At this age the small dimensions of the brain and its high water content make it difficult to restrict tracer injections to a single cerebellar lobule or to a defined olivary subnucleus. This situation allows only a rough estimation of the degree of organization of the projection, but it is sufficient to determine the distribution of olivary fibers within the vermal, intermediate, and hemispheric cortical regions. Thus, the vermal cortex receives olivary projections from neurons located in the caudal half of the contralateral MAO; the intermediate cortex is innervated mainly by neurons in the contralateral DAO, and to a lesser extent in the contralateral rostral half of the MAO. Finally, the hemispheric cortex receives most of its olivary projections from the contralateral PON and from the contralateral rostral half of the MAO (Fig. 1). This highly organized distribution is already identical to the adult olivocerebellar projection.

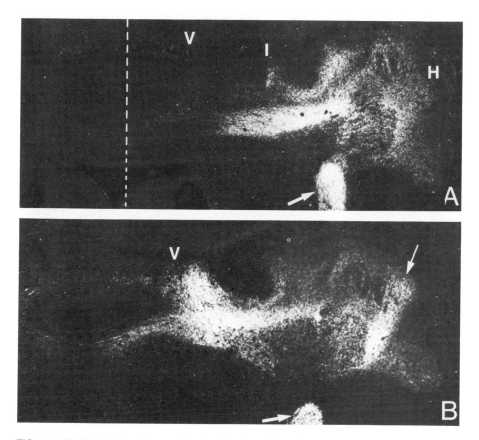

FIG. 1. Darkfield microphotographs obtained from autoradiograms of rat cerebella. The rats received left olivary injections within the first 4 hr after birth and were fixed 20 hr later. **A:** Lateral injection of the olivary complex mainly affecting the PON and the DAO. Labeled fibers penetrate the inferior cerebellar peduncle *(large arrow)* and span the prospective white matter of the hemispheric cortex (H) and part of that of the intermediate cortex (I). The vermis (V) is unlabeled. The dashed line marks the cerebellar midline. (Rat, R3-PO-1, × 36.) **B:** More medial olivary injection; the caudal MAO is partially filled. After entering the cerebellum through the inferior peduncle *(large arrow)*, the labeled fibers extend to the medullary zone. In contrast to **A**, labeling involves mainly the intermediary zone and the vermis (V). In the hemisphere, labeling is uneven and heavier in a sagittal band *(small arrow)* than in other areas. This band represents the initial stage of the sagittally aligned stripes observed in more mature rats. (Rat, R4-PO-1, × 36.)

In newborn rats, the bulk of the olivocerebellar fibers are arrested in the prospective white matter and only a few have invaded the overlying gray matter (Fig. 1). Therefore, these afferent axons reach their proper cerebellar territories before their appropriate targets, the Purkinje cells, have matured. As in other systems, such as the visual pathway (5), the arrival of a projection near a target structure is asynchronous with its definitive distribution to cellular targets. At PO, Purkinje cells have a smooth perikaryon and one or two long dendritic processes which, without penetrating into the external granular layer, can follow a long trajectory parallel to it. At P2

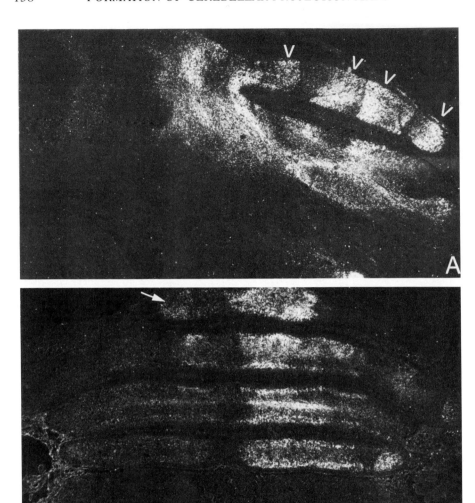

FIG. 2. Darkfield micrographs obtained from autoradiograms of rat cerebella. The rats received left olivary injections on the fourth day after birth and were fixed 20 hr later. **A:** Olivary injection partially involving the PON and the DAO. The MAO was almost unaffected. The most caudal and rostral poles of the olivary complex were free of labeling. Labeled fibers are absent from the medial regions of the vermis, but they are numerous within the hemispherical cortex, where they form bands of unequal width *(arrowheads).* (Rat, R8b-P4-5, × 34.) **B:** Left olivary injection involving almost the entire left caudal MAO and extending through the midline, contaminating the right caudal region. As a result of this contamination, labeled fibers reach the cerebellum through both inferior peduncles *(large arrows),* and a narrow, lightly labeled band is present at the ipsilateral side of the injection *(small arrow).* The massive involvement of the MAO explains the fact that most of the vermal cortex contralateral to the injection site contains heavy labeling. (Rat, R1-P4-5, × 34.)

to P3 these neurons lose their apical dendrites while numerous thin processes are formed and emerge in all directions from the cell body. At this stage of maturation, the climbing fibers establish early synaptic contacts with the Purkinje cells. Thus after arrival into the cerebellum and until their target cells attain certain developmental stages, these climbing fibers "wait" in the subcortical white matter.

By the fifth postnatal day (P5) the olivocerebellar fibers have moved from the prospective white matter towards the interface between the molecular and granular layers (Fig. 2), where Purkinje cells have arranged themselves into a monolayer. Although a more precise analysis of the topography of the olivocerebellar projection in these older rats is possible, no changes in the organizational pattern were observed. In P5 rats it is identical to that of adult animals (Figs. 2 and 3).

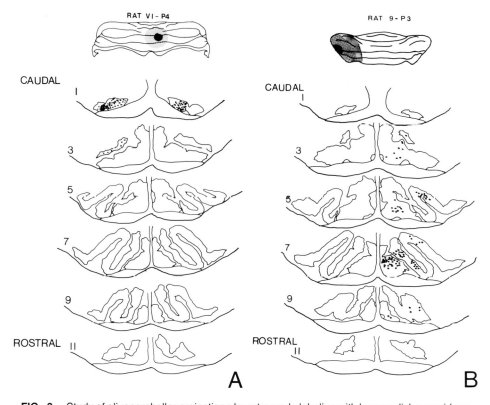

FIG. 3. Study of olivocerebellar projections by retrograde labeling with horseradish peroxidase (HRP). The zones of dense tetramethylbenzidine (TMB) reaction corresponding to the injection sites are indicated in black on the drawings of the cerebellum, whereas the gray areas represent the extension of the blue reaction. The retrograde labeled neurons are plotted on outlines of the inferior olivary complex. **A:** The HRP injection involves the vermis on the right side but also partially affects the left vermis. Consequently, labeled olivary neurons are present at both sides of the most caudal regions of the MAO. The rest of the olive is free of labeled neurons. **B:** In this case, the HRP injection involved the left hemispherical region and spread into the intermediate cortex and most lateral region of the vermis. Retrogradely labeled neurons are present only in the contralateral olive. They are disposed in patches mainly present in the rostral MAO, the ventral lamella of the PON, and the caudomedial part of the DAO.

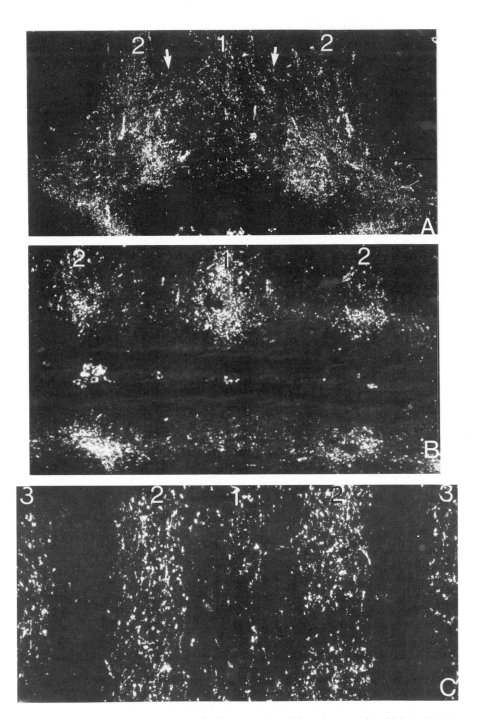

FIG. 4. Development of the spinocerebellar projections. Microphotographs of lobule III of the anterior vermis, in rats which received lectin-conjugated peroxidase (WGA-HRP) in the spinal cord (T12 to L3). (Polarized illumination.) **A:** Injection on P4 and fixation 24 hr later (P5). The WGA-HRP labeled fibers have invaded most of the granular layer and are organized in clearly

Therefore, neither synaptogenesis between climbing fibers and Purkinje cells nor the regression of their multiple innervation influence the acquisition of the topography of the olivocerebellar projection. However, this study is too coarse to provide the final cell-to-cell correlation that characterized this projection. It is possible that olivocerebellar specificity could be refined at the synaptic level within the cerebellar longitudinal zones during the selective processes of synapse stabilization and synapse elimination (11).

THE FORMATION OF SPINOCEREBELLAR TOPOGRAPHY

The spinocerebellar projection has been studied in various mammals, particularly in cats (1,16–18). Spinal axons end almost exclusively in the vermis, where they are distributed within two distinct areas: the anterior target zone, which is the most important and comprises lobules I to V of the anterior lobe; and the posterior target zone, which is restricted to lobule VIII. All spinal fibers terminate as mossy fibers in the granular layer, where they are segregated into five parallel sagittally situated zones varying in width from 200 to 480 μm and separated by terminal-free intervals of 600 to 800 μm (Fig. 4C).

Information on the development of this projection is scanty. Only recently Martin et al. (19) reported the first experimental study of the formation of the spinocerebellar projection. This work was carried out in a marsupial, the opossum, whose ontogenic calendar differs from that of the rat. Accordingly, spinal afferents reach the cerebellum on P7 and acquire their adult topography on P50. The precise stages followed by the intracerebral spinal axons to achieve their adult pattern were not analyzed.

Most of the electrophysiological information on the development of this projection is limited to rats. Analysis of field potentials evoked by white matter stimulation and aimed at disclosing the earliest signs of synaptic activity have failed to demonstrate functional synaptic transmission between spinal mossy fibers and granule cells before P10 (6). However, at P7 it has been possible to activate Purkinje cells after limb stimulation by inputs mediated through spinal mossy fibers (7). These results indicate that synaptogenesis between spinal axons and granule cells is achieved by the end of the first postnatal week.

Anterograde tracer experiments carried out in rats aged 0, 3, 5, 7, and 30 days (20) have permitted the conclusion that spinal axons reach the cerebellum during fetal life and that their ultimate organization is qualitatively attained by P7. Between P0 and P7 these axons must pass through the various developmental stages neces-

---

defined sagittal columns (1 to 2). Note the presence of some dispersion of labeled axons between the columns *(arrows)*. (Rat, × 72.) **B:** Injection on P6 and fixation on P7. The WGA-HRP labeled fibers are disposed in sharply delimited columns (1 to 2) separated by zones almost completely devoid of labeling. (Rat, × 72.) **C:** Injection on P29 and fixation on P30 (adult pattern). The labeled spinocerebellar axons are confined to five clearly delimited columns (1 to 3). (Rat, × 88.)

sary for the establishment of the adult spinocerebellar topography. A summary of these successive stages follows.

The Early Stage of Axonal Growth

During intrauterine life, spinal axons grow rostrally in the ventrolateral aspect of the lower brain stem to the inferior and superior cerebellar peduncles. Once in the cerebellum, these fibers only enter those areas where they are normally present in the adult animal, since transient aberrant projections were not detected. Thus, adult terminal domains correspond nicely with the "attracting" cerebellar zones for ingrowing spinal fibers.

The Intermediate Stage or Waiting Period

From P0 to P3 the ingrowing spinal axons remain in the prospective white matter, where they are distributed more or less uniformly. As is the case for olivocerebellar fibers, those emerging from spinal neurons also reach their appropriate territories before the proper maturation of their target cells (the bulk of granule cell proliferation occurs during the second postnatal week (see ref. 21), and wait in the medullary zone until a distinct granular layer is formed.

The Protocolumnar Stage

By P3 spinal axons begin to invade the cortical gray matter. Although Purkinje cells have not yet reached their final monolayer arrangement at this age, a nascent granular layer containing a noticeable contingent of granule cells already exists. The invasion by spinal fibers does not occur randomly, as they have a tendency to remain clustered within their ultimate terminal domains. However, the typical columnar organization of the adult projection is not yet observed at this early stage, since labeled fibers are dispersed to an important degree between the nascent columns, hence the term protocolumnar stage.

The Columnar Stage

From P3, concomitant with the rapid increase in the amount of labeled spinal fibers entering the granular layer, intercolumnar dispersion diminishes. At P5 the columns have almost acquired their adult appearance, although a low degree of dispersion is still evident (Fig. 4A). From P7, adult topography is totally achieved; the five columns are situated as in P30 rat cerebellum (Fig. 4B). Besides changes in cerebellar size, the only difference in the adult is quantitative (compare Figs. 4B and 4C).

Experiments with retrograde transport techniques indicate that spinal fibers invade the cerebellum in two successive groups. The first one, formed prenatally, contains axons from the central cervical nucleus, Clarke's column, the sacral nucleus of Stilling, and to a lesser degree, some border cells. The second group, which reaches the cerebellum between P1 and P3, emerges from new neurons in these spinal areas, especially from scattered cells of the spinal gray matter. These results indicate that the dorsal spinocerebellar tract matures somewhat earlier than the ventral tract, which mainly originates from the border cells (1F) and are in line with those obtained in the opossum by Martin et al. (1G).

Morphological analysis of synaptogenesis between spinal mossy fibers and granule cells requires the ultrastructural study of immature rat cerebella after tracer injections into the spinal cord, since, contrary to climbing fibers which originate from the inferior olive, mossy fibers are a composite population of which only a small part is of spinal origin. However, ultrastructural examination of the immature lobules II and III of the anterior lobe of the vermis, which permits the analysis of mossy fiber maturation in general, discloses indirect evidence of spinocerebellar synaptogenesis. Using this approach, we have identified mossy fibers establishing synaptic contacts from P5 (20). They appear as axonal varicosities partially covered by one or two postsynaptic dendrites and correspond to the primitive stage of mossy fiber synaptogenesis. By P7 the number of detectable mossy rosettes has increased and maturation has progressed. Here, mossy terminals in the primitive stage and in the cup stage (the most numerous) are intermixed with terminals already in the claw stage (see ref. 22 for the definition of these stages). Thus our results provide indirect evidence that spinocerebellar fibers may start synaptogenesis almost immediately after their invasion of the nascent granular layer, since by P5 primitive mossy rosettes bearing mature synaptic junctions are present in the terminal domains of spinal axons. Comparison of these morphological observations with the results of electrophysiological studies reported above indicates a time lag between the onset of synapse formation and the production of synapse activity, suggesting that synaptogenesis must be rather advanced before global synaptic activity can be detected. More important, the temporal correlation between the columnar organization of spinal axons and the appearance of mossy rosettes with mature synaptic junctions indicates that the process of synapse formation does not interfere with the organization of spinocerebellar topography.

GENERAL CONCLUSIONS

The results of the morphological reading reported here provide the developmental chronology of the olivo- and spinocerebellar projections in the rat. For both systems of afferents, the following conclusions can be made. Extracerebellar afferents invade the cerebellum during intrauterine life. At birth, they are arrested in the prospective white matter in a "waiting" period. Olivocerebellar fibers mature somewhat earlier than spinocerebellar. By P1, the former occupy their ultimate territories according to a topography similar to that of adult rats; thus at this age the longitudinal-zonal organization of the olivocerebellar projection already exists. Later, at P3, the spinocerebellar axons display an almost adult organization. Therefore, both projections undergo organization from the moment they enter the cerebellum, at a still undetermined fetal age, up to the fifth postnatal day. The ultimate topography of both projections is thus attained before the onset of synaptogenesis, indicating that this process does not influence the acquisition of general cerebellar topography.

TRANSIENT BIOCHEMICAL HETEROGENEITY OF IMMATURE PURKINJE CELLS AS A PRESUMPTIVE BASIS FOR CEREBELLAR COMPARTMENTALIZATION

Cytoarchitectonic analysis of the developing cerebellum has shown that the process of Purkinje cell migration and segregation ends in the formation of intracortical clusters. This clustering has been observed in many mammals, such as the mice (23), the rats (24), and humans (25). More recently, Kappel (26) was able to identify in monkey embryos nine longitudinal clusters in each hemicerebellum. She emphasized the topographical similarity between the pattern of Purkinje cell clustering in embryos and the adult longitudinal-zonal organization of corticonuclear and olivocerebellar projections. It is therefore tempting to consider that the embryological clustering of Purkinje cells could be related to the zonal arrangement of the cerebellar afferent and efferent connections in the adult (27).

With the aim of studying this hypothesis, Wassef (28,29) carried out an immunohistochemical analysis of early Purkinje cell clustering and differentiation. Among the known antibodies that selectively stain all Purkinje cells in the adult rat cerebellum, three were used for her study. The antibodies were oriented against: cyclic-GMP-dependent protein kinase (cGK) (kindly provided by Prof. Greengard); vitamin-D-dependent calcium binding protein (kindly provided by Dr. Thomasset); and Purkinje-cell-specific glycoprotein (PSG) (kindly provided by Dr. Zanetta). Between E17 and P5, Wassef observed a period in which each of these markers is expressed in an asynchronous manner by Purkinje cells (Fig. 5). Each antibody gives a reproducible mosaic of positive and negative Purkinje cell clusters, varying with age. Although the pattern of positive and negative clusters differs for each antibody, the clusters have common limits in some cerebellar areas. As in adulthood, all Purkinje cells react with the three antibodies by P5.

These results show that during cerebellar ontogeny a transient biochemical heterogeneity exists among Purkinje cells. Furthermore, they suggest that the synthesis of a whole set of proteins by these neurons is topographically regulated, indicating that the biochemical heterogeneity could represent an intrinsic parcellation of the cerebellar cortex. By definition, a basic cerebellar compartment contains identical Purkinje cells. Owing to the observed overlapping of differently immunostained clusters, the basic compartment must be the result of the intersection of several clusters which are positive or negative for various proteins. Therefore, the algebraic addition of the clusters displayed by the immunohistochemical staining of three proteins reveals that the presumed number of basic compartments must be much

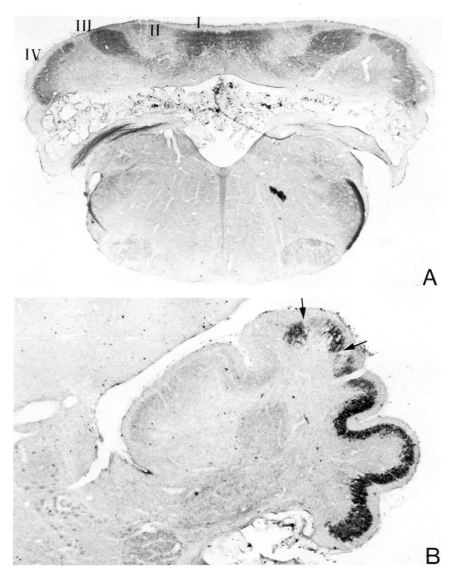

FIG. 5. Immunohistochemical staining of Purkinje cell clusters in the immature cerebellum. **A:** Frontal section of E19 embryo stained with cGK antiserum. This micrograph illustrates the biochemical heterogeneity of developing Purkinje cells as well as the size and distribution of the cGK-containing clusters. The cortical region is occupied by clusters of immunopositive Purkinje cells separated by immunonegative ones. The positive clusters are indicated by Roman numerals. There are four clusters in each hemicerebellum. (Magnification × 26.) **B:** Sagittal section of a newborn rat cerebellum stained with PSG antiserum. The biochemical heterogeneity of immature Purkinje cells is obvious: numerous Purkinje cells are immunostained in the posterior region, whereas the anterior one shows none. The arrows point to the border between positive and negative clusters (Magnification × 47.)

higher than the number of longitudinal zones and that their size, although varying throughout the cortex, must be smaller than that of a longitudinal zone. Therefore Voogd's sagittal zones (1) do not correspond to the intrinsic Purkinje cell compartments.

The fine electrophysiological analysis of Oscarsson (30) has provided evidence for a further subdivision of the longitudinal zones. His analysis, carried out in the cat, showed that according to the functional characteristics of climbing fiber inputs, zone B can be subdivided into five subgroups. Each of them is about 200 μm wide and projects to a different subgroup of Deiter's neurons. This result prompted Oscarsson (30) to postulate the microzone concept, that is, that the cerebellar cortex is composed of an assembly of sagittal microzones, 200 μm or less in width in the cat, defined by their specific efferent and afferent connectivity. Each microzone would represent a structural-functional unit, corresponding to the columns of Mountcastle (31) in the cerebral cortex. Until now the existence of microzones has been shown only in zone B (30) and in the flocculus (for further references, see ref. 32), but they most probably exist throughout the cerebellar cortex. Because of their average size and relatively high number, the microzones could correspond to Purkinje cell basic compartments.

Information obtained from immunohistochemical studies is still fragmentary and does not allow definite conclusions, but it does suggest the following. (a) A temporal relationship exists between the period of Purkinje cell biochemical heterogeneity and the period of cerebellar projection map establishment. As indicated by the analysis of olivo- and spinocerebellar topographical development, the extracerebellar afferents enter the cerebellum during fetal life and acquire their adult pattern by P5. At this age, the biochemical heterogeneity of Purkinje cells disappears. (b) The biochemical heterogeneity of immature Purkinje cells provides a basis for the intrinsic parcellation of the cerebellar cortex resulting from the differential expression of parts of the same genotype by Purkinje cell clusters. (c) The size and number of basic Purkinje cell compartments, as defined by the combination of the differently immunostained clusters, appear to be compatible with the organization of the cerebellar cortex as an assembly of numerous microzones having distinct efferent and afferent connections.

More work is necessary to correlate Purkinje cell compartments and sagittal microzones. However, as a working hypothesis, one can postulate that the intrinsic parcellation of Purkinje cells could provide cues for the afferent axons and orient their growth towards appropriate terminal territories. A possible, although not exclusive, explanation of the mechanism involved in the establishment of cerebellar topography is that the differences observed in Purkinje cell cytoplasmic proteins could indicate differences in plasma membrane proteins that would be reflected on the surface of the Purkinje cells in each compartment in such a way that they would be specifically marked, not only on the somatic plasma membrane but especially on the axolemma. Thus growth cones of the extracerebellar axons in the deep nuclear region could recognize Purkinje cell axons and follow them to their neuron of origin.

This hypothesis considers neither the mechanisms controlling the oriented growth of extracerebellar fibers nor their arrangement in the ascending tracts, the cerebellar peduncles, and the cerebellar central white matter. It supposes, however, that during the ordered growth of extracerebellar axons, they become organized to a certain degree. Once these axons reach the regions occupied either by migrating Purkinje cells or by the specifically displayed bundles of Purkinje cell axons, the somewhat broad topography of the olivo- and spinocerebellar fibers is refined by the above-mentioned mechanism of recognition of appropriate Purkinje cell bundles. Therefore, the ultimate pattern would emerge as the result of the confrontation between two distinct maps, one—related to Purkinje cell parcellation—more precise than the other. In any case, this hypothesis, which attempts to integrate different experimental data, proposes that Purkinje cells are the organizers of cerebellar topography.

REFERENCES

1. Voogd J. The importance of fiber connections in the comparative anatomy of the mammalian cerebellum. In: R Llinas, ed,. *Neurobiology of cerebellar evolution and development*. Chicago: American Medical Association 1969:493–514.
2. Oscarsson O. Functional organization of spinocerebellar paths. In: Iggo A, ed. *Handbook of sensory physiology,* vol 2: *Somatory system,.* Berlin: Springer-Verlag, 1973:339–80.
3. Crepel F. Maturation of climbing fiber responses in the rat. *Brain Res* 1971;35:272–6.
4. Crepel F, Mariani J, Delhaye-Bouchaud N. Evidence for a multiple innervation of Purkinje cells by climbing fibers in the immature rat cerebellum. *J Neurobiol* 1976;7:567–78.
5. Puro DG, Woodward DJ. Maturation of evoked climbing fiber input to rat cerebellar Purkinje cells (I). *Exp Brain Res* 1977;28:85–100.
6. Shimono T, Nosaka S, Sasaki K. Electro-physiological study on the postnatal development of neural mechanisms in the rat cerebellar cortex. *Brain Res* 1976;108:279–94.
7. Puro DG, Woodward DJ. Maturation of evoked mossy fiber input to rat cerebellar Purkinje cells (II). *Exp Brain Res* 1977;28:427–41.
8. Eccles JC, Llinas R, Sasaki K. The excitatory synaptic action of climbing fibers on the Purkinje cells of the cerebellum. *J Physiol (London)* 1966;182:268–96.
9. Crepel F, Delhaye-Bouchaud N, Dupont JL. Fate of the multiple innervation of cerebellar Purkinje cells by climbing fibers in immature control, X-irradiated and hypothyroid rats. *Dev Brain Res* 1981;1:59–71.
10. Mariani J, Changeux JP. Ontogenesis of olivocerebellar relationships. I. Studies by intracellular recordings of the multiple innervation of Purkinje cells by climbing fibers in the developing rat cerebellum. *J Neurosci* 1981;1:696–701.
11. Changeux JP, Danchin A. Selective stabilization of developing synapses, a mechanism for the specification of neuronal networks. *Nature* 1976;264:705–12.
12. Sotelo C, Bourrat F, Triller A. Postnatal development of the inferior olivary complex in the rat. II. Topographic organization of the immature olivocerebellar projection. *J Comp Neurol* 1984;222:177–99.
13. Brodal A, Kawamura K. Olivocerebellar projection: a review. *Adv Anat Embryol Cell Biol* 1980;64:1–140.
14. Campbell NC, Armstrong DM. Topographical localization in the olivocerebellar projection in the rat: an autoradiographic study. *Brain Res* 1983;275:235–49.
15. Rakic P. Prenatal genesis of connections subserving ocular dominance in the rhesus monkey. *Nature* 1976;261:467–71.
16. Brodal A, Grant G. Morphology and temporal course of degeneration in cerebellar mossy fibers following transection of spinocerebellar tracts in the cat. An experimental study with silver methods. *Exp Neurol* 1962;5:67–87.

17. Matsushita M, Hosoya Y, Ikeda M. Anatomical organization of the spinocerebellar system in the cat, as studied by retrograde transport of horseradish peroxidase. *J Comp Neurol* 1979;184:81–106.
18. Robertson B, Grant G, Bjorkeland M. Demonstration of spinocerebellar projection in cats using anterograde transport of WGA-HRP with some observations on spinomesencephalic and spinothalamic projections. *Exp Brain Res* 1983;52:99–104.
19. Martin GF, Culberson JL, Hazlett JC. Observations on the early development of ascending spinal pathways. Studies using the North American opossum. *Anat Embryol Ber* 1983;166:191–207.
20. Arsenio-Nunes ML, Sotelo C. Development of the spinocerebellar system in the postnatal rat. *J Comp Neurol* 1985;237:291–306.
21. Altman J. Autoradiographic and histological studies of postnatal neurogenesis. III. Dating the time of production and onset of differentiation of cerebellar microneurons in rats. *J Comp Neurol* 1969;136:269–94.
22. Larramendi LMH. Analysis of the synaptogenesis in the cerebellum of the mouse. In: Llinas R, ed. *Neurobiology of cerebellar evolution and development*. Chicago: American Medical Association, 1969:803–43.
23. Tello JF. Histogenèse du cervelet et ses voies chez la souris blanche. *Trab Lab Invest Biol Univ Madrid* 1940;32:1–74.
24. Korneliussen HK. On the ontogenic development of the cerebellum (nuclei, fissures, and cortex) of the rat, with special reference to regional variations in corticogenesis. *J Hirnforsch*, 1968;10:379–412.
25. Hayashi M. Einige wichtige Tatsachen aus der ontogenetischen Entwicklung des menschlichen Kleinhirns. *Dtsch Z Nervenheilk* 1924;81:74–82.
26. Kappel RM. *The development of the cerebellum in Macaca Mulatta. A study of regional differences during corticogenesis*. Leiden: University of Leiden, 1981. Thesis.
27. Feirabend HKP, Voogd J. The development of longitudinal subdivision in the cerebellum of the White Leghorn *(Gallus domesticus)*. *Acta Morphol Neerl Scand* 1979;17:238–9.
28. Wassef M, Sotelo C. Asynchrony in the expression of cyclic GMP-dependent protein kinase by clusters of Purkinje cells during the perinatal development of rat cerebellum. *Neuroscience* 1984;13:1219–43.
29. Wassef M, Zanetta JP, Brehier A, Sotelo C. Transient biochemical compartmentalization of Purkinje cells during early cerebellar development. *Devel Biol* 1985;111:129–37.
30. Oscarsson O. Spatial distribution of climbing and mossy fibre inputs into the cerebellar cortex. In: Creutzfeldt, O, ed. *Experimental brain research. Suppl 1. Afferent and intrinsic organisation of laminated structures in the brain*. Berlin: Springer-Verlag, 1976;34–42.
31. Mountcastle VB. Modality and topographic properties of single neurons of cat's somatic sensory cortex. *J Neurophysiol* 1957;20:408–34.
32. Ito M. *The cerebellum and neuronal control*. New York: Raven Press, 1984:189–99.

DISCUSSION

Dr. Roig: Are you suggesting that Purkinje cells can change their own enzymatic machinery, as for instance muscle cells do when differently innervated?

Dr. Sotelo: Not at all. What I am saying is that during differentiation of a given category of cells, you have subgroups of cells which express different proteins at different times. When Purkinje cells differentiate, they go through mitotic events and then migrate to achieve their cortical position, and then they develop dendrites. This is one way of looking at differentiation. What I am proposing is that you look at it with a different set of optics—immunological and chemical optics! Using these techniques it has been shown that within Purkinje cells, which form a big population of neurons, one parameter for differentiation is the genetic expression of a particular set of proteins, and this genetic expression is not synchronous for all Purkinje cells. We see then that proteins begin to differentiate for different sets of Purkinje cells at different times, which have nothing to do with the morphological differentiation. The particular interest of the asynchronous expression of these different proteins is that over a given time period you have biochemical heterogeneity, and this could be very useful in providing cues for the different axons to indicate where they should go in the cerebellum.

Dr. Campagnoni: Could you tell us about the expression of antigens by the Purkinje cells? Are they expressed at a particular time, and then no longer expressed? Or become re-expressed as an adult?

Dr. Sotelo: From postnatal day 5 until death of the rat the three antigens we use are expressed all the time. Our results indicate that when a given cluster of cells becomes positive for protein kinase they stay positive until death. During earlier development we do not know.

From experiments on cultured isolated Purkinje cells in the absence of innervation it can be shown that under these conditions calcium binding is expressed but not protein kinase. It seems that protein kinase is expressed by afferent fibers, mainly climbing fibers.

Dr. Mariani: Immunocytochemistry is a threshold method. Thus it is possible that there could be a quantitative regulation of the level of the protein by the afferents that would not be seen by immunocytochemistry. For example the level of calcium binding increases between postnatal day P5 and P30, but with immunocytochemistry it looks exactly the same.

Dr. Sotelo: If you put an isotope like tritium into an antibody you can use autoradiography and computerized densitometry to give you as effective a degree of quantification as with radioimmunoassay.

Dr. Mariani: It has been proposed that the Purkinje cells are committed by a small number of progenitors very early in development. Do you think that asynchrony in expression of proteins can be related to the different progenitors?

Dr. Sotelo: I think that is too speculative. We are looking at a much later period of development. What we are seeing at this stage is the neuroepithelium of the cerebellum, with much more dispersed stem cells to provide the Purkinje cells. What we want to do next, though I do not yet know how to handle this, is to investigate whether the heterogeneity in expression of these different antibodies has something to do with the columnar organization which is already expressed in the neural epithelium.

Developmental Neurobiology, edited by
Philippe Evrard and Alexandre Minkowski.
Nestlé Nutrition Workshop Series, Vol. 12.
Nestec Ltd., Vevey/Raven Press, Ltd.,
New York © 1989.

Do Serotonin and Other Neurotransmitters Exert a Trophic Influence on the Immature Brain?

*Michel Hamon, *S. Bourgoin, †C. Chanez, and ‡F. De Vitry

INSERM Unité 288, Neurobiologie Cellulaire et Fonctionnelle, Faculté de Médecine Pitié-Salpêtrière, 75634 Paris Cédex 13, France; †INSERM Unité 29, Centre de Recherches de Biologie du Développement Foetal et Néonatal, 75674 Paris Cédex 14, France; ‡Groupe de Neuroendocrinologie Cellulaire, ER CNRS 89, Collège de France, 75231 Paris Cédex 05, France

Monoamines have an important cerebral regulatory function in adult animals. Serotonin (5-hydroxytryptamine, 5-HT), noradrenalin (NA), and dopamine (DA) are central neurotransmitters involved in the regulation of major functions such as nociception, sleeping and waking cycles, thermoregulation, and some types of behavior (e.g., the 5-HT syndrome evoked by 5-HT agonists, or the turning behavior induced by DA agonists in rats with a unilateral lesion of the dopaminergic nigrostriatal pathway). In man, alterations in monoamine metabolism have been shown to occur in various neurological and psychiatric diseases such as Parkinsonism, Huntington's chorea, schizophrenia, and depression, suggesting that altered monoaminergic neurotransmission is causally related to these diseases (1,2).

The anatomical, biochemical, and electrophysiological characteristics of central neurons containing monoamines are now well known owing to the development of appropriate techniques since their discovery 35 years ago. Although serotoninergic, noradrenergic, and dopaminergic neurons are clearly distinct since they have different neurotransmitters and different functional roles in the central nervous system (CNS), the three categories of monoaminergic neurons also exhibit common properties. For example, their cell bodies are all located within nuclei in the brain stem (mesencephalon and metencephalon), and they send axons and collaterals to most brain regions. Thus monoaminergic (particularly serotoninergic and noradrenergic) nerve terminals are diffusely distributed within the whole brain. Such an anatomical organization is not unexpected since physiological studies have indicated that monoaminergic neurons exert a modulatory influence on various central functions but play no crucial role in the executive program of a given function (1,2).

Striking similarities also exist in the biochemical properties of the various classes of monoaminergic neurons since the synthesis of each monoamine requires only 2 to

3 enzymatic steps corresponding first to the hydroxylation of an essential aminoacid (tryptophan for 5-HT, and tyrosine or phenylalanine for NA and DA), and second to the decarboxylation of the hydroxylated product. This second step is catalyzed by the same enzyme, aromatic aminoacid decarboxylase (AADC, EC 4.1.1.28), in all monoaminergic neurons.

Finally, electrophysiological studies have also revealed common characteristics, since a uniform regular nerve impulse flow in the range of 2 to 8 spikes/sec has been reported for the three classes of monoaminergic neurons in the rat brain (3).

All these analogies suggest that monoaminergic neurons have a similar origin, and examination of their appearance during ontogenetic development further supports this concept since serotoninergic, noradrenergic, and dopaminergic neurons differentiate together in the early stage of fetal life in rodents. Histofluorescence and immunohistochemical observations indicate that neurons storing 5-HT or NA are detectable in brain of rats and mice as early as the 12th to 13th day of embryonic life (4,5). In agreement with such findings, De Vitry et al. observed recently that primary cultures from the brain stem of E12 mice embryos contain neurons able to synthesize, store, and take up 5-HT *(unpublished data)*.

Since the differentiation of monoaminergic neurons occurs about two days before that of most brain neurons in the rat fetus (6–8), several authors have postulated that such early maturation may be physiologically relevant, that is, that monoamines play some role in brain growth (8–12). This hypothesis is based mainly on pioneer studies demonstrating that 5-HT exerts a critical role in the early development of the sea urchin, particularly during the stage of gastrulation and for the formation of mesenchyme (13). In the case of the mammalian brain, pharmacological evidence indirectly supports the concept that monoamines, particularly 5-HT, participate in neuronal differentiation during early ontogenesis. Thus Lauder and Krebs (6,7) reported that the blockade of 5-HT synthesis by parachlorophenylalanine (pcpa) during fetal life in rats retards the onset of neuronal differentiation (cessation of germinal cell proliferation) in various brain regions, particularly those innervated by serotoninergic fibers. In addition, complementary pharmacologic studies have confirmed that psychotropic drugs which markedly alter the activity of monoaminergic neurons reduce brain cell replication *in vitro* as well as *in vivo*, even during the early postnatal period (14,15). However, pharmacologic evidence is often questionable since the drugs used may act not only on monoaminergic neurons but also on unknown targets, particularly at the high doses used in the studies mentioned above. This is true, for instance, for pcpa which has been shown recently to depress the rate of protein synthesis in the brain (Jouvet, *personal communication*).

We have reinvestigated the possible role of monoamines, particularly 5-HT, during brain growth by selecting two approaches. Since 5-HT has to act on specific receptors in order to exert any function, we first looked for such entities in the brain during early life, before synaptic serotoninergic neurotransmission is fully established. We observed that 5-HT stimulates two enzyme activities, adenylate cyclase and Na^+/K^+-ATPase, probably via the interaction with specific receptors not involved in the neurotransmitter function of the indoleamine. The second approach consisted of examining the possible effects of 5-HT agonists (acting on these specific receptors) on the maturation of brain neurons *in vitro,* with particular attention to those exhibiting serotoninergic properties.

CHARACTERISTICS AND POSSIBLE FUNCTIONS OF CENTRAL 5-HT RECEPTORS DURING EARLY LIFE

At least five classes of specific 5-HT receptors have been identified in the adult rat brain (16). Studies with labeled ligands have distinguished two categories of postsynaptic binding sites called 5-HT$_1$ and 5-HT$_2$. 5-HT$_1$ sites are characterized by their nanomolar affinity for agonists including 5-HT itself and are poorly recognized by 5-HT antagonists. In contrast, 5-HT$_2$ sites display nanomolar affinity for antagonists and only micromolar affinity for agonists. In addition, a third category of *postsynaptic* 5-HT receptors positively coupled to adenylate cyclase has been characterized. Pharmacological properties of the 5-HT-sensitive adenylate cyclase indicated clearly that it corresponds neither to the 5-HT$_1$ nor to the 5-HT$_2$ sites (17).

At the presynaptic level, two classes of autoreceptors have been demonstrated: A$_1$, located on cell bodies and dendrites, and A$_2$, located on the nerve terminals of serotoninergic neurons. These receptors participate in negative feedback processes controlling the activity of serotoninergic neurons. The stimulation of A$_1$ autoreceptors induces a marked reduction in the nerve impulse flow within serotoninergic neurons (18). Stimulation of A$_2$ autoreceptors causes a decrease in the Ca^{2+}-dependent release of 5-HT (19). These presynaptic autoreceptors are already functional at birth in the rat, suggesting that they participate in the control of serotoninergic neurons even during fetal life. Thus, Lanfumey and Jacobs (20) observed that stimulation of A$_1$ sites by 5-methoxy-*N,N*-dimethyltryptamine reduces the firing rate of serotoninergic neurons within the dorsal raphe nucleus as soon as electrophysiologic recording is possible, that is, on the third postnatal day. On the other hand, stimulation of A$_2$ sites by lysergic acid diethylamide (LSD) results in a marked decrease in the *in vitro* release of 5-HT from brain slices of newborn rats, as has also been observed in tissues from adult animals (19).

Postsynaptic receptors are also detected in the rat brain at birth but the density of 5-HT$_1$ and 5-HT$_2$ sites is rather low compared to that observed in adult brain tissue (17). During the postnatal period, the density (B$_{max}$) of these sites increases in parallel with the progressive formation of functional serotoninergic synapses in various forebrain areas. That these binding sites are directly involved in the neurotransmitter role of 5-HT is illustrated by the fact that their density increases following the selective degeneration of serotoninergic systems in the adult rat brain (supersensitivity phenomenon) (16).

Examination of the evolution of 5-HT-sensitive adenylate cyclase revealed a completely different pattern since the 5-HT receptors coupled to this enzyme are already fully developed at birth in the rat, and even well before birth in the guinea pig

(21). Therefore, in contrast to the 5-HT$_1$ and 5-HT$_2$ binding sites, the 5-HT receptors coupled to adenylate cyclase might mediate 5-HT function(s) different from those directly related to its neurotransmitter role, for instance a trophic effect during brain growth. Indeed, as expected for such a receptor type, 5-HT-sensitive adenylate cyclase is particularly active in the immature brain, and the product of this enzyme, cyclic AMP, is well known to promote neuronal differentiation *in vitro* (22).

In addition to adenylate cyclase, another membrane enzyme is modulated by monoamines. This is Na$^+$/K$^+$-ATPase, the key enzyme ensuring the maintenance

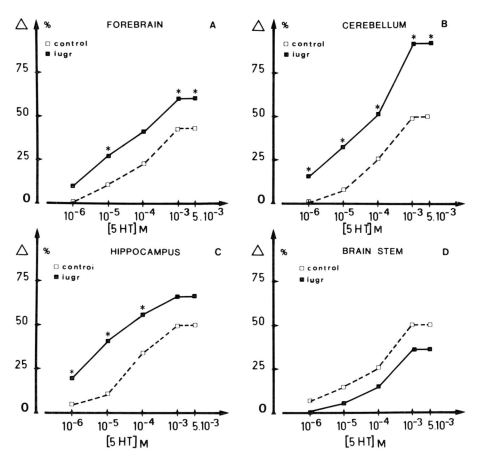

FIG. 1. Stimulatory effect of 5-HT on Na$^+$/K$^+$-ATPase activity in four brain regions from 21 day old control or hypotrophic (IUGR) rats. Intrauterine growth retardation resulted from the ligation of uterine vessels on one side in pregnant rats 5 days before delivery (26). Na$^+$/K$^+$-ATPase was measured in tissue homogenates in the presence of various concentrations of 5-HT as indicated on the abscissa. Each point corresponds to the relative increase (Δ%) over basal enzyme activity due to the addition of 5-HT to the assay mixture. Values are the means of data obtained in three independent experiments. Variations among them were generally less than 5% (24). ($P < 0.05$ when compared to the 5-HT-induced increase of Na$^+$/K$^+$-ATPase activity in the control group.)

of transmembrane potential in living cells (23). Studies on the effects of several 5-HT agonists and antagonists on the Na^+/K^+-ATPase in rat brain membranes have strongly suggested that the 5-HT-induced activation is due to the stimulation of specific receptors possibly coupled to the enzyme (24). In the rat, this putative receptor type is apparently fully functional at birth since 5-HT stimulates Na^+/K^+-ATPase activity in tissues from newborn animals as it does in adults. Dose response curves have even demonstrated that significant activation of the enzyme occurs with markedly lower 5-HT concentrations in newborn (EC50≤50 μM) than in adult (EC50≥150 μM) tissues, suggesting that the putative receptor controlling Na^+/K^+-ATPase activity is supersensitive during early life (24).

The possible functional counterpart of this supersensitivity may well be related to the trophic effect of 5-HT during brain growth, since convergent data suggest that transient alterations in Na^+ and K^+ fluxes (possibly due to changes in the Na^+/K^+-ATPase activity) through the plasma membrane might be involved in neuronal differentiation (22,25). Accordingly, 5-HT-induced stimulation of Na^+/K^+-ATPase activity during a critical period of fetal life would accelerate Na^+ efflux, thus resulting in an appropriate ionic transmembrane gradient for the genetic expression in neuronal 5-HT target cells. In this respect, the recent observation of altered basal and 5-HT-stimulated Na^+/K^+-ATPase activities in the brain of hypotrophic rats is relevant. Both a decrease in basal activity and an enhanced sensitivity of the enzyme to the stimulatory effect of 5-HT in the cerebellum, hippocampus, and the remaining forebrain of young hypotrophic rats born from a mother whose uterine vessels were ligated on one side five days before delivery have been reported (ref. 24.) (Fig. 1). Since brain growth is significantly delayed in these animals, one question to be asked is whether altered basal and 5-HT-stimulated Na^+/K^+-ATPase activities are responsible at least in part for this retardation. Experiments are currently in progress in order to test this possibility.

Thus such studies have confirmed that 5-HT receptors do exist in the rat brain even during early life. Furthermore, two of them, specifically those coupled to adenylate cyclase or to Na^+/K^+-ATPase, are apparently not involved in the neurotransmitter function of 5-HT but might well mediate the trophic effect of the indoleamine during brain growth.

THE POSSIBLE TROPHIC ROLE OF 5-HT DURING BRAIN GROWTH AND MATURATION

In addition to the indirect pharmacological evidence mentioned previously, data have been reported which support more directly the hypothesis of a trophic effect of 5-HT on brain maturation. Ahmad and Zamenhof (9) for instance observed that the weight and protein content of chick embryo brains increased significantly following the direct injection of 5-HT into the egg albumen. However, the 5-HT dose required for evoking such effects was relatively high (1.0 mg per egg) and undoubtedly far above those necessary for maximal saturation of any of the 5-HT receptors detected in the CNS. In contrast, this criticism does not apply to the study by Gromova et al.

(27) since these authors reported that the addition of a moderate concentration (20 μM) of 5-HT to the culture medium of organotypic explants of the dorsal hippocampus of newborn rats was sufficient to cause marked stimulation of neuropil development and synaptogenesis. Electrophysiological activity was recorded in an attempt to characterize the neuronal categories responsive to the differentiating effect of 5-HT, but the preliminary results did not permit precise identification of these 5-HT target cells (27).

This problem was therefore reinvestigated using a well-identified neuronal population (i.e., neurons with serotoninergic capacities) and reasonable concentrations of agonists and antagonists acting selectively on specific 5-HT receptors, in order to reveal any growth-promoting effect of these agents. These conditions were selected because marked alterations of serotoninergic neurons (26) had been found to be associated with significant modifications of the 5-HT-sensitive Na^+/K^+-ATPase activity already described in hypotrophic rats (Fig. 1).

The first experimental model examined the possible effects of chronic administration of metergoline, a potent and rather selective 5-HT antagonist, on the sprouting of additional serotoninergic fibers and terminals in the brain stem of rats treated at birth with the neurotoxin 5,7-dihydroxytryptamine (5,7-HT) (28). This treatment (100 mg/kg of 5,7-HT, subcutaneously on the first and second postnatal days) provokes both a massive degeneration of serotoninergic fibers and terminals in various forebrain areas and, in contrast, hyperinnervation of the brain stem by serotoninergic fibers growing out from cell bodies within the raphe nuclei. Chronic metergoline administration (5 mg/kg day, intraperitoneally for 3 weeks after 5,7-HT treatment) neither accelerates nor delays this phenomenon, indicating that endogenous 5-HT is probably not involved in the regrowth of serotoninergic systems following neonatal 5,7-HT treatment. However, this experiment was carried out during the postnatal period and was therefore of no informative value with respect to the possible action of 5-HT during fetal life.

In order to assess the possible role of 5-HT as a factor promoting the differentiation of neurons in the embryo, we first used a primitive nerve cell line, F_7 initially obtained by viral (SV 40) transformation of hypothalamic cells from mouse fetuses at embryonic day 14 (E14) (29,30). When maintained in the presence of serum (15% heat-inactivated horse serum and 2.5% fetal calf serum), these cells exhibit a flat morphology and are unable to synthesize or take up 5-HT. In contrast, when transferred to a serum-free medium supplemented with various factors including a brain extract from 8 to 10 day old mice, a C_6 glioma cell-conditioned medium, vasopressin, eye-derived growth factor (EDGF) (31), and LSD, the F_7 clonal cells become bipolar or multipolar with short neurites and exhibit the capacity to synthesize 5-HT from 5-hydroxytryptophan (5-HTP) and to take up exogenous 5-HT by an energy-dependent process (Fig. 2). Removal of either LSD or EDGF from the culture medium does not affect the capacity of the cells to synthesize 5-HT but the simultaneous removal of both compounds significantly decreases this capacity (Table 1). Such findings strongly suggest that the interaction of several factors, including

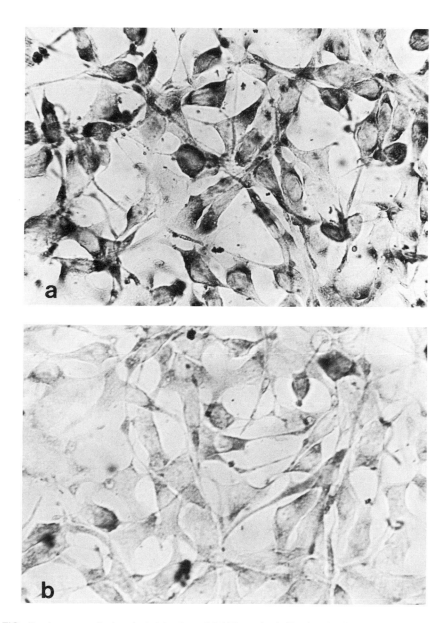

FIG. 2. Immunocytochemical detection of 5-HT uptake in F₇ clonal cells grown in serum-free conditions. Cells were preincubated for 30 min in the presence of 20 μM 5-HT before fixation. **a:** Immunostaining with 5-HT antiserum. **b:** Control with 5-HT antiserum previously adsorbed by 5-HT. (Magnification, ×480.)

TABLE 1. *Expression of AADC activity in F_7 clonal cells grown in serum-free medium (MSN)*[a]

Medium	AADC activity (nCi ^{3}H-5-HT/cult. dish)
+ serum	0 (nd)
− serum (MSN)	29.60 ± 2.06
+ Carbidopa (20 μM)	0.46[b] ± 0.09
− LSD (10 μM)	28.41 ± 2.17
− EDGF (20 μg)	28.18 ± 2.76
− EDGF and LSD	20.01[b] ± 1.12 (− 32%)

[a]Cells were first seeded at 3 to 4×10^4 cells/tissue culture dish and grown for 48 hr in MSN containing ^{3}H-5-HTP (0.45 μM), EDGF (20 μg/ml) and LSD (10 μM). Although removal of EDGF or LSD alone did not affect AADC expression, removal of both compounds resulted in a significant reduction in the enzyme expression. Addition of Carbidopa (20 μM) to the culture medium confirmed that ^{3}H-5-HT was derived from the decarboxylation of ^{3}H-5-HTP by AADC since the indoleamine synthesis was reduced by more than 98% in the presence of the inhibitor.
[b]$p < 0.05$ when compared to AADC activity in F_7 cells grown in complete serum-free medium.
(nd) not detectable.

the 5-HT agonist LSD, plays a critical role in the expression of AADC in F_7 cells.

A similar conclusion was reached from experiments with primary cultures from the hypothalamus of fetal mice (E 12). The serotoninergic pattern of neurons was easily detected by estimating their capacity to synthesize 5-HT from 5-HTP and to take up ^{3}H-5-HT by a specific membrane carrier sensitive to specific inhibitors such as citalopram and fluoxetine. Preliminary data indicated that the addition of a 5-HT agonist to the culture medium tends to increase the number of hypothalamic neurons able to synthesize 5-HT from 5-HTP, therefore suggesting that the stimulation of 5-HT receptors can promote the expression of the monoamine synthesizing enzyme AADC.

Recently, Teitelman et al. (32) observed that AADC is expressed in proliferating cells of the notochord for only a limited period during fetal life in rats. Whether this expression is also mediated by some primary action of 5-HT will deserve further investigation since, curiously, 5-HT is also present at this level for only a short period of time during embryonic development (8).

SUMMARY AND CONCLUSIONS

The early occurrence of monoamines, particularly 5-HT, in the rat brain during fetal life, well before their involvement in synaptic neurotransmission, suggests that these molecules exert some trophic influence on brain growth. In agreement with this hypothesis, two specific 5-HT receptors in the newborn rat, which are probably not involved in the neurotransmitter function of the indoleamine, were found. Stimulation of these receptors triggers the activation of adenylate cyclase and/or of Na^+/K^+-ATPase, thus producing an accumulation of cyclic AMP and/or an alteration of the transmembrane Na^+/K^+ gradients in target cells. Since such effects are likely to induce the differentiation of neurons and glial cells (22), it has been proposed that the 5-HT receptors positively coupled to adenylate cyclase or to Na^+/K^+-ATPase do mediate the trophic effect of the indoleamine during brain growth.

Attempts to demonstrate the participation of 5-HT-dependent mechanisms in neuronal differentiation were made *in vitro* using a clonal primitive nerve cell line (F_7) (29) and primary cultures from fetal mouse hypothalamus. Thus, the capacity of the clone F_7 to express AADC (the second enzyme required for 5-HT-synthesis) seemed to depend more particularly on the stimulation of 5-HT receptors located on these cells. Similarly the differentiation of cultured hypothalamic neurons towards the serotoninergic type appeared to be enhanced when a 5-HT agonist was added to the culture medium. These preliminary data suggest, but do not prove, that 5-HT can exert a trophic influence on the maturation of selected neuronal populations, at least *in vitro*.

Further experiments are necessary for the accurate assessment of the trophic function of the indoleamine during brain growth *in vivo*. For instance, one could examine the possible effects of the selective degeneration of serotoninergic systems at birth (by an intra-raphe injection of 5,7-HT for instance) on the maturation of neurons within central regions which develop principally during the postnatal period (e.g., the cerebellum in the rat). A similar approach has been successfully used recently by Robain et al. (33) who demonstrated the influence of NE upon cerebellum development. These authors observed that the selective degeneration of noradrenergic neurons induced by the administration of the neurotoxin 6-hydroxydopamine directly into the locus ceruleus of 3 day old rats produced a significant retardation in the growth of the cerebellum in subsequent weeks.

Although this chapter focuses exclusively on the possible role of 5-HT and other monoamines as trophic factors during brain maturation, it is clear that other neurotransmitters, such as neuropeptides, can also affect the growth and differentiation of selected neuronal populations during ontogenetic development. Substance P has been shown to exert a stimulatory effect on the outgrowth of noradrenergic fibers following their chemical degeneration by 6-hydroxydopamine (34,35). Convergent observations suggesting that endorphins may be involved as mediators for the control of brain growth in the embryo have also been reported recently (36).

Most neurotransmitters in the CNS thus probably exert a trophic influence on brain tissue, in addition to their well-characterized role in synaptic neurotransmission. Such trophic action corresponds to the main function of neurotransmitters when synaptic contacts are poorly differentiated, that is, in the immature brain; however, in the adult brain, the trophic function very probably persists and may account for the permanent remodeling of neuronal networks within the CNS.

ACKNOWLEDGMENTS

This research was supported by grants from INSERM (CRE to F. De Vitry) and CNRS (ATP to M. Hamon).

REFERENCES

1. Haber B, Gabay S, Issidorides MR, Alivisatos SGA, eds. Serotonin—current aspects of neurochemistry and function. *Adv Exp Med Biol* 1981;133.
2. Roberts PJ, Woodruff GN, Iversen LL, eds. Dopamine. *Adv Biochem Psychopharmacol* 1979; 19.
3. Svensson TH, Bunney BS, Aghajanian GK. Inhibition of both noradrenergic and serotonergic neurons in brain by the α-adrenergic agonist clonidine. *Brain Res* 1975;92:291–306.
4. Lidov HGW, Molliver ME. Immunohistochemical study of the development of serotonergic neurons in the rat CNS. *Brain Res Bull* 1982;9:559–604.
5. Hamon M, Bourgoin S. Ontogénèse des neurones monoaminergiques centraux chez les mammifères. In: Minkowski A, ed. *Biologie du développement*. Paris: Flammarion-Médecine-Sciences, 1981:118–51.
6. Lauder JM, Krebs H. Effects of p-chlorophenylalanine on time of neuronal origin during embryogenesis in the rat. *Brain Res* 1976;107:638–44.
7. Lauder JM, Krebs H. Serotonin as a differentiation signal in early neurogenesis. *Dev Neurosci* 1978;1:15–30.
8. Lauder JM, Wallace JA, Krebs H, Petrusz P, McCarthy K. *In vivo* and *in vitro* development of serotonergic neurons. *Brain Res Bull* 1982;9:605–25.
9. Ahmad G, Zamenhof S. Serotonin as a growth factor for chick embryo brain. *Life Sci* 1978;22:963–70.
10. Hamon M, Bourgoin S. Possible role of serotonin and other monoamines as growth factors during brain development. In: Monset-Couchard M, Minkowski A, eds. *Physiological and biochemical basis for perinatal medicine*. Basel: Karger, 1981:286–95.
11. Hamon M, Bourgoin S. Characteristics of 5-HT metabolism and function in the developing brain. In: Osborne NN, ed. *Biology of serotonergic transmission*. Chichester: John Wiley & Sons, 1982:197–220.
12. Lauder JM, Krebs H. Humoral influences on brain development. *Adv Cell Neurobiol* 1984;5:3–51.
13. Buznikov GA, Shmukler YB. Possible role of "prenervous" neurotransmitters in cellular interactions of early embryogenesis: a hypothesis. *Neurochem Res* 1981;6:55–68.
14. Patel AJ, Barochovsky O, Lewis PD. Psychotropic drugs and brain development: effects on cell replication *in vivo* and *in vitro*. *Neuropharmacology* 1981;20:1243–9.
15. Barochovsky O, Patel AJ. Effect of central nervous system acting drugs on brain cell replication *in vitro*. *Neurochem Res* 1982;7:1059–74.
16. Hamon M, Bourgoin S, El Mestikawy S, Goetz C. Central serotonin receptors. In: Lajtha A, ed. *Handbook of neurochemistry,* 2nd ed, vol 6. New York: Plenum Press, 1984:107–43.
17. Nelson DL, Herbet A, Adrien J, Bockaert J, Hamon M. Serotonin-sensitive adenylate cyclase and (^{3}H) serotonin binding sites in the CNS of the rat. II. Respective regional and subcellular distributions and ontogenetic developments. *Biochem Pharmacol* 1980;29:2455–63.
18. Aghajanian GK. The modulatory role of serotonin at multiple receptors in brain. In: Jacobs BL, Gelperin A, eds. *Serotonin neurotransmission and behavior*. Cambridge, MA: MIT Press, 1981: 156–85.
19. Bourgoin S, Artaud F, Enjalbert A, Héry F, Glowinski J, Hamon M. Acute changes in central serotonin metabolism induced by the blockade or stimulation of serotoninergic receptors during ontogenesis in the rat. *J Pharmacol Exp Ther* 1977;202:519–31.
20. Lanfumey L, Jacobs BL. Developmental analysis of raphe dorsalis unit activity in the rat. *Brain Res* 1982;242:317–20.
21. Enjalbert A, Bourgoin S, Hamon M, Adrien J, Bockaert J. Postsynaptic serotonin-sensitive adenylate cyclase in the central nervous system. I. Development and distribution of serotonin- and dopamine-sensitive adenylate cyclases in rat and guinea pig brain. *Mol Pharmacol* 1978;14:2–10.

22. McMahon D. Chemical messengers in development: a hypothesis. *Science* 1974;185:1012–21.
23. Schwartz A, Lindenmayer GE, Allen JC. The Na$^+$/K$^+$-ATPase membrane transport system: importance in cellular function. In: *Current topics in membranes and transport,* vol 3. New York: Academic Press, 1972:1–82.
24. Chanez C, Flexor M-A, Hamon M. Long lasting effects of intrauterine growth retardation on basal and 5-HT-stimulated Na$^+$/K$^+$-ATPase in the brain of developing rats. *Neurochem Int* 1985;7:319–29.
25. Messenger EA, Warner AE. The function of the sodium pump during differentiation of amphibian embryonic neurones. *J Physiol (London)* 1979;292:85–105.
26. Chanez C, Priam M, Flexor M-A, Hamon M, Bourgoin S, Kordon C, Minkowski A. Long lasting effects of intrauterine growth retardation on 5-HT metabolism in the brain of developing rats. *Brain Res* 1981;207:397–408.
27. Gromova HA, Chubakov AR, Chumasov EI, Konovalov HV. Serotonin as a stimulator of hippocampal cell differentiation in tissue culture. *Int J Dev Neurosci* 1983;1:339–49.
28. Hamon M, Nelson DL, Mallat M, Bourgoin S. Are 5-HT receptors involved in the sprouting of serotoninergic terminals following neonatal 5,7-dihydroxytryptamine treatment in the rat? *Neurochem Int* 1981;3:69–79.
29. De Vitry F. Growth and differentiation of a primitive nervous cell line after *in vivo* transplantation into syngenic mice. *Nature* 1977;267:48–50.
30. De Vitry F, Catelon J, Dubois M, et al. Partial expression of monoaminergic (serotoninergic) properties by the multipotent hypothalamic cell line F7. An example of learning at the cellular level. *Neurochem Int* 1986;9:45–53.
31. Barritault D, Plouet J, Courty J, Courtois Y. Purification, characterization and biological properties of the eye-derived growth factor from retina: analogies with brain-derived growth factor. *J Neurosci Res* 1982;8:477–90.
32. Teitelman G, Jaeger CB, Albert V, Joh TH, Reis DJ. Expression of amino acid decarboxylase in proliferating cells of the neural tube and notochord of developing rat embryo. *J Neurosci* 1983;3:1379–88.
33. Robain O, Lanfumey L, Adrien J, Farkas, E. Developmental changes in the cerebellar cortex after locus ceruleus lesion with 6-hydroxydopamine in the rat. *Exp Neurol* 1985;88:150–64.
34. Jonsson G, Hallman H. Substance P modifies the 6-hydroxydopamine-induced alteration of postnatal development of central noradrenaline neurons. *Neuroscience* 1982;7:2909–18.
35. Nakai K, Kasamatsu T. Accelerated regeneration of central catecholamine fibers in cat occipital cortex: effects of substance P. *Brain Res* 1984;323:374–9.
36. Haynes LW. Opioid systems and the developing brain. *Trends Pharmacol Sci* 1984 Sept:364.
37. Hamon-Bourgoin S. *Evolution du métabolisme cérébral de la sérotonine chez le rat au cours du développement [Thèse de doctorat es Sciences] Université Paris VII, 1976.*

DISCUSSION

Dr. Minkowski: In early life we are very much concerned with serotonin. It was through reading your wife's thesis on tryptophan (37) that pediatricians discovered that tryptophan was so high in fetal life, about eight times higher than in later life. Tryptophan is, of course, the precursor of serotonin, so I would like to hear your comments on why tryptophan is so high.

Second, the many actions of serotonin make an important field of study in human neurophysiology. Although it is very difficult to draw reliable inferences from measurements made in blood and CSF, there have been numerous if not very convincing articles in pediatric journals which claim that blood and CSF serotonin measurements are useful in various types of brain dysfunction. I do not think we have much idea at the moment of how to use serotonin measurements in the human. It would be nice to hear your comments.

Dr. Hamon: Tryptophan levels are very high in the brain and in other tissues in early life, but we have shown that this is merely the result of low serum albumin binding capacity.

Tryptophan is not transported free in the plasma. It is largely bound to albumin (about 80% bound in adults) and is the only amino acid in the blood that is transported in this way. In neonates, including human infants, albumin binding capacity is reduced for a number of reasons; as a result tryptophan is mainly unbound during this period, and increased concentrations are found in the brain and other tissues because of facilitated transport.

What is the importance of this? We know that tryptophan hydroxylase is the limiting enzyme for serotonin synthesis and also that serotonin synthesizing capacity is at a maximum in the neonate, perhaps because it may be an important trophic factor at this period. The ready availability of tryptophan ensures that tryptophan hydroxylase is always fully saturated and that serotonin synthesis can proceed as fast as possible. Tryptophan is also one of the rate-limiting amino acids for protein synthesis, so at a time when synthesis is very active it must be an advantage to have an abundance of this particular substrate.

Concerning the measurement of serotonin in blood, CSF, and so on, we know that any measurement at the periphery has absolutely no meaning, since serotonin is synthesized in tissues outside the CNS, in particular the gut. Platelets store serotonin; indeed, the serotonin in platelets may well be derived largely from the gastrointestinal tract. It is likely that about 95% of whole body serotonin is at the periphery, and thus peripheral measurements have no real meaning in terms of 5-HT in the brain. As far as CSF is concerned it is true there is a suggestion that the measurement of 5-HIAA in the CSF may reflect activity of the 5-HT systems in areas just below the surface of the ventricles or the ependymal canal. This kind of measurement may thus have some meaning, though it has not been well linked to pathology.

When you examine the topography of the 5-HT systems you find them located mainly in the midline of the brain stem. Since almost all areas of the brain are innervated from this region it is quite possible that serotoninergic neurons, and perhaps all monoaminergic neurons, are involved in modulatory actions and could affect other circuits which are directly involved in the execution of a given function. Thus the 5-HT system may modulate many functions without being directly concerned with the executive program of the function.

Dr. Mariani: I believe there have been some studies suggesting that serotonin may be a trophic factor in the development of the inferior olive.

Dr. Hamon: And probably also in the cerebellum although this structure has little 5-HT innervation. An important experiment yet to be done is to make a selective lesion of the 5-HT system just in advance of the arrival of the 5-HT projections in the cerebellum and then examine the effect on cerebellar maturation.

Dr. Sotelo: We have a better experiment. We have been transplanting pieces of embryonic cerebellum before serotoninergic innervation into a cavity in adult brain. We find no interaction between transplant and host, yet a beautiful mini-cerebellum grows, with foliated structure, laminated cortex, and deep nuclei, all in the complete absence of serotonin (checked with immunochemistry). If you transplant cerebellar tissue close to the hippocampus, there is massive invasion of the transplant by serotoninergic innervation, much more than in normal conditions. However we do not find any difference in differentiation of the transplant in the two sites.

Dr. Hamon: But maybe the differences are quite discreet. Experiments have been performed in Paris in which a low dose of 6-hydroxydopamine was injected locally in the locus ceruleus of 3 day old rats. This produced complete denervation of NE-containing neurons in the whole brain, including the cerebellum. The study showed that one week after the injection there was alteration in maturation of the cerebellum, particularly the Purkinje cells and the dendritic tree from these cells. I know there is a possibility of a nonspecific effect, but there was no evidence of alteration of blood–brain barrier permeability in this experiment, which is the most typical nonspecific effect of 6-hydroxydopamine, so I think the results strongly suggest an effect of selective disappearance of specific fibers.

Dr. Hanson: I agree partially, but do not forget that Purkinje cells need their inputs of whatever kind to build up the dendrite, and the absence of one of these inputs will interfere with normal dendritic development. This does not occur because of the release of substances acting as trophic factors but because of the interaction between the growth cones of the dendrites of the Purkinje cells and the climbing fibers, which molds the Purkinje dendrites.

Dr. Guesry: There is a proposal that the use of tryptophan and carbohydrate together in the diet will increase transport of tryptophan into the brain through effects on competitive transport, and that this will help young infants sleep by inducing serotonin formation. Since you have mentioned the possibility of trophic effects on the brain, what do you think of the idea of giving tryptophan and carbohydrate to neonates, particularly premature babies?

Dr. Hamon: As I mentioned before, in the young animal tryptophan is unbound in the periphery so the level of tryptophan in the brain is already quite high. We have shown that there is almost no effect on serotonin synthesis of injecting tryptophan in newborn animals to increase brain levels.

Developmental Neurobiology, edited by
Philippe Evrard and Alexandre Minkowski.
Nestlé Nutrition Workshop Series, Vol. 12.
Nestec Ltd., Vevey/Raven Press, Ltd.,
New York © 1989.

Biochemical Changes During Early Myelination of the Human Brain

Manuela Martínez

*Autonomous University of Barcelona, Hospital Infantil Vall d'Hebron,
Barcelona 08033, Spain*

The onset of myelination is of great interest in the field of pediatric nutrition because it is one of the critical periods of brain development during which nutritional influences may lead to neurological deficiencies. This is so because fundamental processes are proceeding at high speed in the developing brain during this period. Although myelination starts when the processes of neuronal proliferation and migration are well over, it coincides in part with the period of synaptogenesis. Therefore, although the basic ontogenic changes such as the number of neurons have already been completed by this time, the finest neuronal development and the formation of the elaborate circuitry characteristic of the more advanced species are still under way when myelination begins. Given the high velocity at which these processes take place and the high lipid content of brain, especially myelin, it is easy to imagine a special vulnerability of these structures to nutritional insults.

The enormous velocity of myelinogenesis during the period of maximum myelin synthesis is shown by the fact that in the rat each oligodendrocyte makes on average an amount of myelin more than three times its own weight per day (1,2). Since about 70% of myelin weight is lipid, there is no need to emphasize how important the lipid requirements of the myelinating oligodendrocyte must be to provide for such accelerated synthesis of myelin. It is therefore easy to understand that a nutritional restriction may result in a myelin deficit that may even be lasting, and such deductions have been repeatedly confirmed in the experimental animal (3–14).

The comparative scarcity of human data (15–17), even during normal development (18), prompted a biochemical study of the developing human brain during the vulnerable period in as comprehensive a way as possible. The initial objective was to trace the biochemical changes underlying the period of the brain "growth spurt" (19) in order to determine the precise moment at which the vulnerable period starts at a biochemical level. Cerebrum and cerebellum were studied separately so that data could be compared with those in the experimental animal. Since the animal studies suggested a preferential vulnerability of myelin lipids on account of their faster rate of accretion, myelination was studied in more detail, culminating in the isolation of the pure myelin fraction from the developing human brain. These stud-

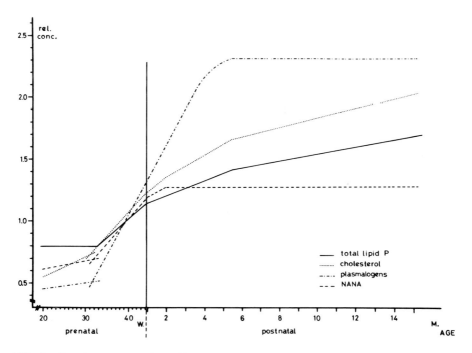

FIG. 1. Developmental profiles of four lipids in the human cerebrum. All the values are relative to the concentration reached at average term of gestation (the concentration of all the lipids is 1.00 at about 39 weeks). Note that plasmalogens are the lipids that increase fastest perinatally, multiplying their concentration by a factor of 5 in a very short period. (From ref. 22.)

ies revealed some interesting differences between brain development in the human and in the experimental animal. This chapter summarizes the main findings, with special reference to myelin lipids and myelin.

PERINATAL PROFILES OF MEMBRANE LIPIDS

Although the study of limited areas may be the method of choice in some situations, in the case of a developmental study in which profiles of several substances are to be obtained to trace the development of a whole region, the use of a total homogenate of that region is preferable. This was, therefore, the procedure chosen to investigate the developmental profiles of different lipids in the human cerebrum and cerebellum. The following were chosen for study: phospholipids and cholesterol as general membrane lipids, gangliosides as neuronal lipids enriched in synaptic membranes, and plasmalogens as membrane lipids relatively enriched in myelin.

Of the main parts of the human central nervous system (CNS) only the cerebrum showed a definite point at which the velocity of lipid deposition started to increase rapidly. The timing of this take-off point was eventually localized to 32 weeks of

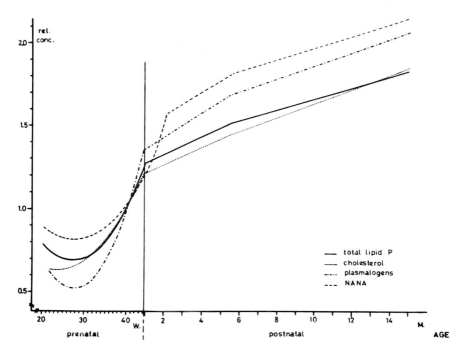

FIG. 2. Developmental profiles of four lipids in the human cerebellum. As in Fig. 1, all the values are relative to the concentration reached at term (1.00 at 39 weeks). (From ref. 22.)

gestational age (20–22). It can be said, therefore, that the "spurt" of membrane lipids starts at 32 weeks of gestation in the human forebrain. There is remarkable agreement between these biochemical data and the morphological and physiological findings of Purpura (23) in the human developing cortex, where this author found an explosive proliferation of dendrites, axons, and dendritic spines, reflected in a clear electroencephalographic change at precisely 32 weeks of gestational age.

By plotting the concentrations of these lipids in relation to those reached at term (Fig. 1) it can be seen that, although all four lipids start to increase at 32 weeks of gestation, their speed of accretion varies, being maximum for plasmalogens which are recognized as myelin lipids, although they are also present in many other cellular membranes. The lipid changes in the cerebellum are more gradual, showing a curvilinear profile of the parabolic type, without any definite point of inflexion, but starting to increase at about the same time (Fig. 2).

MYELINATION IN THE HUMAN BRAIN

To trace the profiles of myelination in the different parts of the human CNS some more specific myelin markers are necessary. Among myelin constituents, the most myelin specific are cerebrosides, the enzyme 2′,3′-cyclic nucleotide 3′-phospho-

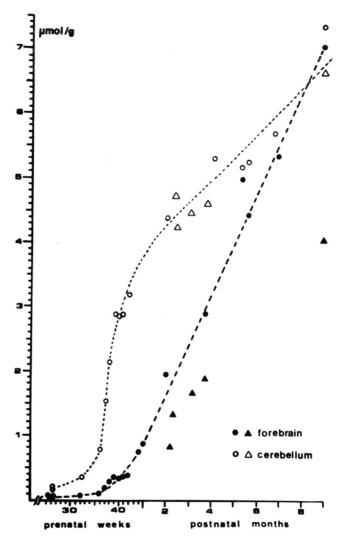

FIG. 3. Concentration of galactolipids in the human forebrain and cerebellum. The open symbols represent the cerebellum and the closed ones, the cerebrum. The circles (○, ●) represent normal, well-nourished cases, and the triangles (△,▲) represent the undernourished cases. Note the clear decrease in the cerebral concentration of galactolipids caused by undernutrition, especially marked in the most severely undernourished child.

diesterase (CNP) (EC 3.1.4.37), and myelin basic protein (MBP). The two first myelin markers were chosen because they could readily be determined in total brain tissue with a high degree of accuracy. Cerebrosides (together with sulfatides) were measured by gas-liquid chromatography of lipid galactose (24), and CNP was assayed by the procedure of Prohaska et al. (25).

These two measures (Figs. 3 and 4) show very similar developmental profiles in the forebrain as well as in the cerebellum, indicating their value as myelin markers. In the forebrain, galactolipids do not increase their accretion until very near term, the postnatal increase being enormous (more than 100 times between 36 weeks of gestation and 14 months of age). The cerebellar values are initially higher, as they should be in a CNS region that myelinates earlier, but after a fast increase before term the postnatal accretion is much slower than in the cerebrum. The CNP profiles also show a much higher postnatal rate of myelinogenesis in the forebrain than in the

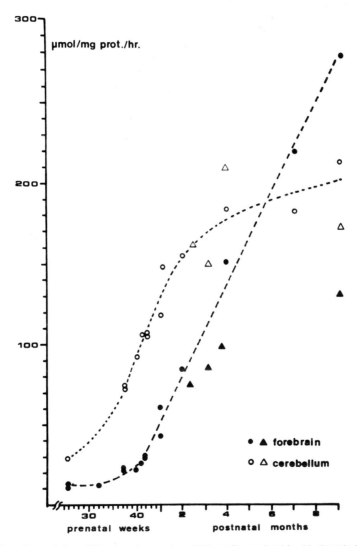

FIG. 4. Specific activity of the myelin marker 2′,3′-cyclic nucleotide 3′-phosphohydrolase (CNP) in the human forebrain and cerebellum. For definition of symbols, see Fig. 3.

cerebellum. These graphs seem to suggest that the cerebrum is more vulnerable than the cerebellum to disturbances of myelination in the early postnatal period. These deductions were checked in a few cases of undernutrition.

EFFECT OF EARLY UNDERNUTRITION
ON HUMAN BRAIN DEVELOPMENT

Ten cases of undernutrition were studied (26): three cases of intrauterine undernutrition (small for dates) and seven postnatally undernourished infants. Three of the latter were premature babies undernourished for a few weeks that died before reaching 43 weeks of gestation, and the other four were full-term infants undernourished as a result of chronic diarrhea for periods ranging between 2 and 4 postnatal months. Of all the parameters studied only those related to myelination, especially in the forebrain, were clearly affected by undernutrition. Thus plasmalogens were decreased in the cerebrum (Fig. 5) in all children suffering from undernutrition during the period of "biochemical spurt," to a degree directly proportional to the duration of the nutritional insult. The effect on the cerebellum was less than in the cerebrum and in the case of galactolipids it is remarkable that only the cerebrum was affected (26), in contrast to findings in the experimental animal (27–29). The values of the myelin marker CNP confirmed these findings, and Figs. 3 and 4 show the effects of early postnatal undernutrition on the developmental profiles of galactolipids and CNP in cerebrum and cerebellum.

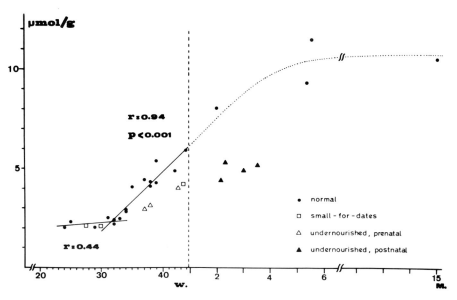

FIG. 5.   Normal values and effect of undernutrition on the cerebral concentration of plasmalogens. "Undernourished, prenatal" refers specifically to children born prematurely and undernourished *ex utero* during a period that in normal conditions corresponds to the prenatal period. (From ref. 26.)

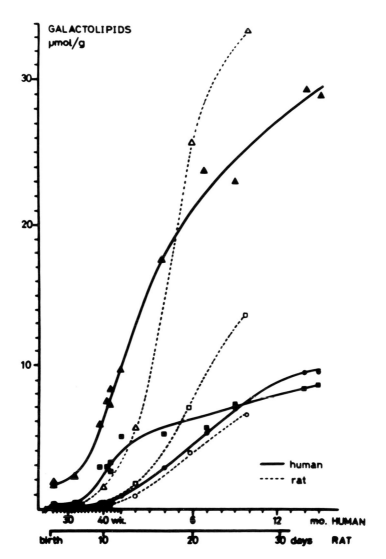

FIG. 6. Developmental profiles of brain galactolipids in the human and the rat. ●, human cerebrum ; ■, human cerebellum; ▲, human brain stem; ○, rat cerebrum; □, rat cerebellum; △ rat brain stem. (From ref. 26.)

These results are therefore consistent with the developmental profiles obtained in the normal human in that myelin lipids, which are the measures that increase most dramatically, are correspondingly the most affected by a period of coinciding undernutrition and proportionally more so in those parts of the CNS where the increase is fastest. However, why is there such disagreement with regard to the data obtained in experimental animals? It might simply be a matter of the different timing of myelination in different species. To answer this question the myelin lipid profiles of human and rat brain were compared.

MYELIN LIPIDS IN HUMAN AND RAT BRAIN

Figure 6 shows a comparison of the galactolipid profiles in human and rat brain, taking into account the different timing of brain growth spurt in the two species. There is excellent agreement between the cerebral profiles, but two important differences exist in the two other CNS regions. First, in the rat all the regions, not only the cerebrum, have very low values of galactolipids at birth (equivalent to 25 weeks of gestation in the human); and second, the other brain regions show an even faster accretion of galactolipids than the cerebrum. Consequently, it is not surprising that in the rat all the regions, and not only the cerebrum, have been shown to be vulnerable to nutritional deprivation (29). In the human, on the other hand, the forebrain is the only region that myelinates in an explosive way during the perinatal period, passing from negligible values in prenatal life to a fairly advanced degree of myelination, equivalent to that of the cerebellum, at about 6 to 8 postnatal months. Consequently, in the human species the cerebrum is much more vulnerable to nutritional insults occurring during the perinatal period than the cerebellum which, being quite advanced in myelination at this time, is relatively spared. This indicates that species differences are probably more important than has commonly been accepted and that simple extrapolation from one species to another is not always valid.

DEVELOPING HUMAN MYELIN

After tracing the timing of myelination and its vulnerability in the human brain the myelinating process was studied in more detail in an attempt to clarify the following: How does myelinogenesis proceed in the human being? Is the first myelin formed by the human oligodendrocyte qualitatively different from mature, compact myelin, as has been postulated for rat "early myelin" and the "myelin-like" fraction? The few researchers who have studied developing human myelin have provided very different answers to these questions. In particular, there is striking disagreement over the protein composition of human myelin at birth. According to Savolainen et al. (30) there is no basic protein at all in human myelin until about 6 months of age, and Banik et al. (31) find that only 0.5% of the total protein of newborn cerebral myelin is basic protein. On the other hand, Fishman et al. (32) report a value of MBP in the human neonate of 8.5% of total myelin protein, and Eng et al. (33) find that at 2 months of age MBP amounts to 16% of total myelin protein. As a consequence, all these investigators describe more or less conspicuous developmental changes in the protein patterns of human myelin.

The agreement is not much better regarding the lipid composition. Whereas some investigators (33–35) find clear developmental changes in the lipid composition of human myelin, similar to those reported in rat myelin (1,36–38), others (32,39) describe very little variation in the lipid composition throughout development. It is therefore of some importance to try to resolve these differences, particularly in the case of MBP in the human newborn.

Myelin basic protein is extremely labile, so one possible explanation for these discrepancies is variations in conditions and time periods of storage of the postmortem material used by different investigators. Another factor may be the methodological differences in myelin isolation. We studied these variables in depth (40,41) to try to determine the true composition of human myelin at the earliest stages of myelination.

Myelin was isolated from the cerebrum of three full-term newborns, a 2 month old infant, a 9 month old infant and an 8 year old child. Myelin from the forebrain of a 9 month old severely undernourished infant was also studied. Myelin was isolated from fresh brain in all cases.

We used three different methods of myelin isolation to determine whether the compositional differences in immature human myelin described by different authors could be attributable to methodological variation. Briefly, the procedures used were (a) the method of Norton and Poduslo (42); (b) the method of Agrawal et al. (43), with the purification steps as in the Norton and Poduslo method; and (c) a procedure consisting of two simple flotation steps from 0.85M sucrose (41), plus all the purification steps used in the Norton and Poduslo method. Since the main object was to obtain a myelin fraction as pure as possible from the newborn cerebrum, 1 mM ethyleneglycol-bis (β-aminoethyl ether)N,N'-tetraacetic acid (EGTA) was used throughout the procedure of myelin isolation from the most immature brains in order to minimize microsomal contamination.

A parallel study was performed with one of the brains (9-month-old infant) in which myelin was isolated both from fresh tissue and from tissue which had been stored frozen for varying lengths of time to look for possible degradative changes due to freezing and storing the brain tissue.

Morphological Appearance of Immature Human Myelin

The purity of the myelin fractions was of an equivalent, very high degree in all cases, including newborn cerebral myelin, the estimated microsomal contamination being always less than 5%, as shown in the extensive field of newborn myelin in Fig. 7. With high power electron microscopy profuse multilamellar images of compact myelin, with evident period and intraperiod lines (Fig. 8), were readily apparent in preparations of cerebral myelin from the human newborn. On the other hand, there were no loose membrane images of the myelin-like type, as described by Banik et al.(31).

Biochemical Composition of Developing Human Myelin

We found no differences in the composition of myelin attributable to the different isolation methods.

In concordance with the electron microscopy images, the biochemical composition of the myelin is characteristic of well-organized, compact myelin from the earli-

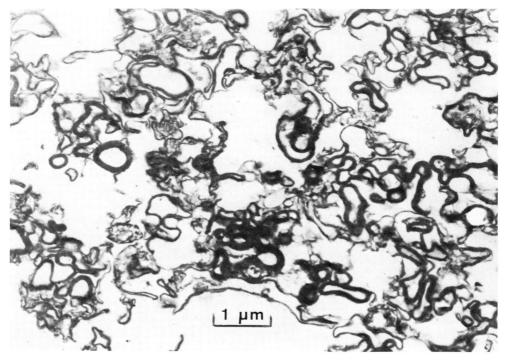

FIG. 7. Low power electron micrograph (magnification × 14,625) of newborn cerebral myelin.

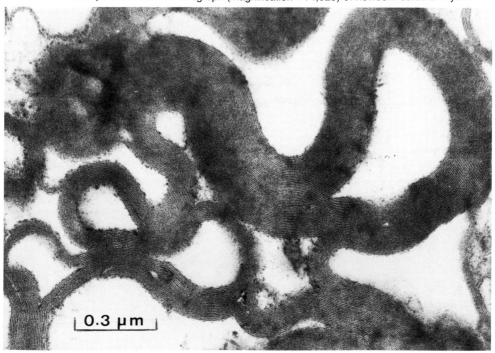

FIG. 8. High power electron micrograph (magnification × 80,250) of newborn cerebral myelin. Note the profuse multilamellar images of compact myelin, with evident period and interperiod lines.

est stages of myelination. Table 1 shows that the most myelin-specific components, such as galactolipids and CNP, are present in newborn myelin at substantially the same concentration as in more mature myelin. Although adult myelin is only present in one case, the only discernible trend is perhaps a decrease in phospholipids (including plasmalogens) and gangliosides in older myelin, in agreement with the tendency described by Fishman et al. (32).

Protein Patterns of Developing Human Myelin

The protein composition is also characteristic of compact myelin at all stages of development (Table 1). In particular, the high level of basic protein already present in newborn cerebral myelin is remarkable. This is illustrated in Fig. 9, which shows the disc gel electrophoretic patterns of myelin from three different regions of newborn brain. It is apparent that the level of MBP is very similar in myelin from the three regions, despite the very different stages of myelination of these regions at birth. This is further proof that compact myelin is formed from the start in the developing human brain. Thus it appears that developmental changes in the protein patterns of human myelin are very subtle, in contrast to findings in previously published work.

TABLE 1. *Composition of human cerebral myelin during development*

Component[a]	Birth,[b] well-nourished	2 months, well-nourished	9 months, well-nourished	9 months, under-nourished	8 years, well-nourished
Phospholipids	454	487	437	472	354
Cholesterol	458	489	465	482	527
Galactolipids	194	207	196	232	196
Plasmalogens	152	169	153	136	114
Sulfatides	46	44	52	44	48
Gangliosides	2.8	2.4	2.7	2.7	1.7
CNP	1214	1481	1306	652	1164
AChE	414	261	194	212	97
Total protein	24.6	25.2	24.6	26.0	29.8
MBP	40.0	38.9	46.0	47.5	54.7
Intermediate protein (DM-20)	14.3	10.6	5.3	5.9	4.0
Proteolipid protein	28.8	33.0	29.2	31.6	26.8
Wolfgram protein	16.8	17.5	19.5	15.0	14.5

[a]All lipid values are expressed as μmol per gram of dry weight (gangliosides, as lipid sialic acid); CNP, as μmol/mg protein/hour; AChE, as nmol/mg protein/hour; total protein, as a percentage of dry weight of myelin; and individual proteins, as percent of total myelin protein (percent of dye-binding).
[b]The values for newborn myelin are the mean of two cases. Myelin from the other newborn was used mainly to compare different methods, and the small amount obtained did not allow all the analyses to be performed with enough accuracy.

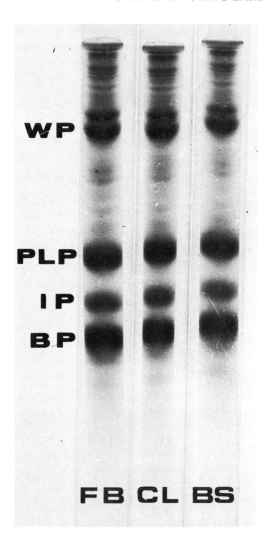

FIG. 9. Polyacrylamide gel electrophoresis of newborn myelin proteins. FB, myelin from the forebrain; CL, myelin from the cerebellum; BS, myelin from the brain stem; WP, Wolfgram protein; PLP, proteolipid protein; IP, intermediate protein (DM-20); BP, basic protein. (From ref. 41.)

We sought the reason for these discrepancies in problems connected with values of MBP.

Degradation of MBP During Brain Storage

Table 2 demonstrates that degradation of MBP starts very soon and that after only one month of brain tissue storage at $-60°C$ the MBP decreases by 15%. After one year of brain storage at $-60°C$ the level decreases to about one third of its original value, a figure corresponding very closely to values given for basic protein in human

TABLE 2. Changes in the protein patterns of human myelin after increasing times of brain storage at −60°C[a]

Months of storage	Tissue[b]	MBP	Intermediate protein (DM-20)	Proteolipid protein	Wolfgram protein
0	WM	46.0	5.3	29.2	19.5
1	WM	38.7	8.3	36.2	16.8
4	TH	35.6	11.3	36.1	17.0
12	TH	15.3	12.5	46.0	26.2
14	WM	18.8	6.5	47.4	27.3

[a]All the values represent percent of dye-binding, roughly corresponding to percent of total myelin protein.
[b]WM, white matter; TH, total homogenate of brain tissue.

myelin at one year of age (32). This seems to indicate that one of the main causes of the very low and variable figures published to date for basic protein in human myelin is the fact that all investigators working with the human postmortem brain have isolated myelin from brain tissue stored frozen for more or less prolonged periods.

Freezing and thawing causes disruption of membranes and separation of myelin lamellae (44), rendering MBP more vulnerable to proteolysis. Disruption of subcellular organelles can also cause greater microsomal contamination, and the hydrolytic enzymes liberated can alter the apparent composition of myelin. It is therefore very important that myelin be isolated from fresh brain if reliable data are to be obtained.

Effect of Undernutrition on the Composition of Human Myelin

Myelin from a very severely undernourished infant was studied. This child was born at 37 weeks of gestation with a body weight appropriate for gestational age (2,600 g) and died at 9 months of age in a state of extreme marasmus (body weight at death, 2,220 g). The cause of such severe undernutrition was prolonged severe diarrhea, starting immediately after birth and not responding to treatment. In this case, therefore, the nutritional insult impinged upon the whole vulnerable period, causing a reduction in brain weight of about 50% and a decrease in cerebral myelin to about half the normal levels (see Figs. 3 and 4). However, the quality of myelin was basically preserved, showing a high level of galactolipids and MBP (Table 1). The only alteration was a low value of the enzyme CNP, a finding that must await confirmation before trying to evaluate its significance. It is highly significant that despite the severity of undernutrition in this child no alteration in the lipid or protein composition of the myelin was found, especially since this agrees with the lack of lipid alterations found by Fox et al. (45) in myelin from three cases of undernutrition of a much more moderate degree.

CONCLUSIONS

The biochemical development of the human brain has some unique characteristics that must be taken into account before extrapolating from animal experiments. In contrast to what happens in the rat, in the human species myelination is much more rapid and thus more vulnerable in the cerebrum than in the cerebellum.

At 32 weeks of gestation a sudden surge of membrane lipids in the human forebrain coincides with the spurt of synaptogenesis found in histological studies. After that comes myelinogenesis, which in the human cerebrum is an explosive perinatal process that starts just before term and progresses very rapidly during the first year of life.

In contrast to the findings in the laboratory animal, no early myelin exists in the human cerebrum at birth, but well-organized, compact myelin forms at this earliest stage of myelinogenesis. Therefore myelination in the human forebrain is primarily a quantitative rather than qualitative process, consisting of rapidly progressive apposition of myelin lamellae with a biochemical composition substantially similar to that of adult myelin. Consequently, the depression of myelinogenesis caused by undernutrition is also a quantitative process.

REFERENCES

1. Norton WT, Poduslo SE. Myelination in rat brain: changes in myelin composition during brain maturation. *J Neurochem* 1973;21:759–73.
2. Norton WT. Formation, structure, and biochemistry of myelin. In: Siegel GJ, Albers RW, Agranoff BW, Katzman R, eds. *Basic neurochemistry*. Boston: Little, Brown, 1981:63–92.
3. Dobbing J. The influence of early nutrition on the development and myelination of the brain. *Proc R Soc London (Biol)* 1964;159:503–9.
4. Culley WJ, Mertz ET. Effect of restricted food intake on growth and composition of preweanling rat brain. *Proc Soc Exp Biol Med* 1965;118:233–5.
5. Benton JW, Moser HW, Dodge PR, Carr S. Modification of the schedule of myelination in the rat by early nutritional deprivation. *Pediatrics* 1966;38:801–7.
6. Chase HP, Dorsey J, McKhann GM. The effect of malnutrition on the synthesis of a myelin lipid. *Pediatrics* 1967;40:551–9.
7. Dickerson JWT, Dobbing J, McCance RA. The effect of undernutrition on the postnatal development of the brain and cord in pigs. *Proc R Soc London (Biol)* 1967;166:396–407.
8. Fishman MA, Madyastha P, Prensky AL. The effect of undernutrition on the development of myelin in the rat central nervous system. *Lipids* 1971;6:458–65.
9. Chase HP, Carol S, Dabiere CS, Welch NN, O'Brien D. Intra-uterine undernutrition and brain development. *Pediatrics* 1971;47:491–500.
10. Schain RJ, Watanabe K, Harel S. Effects of brief postnatal fasting upon brain development of rabbits. *Pediatrics* 1973;51:240–50.
11. Kerr GR, Helmuth AC. Malnutrition studies in *Macaca mulatta*. 3. Effect on cerebral lipids. *Am J Clin Nutr* 1973;26:1053–9.
12. Krigman MR, Hogan EL. Undernutrition in the developing rat: effect upon myelination. *Brain Res* 1976;107:239–55.
13. Wiggins RC, Miller SL, Benjamins JA, Krigman MR, Morell P. Myelin synthesis during postnatal nutritional deprivation and subsequent rehabilitation. *Brain Res* 1976;107:257–73.
14. Wiggins RC, Fuller GN. Early postnatal starvation causes lasting hypomyelination. *J Neurochem* 1978;30:1231–7.
15. Fishman MA, Prensky AL, Dodge PR. Low content of cerebral lipids in infants suffering from malnutrition. *Nature* 1969;221:552–3.

16. Rosso P, Hormazébal J, Winick M. Changes in brain weight, cholesterol, phospholipid, and DNA content in marasmic children. *Am J Clin Nutr* 1970;23:1275–9.
17. Chase HP, Welch NN, Dabiere CS, Vasan NS, Butterfield LJ. Alterations in human brain biochemistry following intrauterine growth retardation. *Pediatrics* 1972;50:403–11.
18. Svennerholm L, Vanier MT. The distribution of lipids in the human nervous system. II. Lipid composition of human fetal and infant brain. *Brain Res* 1972;47:457–68.
19. Dobbing J. Vulnerable periods in developing brain. In: Davison AN, Dobbing J, eds. *Applied neurochemistry*. Oxford: Blackwell, 1968:287–316.
20. Conde C, Martínez M, Ballabriga A. Some chemical aspects of human brain development. I. Neutral glycosphingolipids, sulfatides, and sphingomyelin. *Pediatr Res* 1974;8:89–92.
21. Martínez M. Conde C, Ballabriga A. Some chemical aspects of human brain development. II. Phosphoglyceride fatty acids. *Pediatr Res* 1974;8:93–102.
22. Martínez M, Ballabriga A. A chemical study on the development of the human forebrain and cerebellum during the brain "growth spurt" period. I. Gangliosides and plasmalogens. *Brain Res* 1978;159:351–62.
23. Purpura DP. Morphogenesis of the visual cortex in the preterm infant. In: Brazier MAB, ed. *Growth and development of the brain*. New York: Raven Press, 1975:33–49.
24. Sweeley CC, Walker B. Determination of carbohydrates in glycolipids and gangliosides by gas chromatography. *Anal Chem* 1964;36:1461–6.
25. Prohaska JR, Clark DA, Wells WW. Improved rapidity and precision in the determination of brain 2',3'-cyclic nucleotide 3'-phosphohydrolase. *Anal Biochem* 1973;56:275–82.
26. Martínez M. Myelin lipids in the developing cerebrum, cerebellum, and brain stem of normal and undernourished children. *J Neurochem* 1982;39:1684–92.
27. Chase HP, Lindsley WFB, O'Brien D. Undernutrition and cerebellar development. *Nature* 1969;221:554–5.
28. Fish I, Winick M. Effect of malnutrition on regional growth of the developing rat brain. *Exp Neurol* 1969;25:534–40.
29. Wiggins RC, Fuller GN. Relative synthesis of myelin in different brain regions of postnatally undernourished rats. *Brain Res* 1979;162:103–12.
30. Savolainen H, Palo J, Riekkinen P, Mörönen P, Brody LE. Maturation of myelin proteins in human brain. *Brain Res* 1972;37:253–63.
31. Banik NL, Davison AN, Ramsey RB, Scott T. Protein composition in developing human brain myelin. *Dev Psychobiol* 1974;7:539–49.
32. Fishman MA, Agrawal HC, Alexander A, Golterman J. Biochemical maturation of human central nervous system myelin. *J Neurochem* 1975;24:689–94.
33. Eng LF, Chao F-C, Gerstl B, Pratt D, Tavaststjerna MG. The maturation of human white matter myelin. Fractionation of the myelin membrane proteins. *Biochemistry* 1968;7:4455–65.
34. O'Brien JS, Sampson EL. Lipid composition of the normal human brain: gray matter, white matter, and myelin. *J Lipid Res* 1965;6:537–44.
35. Svennerholm L, Vanier MT, Jungbjer B. Changes in fatty acid composition of human brain myelin lipids during maturation. *J Neurochem* 1978;30:1383–90.
36. Cuzner ML, Davison AN. The lipid composition of rat brain myelin and subcellular fractions during development. *Biochem J* 1968;106:29–34.
37. Eng LF, Noble EP. The maturation of rat brain myelin. *Lipids* 1968;3:157–62.
38. Agrawal HC, Banik NL, Bone AH, Davison AN, Mitchell RF, Spohn M. The identity of a myelin-like fraction isolated from developing brain. *Biochem J* 1970;120:635–42.
39. Poduslo SE, Jang Y. Myelin development in infant brain. *Neurochem Res* 1984;9:1615–26.
40. Martínez M. Myelin in developing human central nervous system. *Trans Am Soc Neurochem* 1983;14:213.
41. Martínez M. Myelin in the developing human cerebrum. *Brain Res* 1986;364:220–32.
42. Norton WT, Poduslo SE. Myelination in rat brain: method of myelin isolation. *J Neurochem* 1973;21:749–57.
43. Agrawal HC, Burton RM, Fishman MA, Mitchell RF, Prensky AL. Partial characterization of a new myelin protein component. *J Neurochem* 1972;19:2083–9.
44. Ansari KA, Hendrickson H, Sinha AA, Rand A. Myelin basic protein in frozen and unfrozen bovine brain: A study of autolytic changes *in situ*. *J Neurochem* 1975;25:193–5.
45. Fox JH, Fishman MA, Dodge PR, Prensky AL. The effect of malnutrition on human central nervous system myelin. *Neurology* 1972;22:1213–6.

DISCUSSION

Dr. Bourre: You mentioned that the composition of myelin changes during maturation, older myelin containing more short chain fatty acids in its sphingolipids than early myelin. Do you have any ideas about the composition of sphingolipids in human undernutrition in terms of the fatty acid profile?

Dr. Martinez: We are planning this work. I am sure we shall find some subtle changes, but we have no data as yet.

Dr. Volpe: I am interested in the effect of undernutrition on the composition of myelin lipids. Do you think some or perhaps all of the effect relates to an influence on glial cell proliferation, which is very active during this period in human brain development? Have you expressed your data as a function of DNA concentration in the brain, and do you have any insight into whether this is an effect on the number of oligodendrocytes rather than on the amount of myelin per se?

Dr. Martinez: It is very possible that it is an effect on oligodendrocytes because as you say it is proliferating very fast. However, I have no data expressing the result on a DNA basis.

Dr. Ballabriga: We have data which show that DNA is decreased compared with normally nourished infants.

Dr. Minkowski: What is the role of hormones in myelin synthesis? As you know corticosteroids are supposed to suppress myelin formation in experimental animals. This is a matter of concern because steroids are widely used throughout the world to accelerate the production of surfactant by the fetus.

Dr. Martinez: We have not studied the effect of corticosteroids.

Dr. Volpe: There are data which indicate that pharmacological quantities of glucocorticoids given to the prenatal animal do diminish myelin lipid synthesis in several animal models, particularly in tissue culture. Glucocorticoids also have an interesting inhibitory effect on the cholesterol biosynthetic pathway, changing the flux in that pathway into the segment of the pathway involved in glycoprotein synthesis. Glycoproteins are of course very important in a number of aspects of the differentiation of cells, so it is likely that glucocorticoids have complex and possibly profound effects when given in pharmacological doses which must have a bearing on their use in obstetric practice.

Dr. Minkowski: That was one of the important statements of this meeting. Corticosteroids are used all over the world because of their demonstrated effectiveness in reducing the incidence of hyaline membrane disease. However, there are other ways to reduce the incidence of this disease, such as good obstetric practices, and the adverse effects of corticosteroids are not considered carefully enough. Strang in London does not use them at all for the specific reason that they may interfere with myelin formation.

Developmental Neurobiology, edited by
Philippe Evrard and Alexandre Minkowski.
Nestlé Nutrition Workshop Series, Vol. 12.
Nestec Ltd., Vevey/Raven Press, Ltd.,
New York © 1989.

Visual Function in the Normal and Neurologically Compromised Newborn Infant

Lilly M. S. Dubowitz, J. Mushin, and L. De Vries

Department of Pediatrics and Neonatal Medicine, Royal Postgraduate Medical School, Hammersmith Hospital, London W12 OHS, England

In the adult, vision is a cortical function and thus it has always been assumed that this would also hold true for the newborn infant. This view received support from the findings that behavioral and electrophysiological evidence of vision is first recorded around the same gestation in the premature infant as arborization of the dendrites is observed in the visual cortex (1). This assumption led to the belief that good visual function might be a marker for the integrity of cortical function in the neonate and in particular a better predictor for future intellectual outcome than formal neurological assessment (2). Thus in the last decade great interest has developed in the evolution of visual function in the newborn and its assessment.

During the same period the advent of new imaging techniques—computerized tomography (CT), nuclear magnetic resonance (NMR) scanning, and especially cranial ultrasonography—provided for the first time a window on the brain and made possible the recognition and accurate localization of lesions during life, which in the past could only be made at postmortem. These allowed a better correlation of visual function with anatomical lesions.

The aim of this chapter is to evaluate the current methods used to assess visual function in the neonate and to illustrate how correlative studies of imaging and function can widen understanding of the development of the neonatal nervous system.

METHODS OF ASSESSING VISUAL FUNCTION IN THE NEWBORN

Behavioral Testing

Tracking

The infant's ability to fixate on and track an object can be tested by propping him or her at about 30° in the supine position and observing the infant's ability to focus on and follow a red woolly ball held at approximately 20 to 25 cm away from his or her face, moving it slowly horizontally, vertically, and in an arc (3,4). This test can be used in the neonatal unit inside and outside an incubator. Even better responses can be obtained by watching the infant's response to the mother's face, but this cannot be tested inside the incubator.

Pattern Preference

Fantz in 1963 demonstrated that newborn infants have a definite preference for patterns of different shape, size, and complexity (5). To test this the infant is presented with sequential pairs of patterns on a uniformly illuminated stage and preference for one of the patterns is judged by deviation and fixation of his eyes in the direction of the preferred pattern.

Measuring Visual Acuity

This can be studied in infants by optokinetic nystagmus (6) and visually evoked potentials (7), and by discriminating vertical stripes of various widths from a gray area matched for luminance (8–10). The latter test is best suited for preterm and full-term newborns (10).

Electrophysiologic Tests

Visual Evoked Responses

Visual evoked responses (VER) can be elicited by a flash of light or by a pattern stimulus, but as the latter requires the maintenance of fixation during testing it is not suitable for preterm infants. The source of light can be either a stroboscope (11–17) or a stimulator consisting of an array of light emitting diodes (LEDs) which has been found to have certain advantages over the conventional discharge stroboscope (18). Single-channel recordings are made with a single electrode in the midline over the inion or the activity obtained simultaneously from each occipital lobe on a two-channel recorder from electrodes placed 2 cm lateral to the inion.

IMAGING TECHNIQUES

Cranial Ultrasonography

This allows the diagnosis of ischemic/hypoxic lesions such as intracranial hemorrhage and periventricular leukomalacia, and of congenital anomalies and infections (19). Not only can these lesions be diagnosed with remarkable accuracy as long as the fontanelle remains open, but one can also follow their evolution into cysts or to ventricular dilatation. Figure 1 shows the grading of periventricular hemorrhages

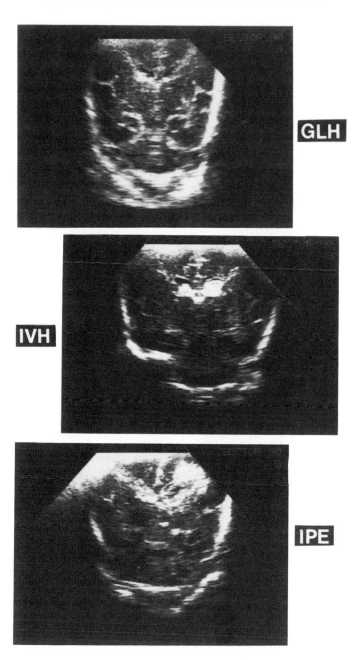

FIG. 1. Coronal view showing small germinal left hemorrhage (GLH) on the left (**top**), bilateral intraventricular hemorrhage (IVH) (**middle**), and intraparenchymal extension (IPE) on the right (**bottom**).

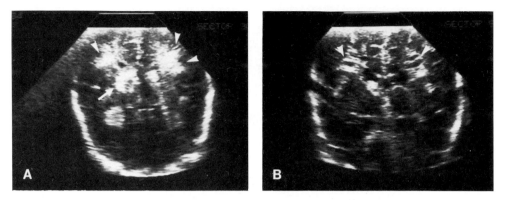

FIG. 2. Note multiple cysts in brain parenchyma adjacent to ventricles (**right**) in previously echodense areas (**left**). Cysts do not communicate with the ventricles.

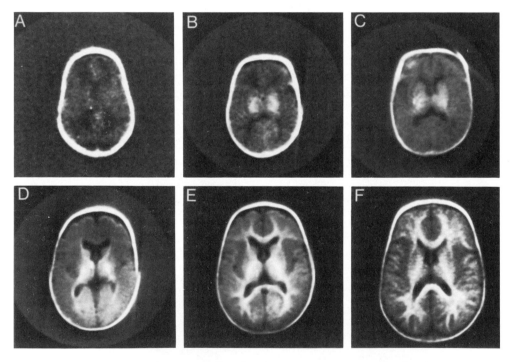

FIG. 3. Nuclear magnetic resonance imaging. Inversion recovery scan showing development of myelination. **A:** 36 weeks PMA; no myelin is visible. **B:** 42 weeks PMA; early myelination in the thalami and posterior limb of the internal capsule. **C:** Early myelination extending into the opticothalamic radiation. **D:** Full-term infant at 6 months showing extension of myelin into the opticothalamic radiation. **E:** Full-term infant at 10 months; myelin is now present in forceps minor and major, and myelin is more prominent posteriorly. **F:** Full-term infant at 20 months; further extension of myelin anteriorly and posteriorly.

(PVH) whereas Fig. 2 shows the evolution of periventricular leukomalacia (PVL) from densities to cysts. This method of imaging has been found not only the most convenient and least invasive for neonatal use, but also most accurate in many instances, as hemorrhages become isodense on CT scannings and cysts are poorly visualized.

Computerized Tomography Scanning

Cranial ultrasonography is limited by the penetration of the beam through the anterior fontanelle, and thus lesions in the posterior fossa and those involving convexities are better demonstrated by CT scanning.

Nuclear Magnetic Resonance Imaging

This new modality is not only able to give an excellent image of normal and abnormal anatomy but also allows the study of the process of myelination and the effect of neonatal insults on this process (20,21). Figure 3 shows the evolution of myelination in the infants brain from 34 weeks postmenstrual age (PMA) to 20 months postterm.

DEVELOPMENT OF VISUAL FUNCTION IN NEUROLOGICALLY NORMAL NEWBORNS

Fixating and Tracking an Object

Neurologically normal infants persistently show the ability to fixate on and track an object during the first week of life from 31 to 33 weeks gestation onward. When these infants reach 40 weeks PMA their ability to track is superior to full-term infants during the first week of life (Fig. 4).

Pattern Preference

Pattern preference can be successfully tested in 60% to 70% of the infants above 32 weeks gestation who are well enough to be taken out of the incubator. Using the four pairs of patterns shown in Fig. 5, preterm infants of 34 weeks gestation or less are able to discriminate between pattern pairs 2 and 4 in 60% and 70% of the tests performed under 1 week of age. Very few of these immature infants are able to differentiate the other two pairs, but over 70% of full-term infants discriminate among all four pairs. The evolution of pattern preference with increasing gestational age (GA) is illustrated in Fig. 6.

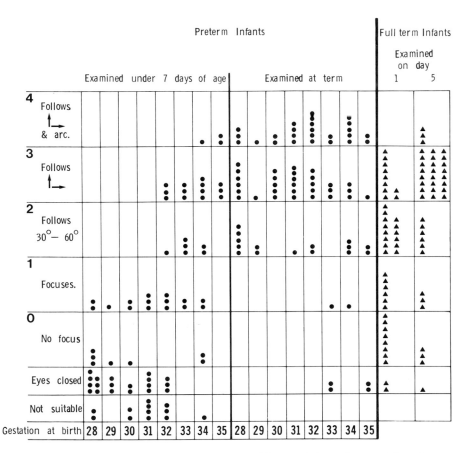

FIG. 4. Evolution of visual orientation in preterm and full-term infants. Preterm infants born at 28 to 34 weeks examined during the first week of life and again at 40 weeks PMA compared to full-term infants on the first and fifth day.

Visual Acuity

When tested by pattern preference technique it is found again that visual acuity matures with increasing GA. At 32 weeks more than 90% of infants have a visual acuity of at least 160' arc, but only one third have more than 80' arc. The increase in acuity with gestational age is shown in Fig. 7.

Visually Evoked Responses

Visually evoked responses have been reported in infants from 24 weeks gestation onward (15). With increasing GA there is a shortening of the latency of the main negative component and an increase in the complexity of the wave form. Ellingson

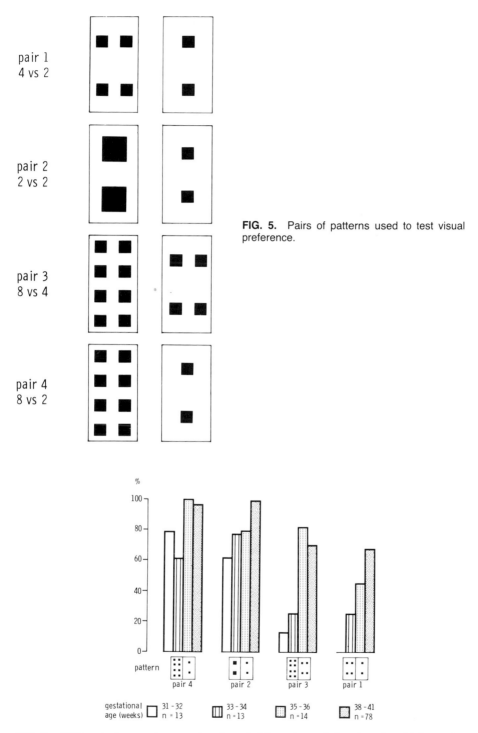

FIG. 5. Pairs of patterns used to test visual preference.

FIG. 6. Pattern preference in normal preterm (<36 weeks gestational age) and full-term infants (>38 weeks gestational age) examined during the first week of life.

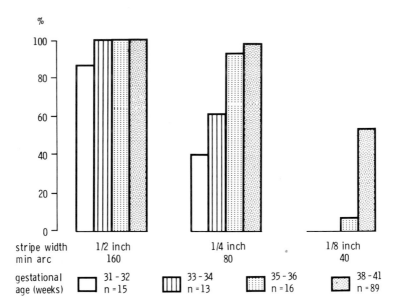

FIG. 7. Visual acuity in normal preterm (<36 weeks gestational age) and full-term infants (>38 weeks gestational age) examined during the first week of life.

(11) has described a bimodal curve relating latency to age, with a steep reduction of latency between 1 to 2 months of age in infants born at term.

In normal preterm infants below 32 weeks gestation the VER consists of a broad negative deflection only. At 32 to 35 weeks PMA a small positive deflection appears before the negativity which increases in amplitude with increasing PMA. By 40 weeks a preceding negativity appears giving rise to the negative-positive-negative (N-P-N) complex. A nearly adult configuration is reached 6 months postterm with a prominent surface positive component peaking 100 to 150 msec after the flash. The development of the VER configuration is a more reliable indication of maturation than either latency or amplitude measurements (14).

VISUAL DEVELOPMENT IN THE NEUROLOGICALLY DEVIANT NEWBORN INFANT

The development of focusing and tracking, pattern preference, acuity, and maturation of VER are all delayed in the neurologically compromised newborn infant. However, not all modalities of visual function are equally affected by different lesions.

Periventricular Hemorrhage and Posthemorrhagic Ventricular Dilatation

Infants with periventricular/intraventricular hemorrhage (PVH/IVH) are delayed in their ability to focus on and track an object (22). There is a weak correlation be-

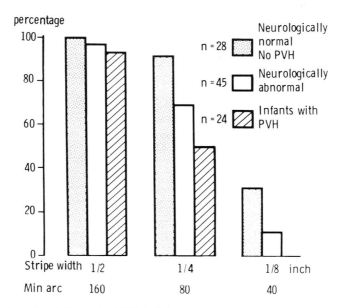

FIG. 8. Visual acuity at 40 weeks PMA in infants who were initially neurologically normal (*n* = 28) and in neurologically abnormal infants without periventricular hemorrhage (PVH) (*n* = 45) and with PVH (*n* = 24).

tween this delay and the size of the hemorrhage. Similarly there is a delay in the maturation of pattern preference, but this delay is of the same magnitude as the delay in other neurologically abnormal infants (10). However, the delay in maturation of visual acuity is much more marked in infants with a hemorrhage than in those without (Fig. 8). A difference in the maturation of the wave forms of the VER has also been noted. Again there is a tendency for the delay to be more marked in the larger hemorrhages, but the difference between larger and smaller hemorrhages is not significant (23). Figure 9 demonstrates the difference in the maturation of VER waveform in a neurologically normal premature infant and one with PVH-IVH.

The presence of ventricular dilatation in these premature infants did not seem to have any effect on the wave form. The VER was symmetrical even in the presence of grossly asymmetrical dilatation of the occipital horn in neonates up to 44 to 48 weeks PMA. However, at about 48 weeks the VER became asymmetrical in these infants. The asymmetry usually did not involve the large negative deflection but the more early positive waves. (Fig. 10).

Cystic Periventricular and Subcortical Leukomalacia

Below and at 36 weeks PMA many of these infants are still too ill to be assessed. Later on marked irritability often interferes with testing, but when a suitable state is achieved, most are able to track well (Fig. 11) in spite of apparently near complete destruction of the visual cortex (present in 3 out of 8 of the series). In these infants

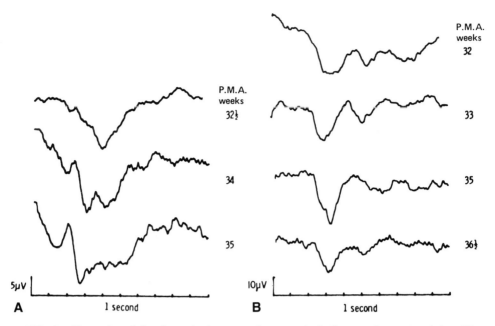

FIG. 9. Maturation of visually evoked response in a neurologically normal premature infant (**A**) and in a neurologically abnormal infant with periventricular hemorrhage/intraventricular hemorrhage (**B**). Note the difference in the maturation of the latency of the negative component and the delay in the appearance of the early positivity upwards. PMA, postmenstrual age.

the ability to track was lost around 48 weeks PMA though there was no apparent progression of the condition.

The evolution of pattern preference and acuity was delayed, but surprisingly around 40 weeks PMA some preference was recorded for the most striking patterns in all infants who later became cortically blind.

Three of four infants with cystic PVL had a VER recorded at 36 weeks PMA; two had a normal recording, the third had an abnormal recording which normalized by 40 weeks PMA. Infants who also had subcortical leukomalacia, mainly involving the frontal region, had very abnormal low amplitude VERs.

Nuclear magnetic resonance imaging in infants with this condition showed marked delay in myelination, particularly in the opticothalamic radiation (Fig. 12). All those who exhibited this lesion had severe spastic diplegia or quadriplegia at follow-up examination, but cortical blindness was only found in the infants who also had frontal subcortical lesions (Fig. 13).

The diagnosis of holoprosencephaly was made in one infant soon after birth by ultrasonography and CT scanning (Fig. 14A). Complete absence of the occipital cortex was confirmed at autopsy. During the first two days of life the infant was able to fixate and track briefly. Pattern preference could not be elicited. An abnormal but consistent VER was recorded from this infant (Fig. 14B).

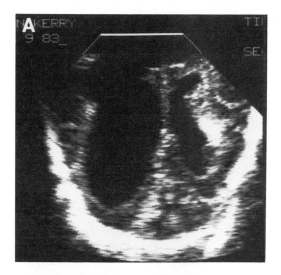

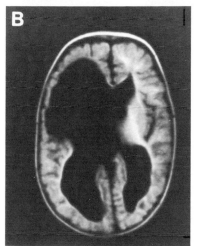

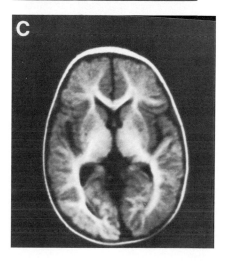

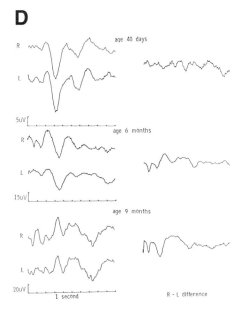

FIG. 10. Infant born at 27 weeks gestational age. **A:** Semiaxial ultrasound scan showing asymmetrical ventricular dilatation at 31 days. **B:** NMR image of the same infant at 1 year of age compared to normal twin (**C**). **D:** Serial visually evoked response in the abnormal twin. Note the asymmetry in the early positive wave at 6 months, becoming more marked at 9 months.

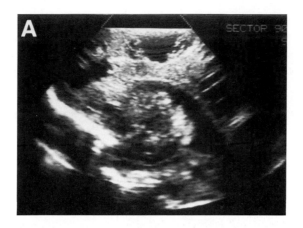

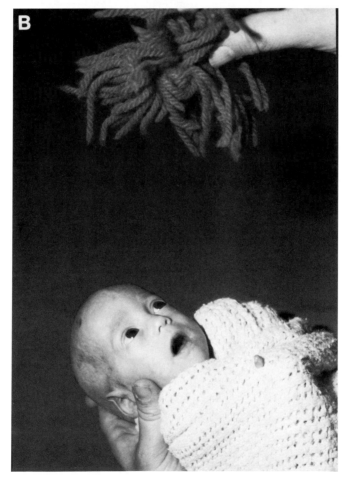

FIG. 11. Infant born at 31 weeks gestation, examined at 37 weeks postmenstrual age. **A:** Ultrasound image showing subcortical cystic leukomalacia in occipital and frontal areas. **B:** Infant visually tracking an object.

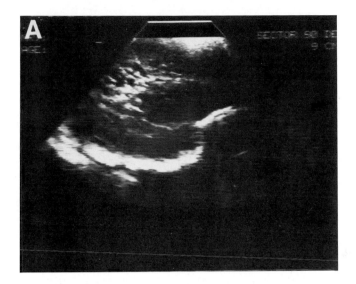

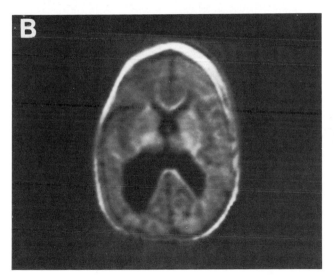

FIG. 12. Infant born at 30 weeks gestational age. **A:** Ultrasound showing cystic lesion adjacent to occipital bone at 5 weeks of age. **B:** NMR image at 11 months chronological age showing asymmetrical dilatation of lateral ventricles posteriorly more marked on the left. Note also the delay in myelination, particularly posteriorly. The infant has spastic diplegia, right more than left, and squint, but normal vision.

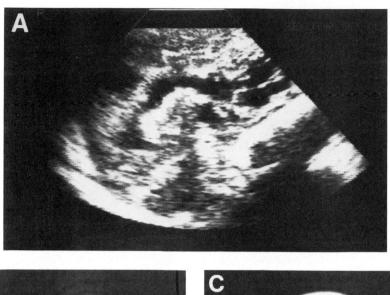

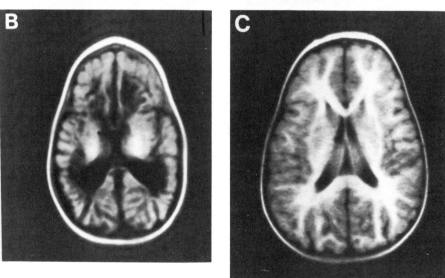

FIG. 13. Infant with cystic leukomalacia and cortical blindness. **A:** Ultrasound image at 40 weeks postmenstrual age. **B:** NMR image at 18 months compared with normal twin (**C**). Note the prominent frontal lesions and delayed myelination.

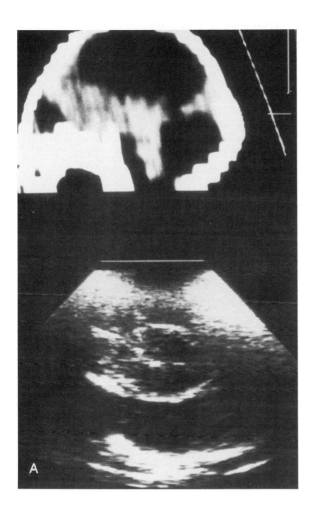

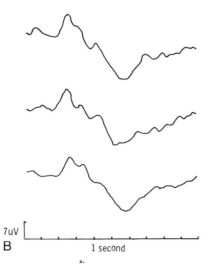

7uV

B

1 second

FIG. 14. Infant with holoprosencephaly. **A:** Computerized tomography scan and ultrasound showing absent occipital cortex (confirmed at autopsy). **B:** Abnormal but persistent visually evoked responses.

DISCUSSION

Methods evolved during the last two decades have demonstrated that many aspects of visual function are already present in very young premature infants. Because many of these responses qualitatively resemble those in older infants and adults, it has been assumed that they are mediated through the same pathways. Recent correlative studies with imaging and function, however, have cast doubt on some of these assumptions.

Fixation, tracking, and pattern preference can all be elicited in premature infants, but it is unlikely that these are mediated through the cortex at this stage. This is supported by the fact that up to 44 weeks PMA the behavioral and electrophysiological functions are more affected by IVH/PVH, which are known to be associated with hypoxic ischemic lesions in the basal ganglia, thalami, and colliculi, than by lesions associated with widespread involvement of the occipital cortex, such as ventricular dilatation and leukomalacia (23).

It has been thought that VERs, even in the youngest premature infants, were generated from the cortex, as the characteristic wave shapes of the response are sharply localized over the occipital scalp (24). Against this theory are the observations that symmetric evoked responses can be recorded from the two hemispheres up to 44 to 48 weeks PMA in infants having very asymmetrical lesions affecting the occipital region. We have also recorded an abnormal but persistent response to visual stimulation from the occipital scalp in an infant with complete absence of the visual cortex.

There are a number of concomitant changes occurring at 44 to 48 weeks PMA suggesting that there is a developmental shift in physiological locus and control of the infant's visual function. Optical pursuit becomes much smoother (25). Pattern preference develops for elements of greater complexity, which in turn has been found to be more predictive for neurological outcome than the ability to discriminate more simple forms (26). There is a marked reduction in the latency of the flash VER (11). Acuity determined by the pattern VER begins to increase (27). This is also the age when it becomes possible to elicit binocular stereopsis for the first time (28). It is thus possible that some sort of control might be exerted by a subcortical locus over a cortical locus at this age.

These observations would suggest that whereas early assessment of visual function and its correlation with imaging might greatly increase our knowledge about visual function and its development, its predictive value as a marker of higher cerebral function in the newborn is questionable.

ACKNOWLEDGMENTS

We wish to acknowledge the help of the Nuclear Magnetic Resonance Unit, Department of Diagnostic Radiology, at the Hammersmith Hospital, London, for the NMR images and Miss Lisa Usher for secretarial help.

J. Mushin was supported by a grant from the Medical Research Council. L.M.S. Dubowitz and L. De Vries were supported by grants from the National Fund for Research into Crippling Diseases (Action Research for the Crippled Child).

REFERENCES

1. Purpura DP. Developmental pathobiology of cortical neurons in immature human brain. In: Gluck L, ed. *Intrauterine asphyxia and the developing fetal brain.* Chicago: Year Book National, 1977.
2. Hack M, Fantz RL, Fanaroff AA, Klaus MH. Neonatal pattern vision: a predictor of future mental performance. *J Pediatr* 1977;91:642–7.
3. Brazelton TB. Neonatal behavioural assessment scale. *Clinics in developmental medicine no. 50.* London: SIMP/Heinemann; Philadelphia: Lippincott, 1973.
4. Dubowitz LMS, Morante A, Verghote M. Visual function in the preterm and full-term Newborn infant. *Dev Med Child Neurol* 1980;22:465–75.
5. Fantz RL. Pattern vision in newborn infants. *Science* 1963;140:296–7.
6. Kiff RD, Lepard C. Visual response of premature infants: use of the optokinetic nystagmus to estimate visual development. *Arch Ophthalmol* 1966;75:631–3.
7. Sokol S. Measurement of infant visual acuity from pattern reversal evoked potentials. *Vision Res* 1978;18:33–9.
8. Ordy JM, Udlef MS. Maturation of pattern vision in infants during the first six months. *J Comp Physiol Psychol* 1962;55:907–17.
9. Miranda SB. Visual abilities and pattern preferences of premature infants and full-term neonates. *J Exp Child Psychol* 1970;10:189–205.
10. Morante A, Dubowitz LMS, Levene M, Dubowitz V. The development of visual function in normal and neurologically abnormal preterm and full-term infants. *Dev Med Child Neurol* 1982;24:771–84.
11. Ellingson RJ. Cortical electrical responses to visual stimulation in the human infant. *Electroencephalogr Clin Neurophysiol* 1960;12:663–77.
12. Feriss GS, Davis GD, Dorsen MM, Hackett ER. Changes in latency and form of one photically induced averaged evoked response in human infants. *Electroencephalogr Clin Neurophysiol* 1967;22:305–12.
13. Umezaki H, Morrell F. Development study of photic evoked responses in premature infants. *Electroencephalogr Clin Neurophysiol* 1970;28:55–63.
14. Watanabe K, Iwase K, Hara K. Maturation of visual evoked responses in low birthweight infants. *Dev Med Child Neurol* 1972;14:425–35.
15. Hrbek A, Karlberg P, Olsson T. Development of visual and somatosensory evoked responses in low birthweight infants. *Electroencephalogr Clin Neurophysiol* 1973;34:225–32.
16. Barnet AB, Friedman SL, Weiss IP, Ohlirich ES, Shanks B, Lodge A. VEP development in infancy and early childhood: a longitudinal study. *Electroencephalogr Clin Neurophysiol* 1980;49:476–89.
17. Blom JL, Barth PG, Visser SL. The visual evoked potential in the first six years of life. *Electroencephalogr Clin Neurophysiol* 1980;48:395–405.
18. Mushin J, Hogg CR, Dubowitz LMS, Skouteli H, Arden GB. Visual evoked responses to LED photostimulation in newborn infants. *Electroencephalogr Clin Neurophysiol* 1984;58:317–20.
19. Levene MI, Williams JL, Fawer CL. Ultrasound of the infant brain. *Clinics in developmental medicine no. 92.* Oxford: SIMP/Blackwell. Philadelphia: Lippincott, 1985.
20. Johnson MA, Pennock JM, Bydder GM. Clinical NMR imaging of the brain in children: normal and neurological disease. *Am J Neurol Radiol* 1983;4:1013–26.
21. Dubowitz LMS, Bydder GM. Nuclear magnetic resonance imaging in the diagnosis and follow up of neonatal cerebral injury. *Clin Perinatol* 1985;12:243–60.
22. Dubowitz LMS, Levene MI, Morante A, Palmer P, Dubowitz V. Neurological signs in newborn intraventricular hemorrhage: a correlation with real-time ultrasound. *J Pediatr* 1981;99:127–33.
23. Placzek M, Mushin J, Dubowitz LMS. Maturation of the visual evoked response and its correlation with visual acuity in preterm infants. *Dev Med Child Neurol* 1985;27:448–54.
24. Kurtzberg D. Vaughan HG. Electrophysiological assessment of auditory and visual function in the newborn. *Clin Perinatol* 1985;12:277–98.
25. Mavrer D, Lewis TL. A physiological explanation of infants' early visual development. *Can J Psychol* 1979;33:232–52.
26. Harmant K, Roucoux M, Culee C, Lyon G. Vision attention and discrimination in infants at risk and neurological outcome. *Behav Brain Res* 1983;10:203–7.

27. Atkinson J, Braddick O. Acuity, contrast sensitivity and accommodation in infancy. In: Aslin RN, Alberts JR, Petersen MR, eds. *The development of perception: psychobiological perspectives. vol. 2, The visual system.* New York: Academic Press, 1981.
28. Moskowitz A, Sokol S. Developmental changes in the human visual system as reflected by the latency of the pattern reversal VEP. *Electroencephalogr Clin Neurophysiol* 1983;56:1–15.

DISCUSSION

Dr. Williams: Years ago I had the opportunity to examine the brain of a child with hydranencephaly who had been seen by many people at an academic neurological center. This was before the days of visually evoked responses, but the child was documented to have visual fixation and following, and opticokinetic nystagmus had been observed. It was also the opinion of the family and of those who looked after the child that there was response to voice. In the second or third month the head began to enlarge abnormally, and by the end of the first year the child no longer had any visual response. There was optic atrophy due to compression of the optic chiasma. The postmortem contrasted with the typical appearances of hydranencephaly, that is, an absence of cortex supplied by the carotid vessels but a relatively intact cortex in the vertebrobasilar distribution; in this child there was no neocortex at all.

In a study on adult monkeys that were trained to a visual task, ablation of the posterior halves of both hemispheres caused apparent blindness until the collicular commissure was sectioned. When this was done the monkeys, although still behaving as if blind, were able to engage again in the visually mediated trained behavior. This is the phenomenon of collicular vision; there may also be a phenomenon of collicular hearing.

Dr. Dubowitz: I agree with this. I now have ten infants on record with similar lesions who have been noted to see in the neonatal period but who later became cortically blind, probably due to major occipital involvement. I believe that all these infants have collicular lesions. You may even get pattern preference in these cases, which therefore is not a good predictor of later performance, though preference for more complicated patterns may be better. Simple patterns may be mediated through the colliculi, but more complicated ones perhaps need the cortex.

Dr. Evrard: A member of our department, K. Armand, did a study that convinced us that one of the best predictive factors is preference by the 6 week old infant for irregular shapes. However, we must wait for a year or two before we can be sure of the long-term predictive value of this finding.

Dr. Volpe: Several reports show acute improvement in visually evoked responses after ventricular drainage in posthemorrhagic hydrocephalus, occurring within hours or perhaps even sooner. Do you think this is an effect of decreasing the size of the occipital poles of the ventricles, which occurs acutely with ventricular drainage in such patients?

Dr. Dubowitz: I think it is likely to be due to relief of pressure on the colliculi because you can get the same improvement with brain-stem responses which are definitely not cortical.

Dr. Ballabriga: Do you have any experience with visual responses in infants who, after an initial light stimulation, have had their eyes covered for 6 or 7 days because they are receiving phototherapy?

Dr. Dubowitz: We have not been able to identify any effect of covering the eyes for a period as short as this. Admittedly we do not cover the eyes continuously so it is difficult to be sure, and preterm infants often have other problems which makes the population too variable for analysis. We have definitely found no effect of eye covering in jaundiced full-term infants.

Dr. Williams: We must not fall into the trap of assuming that because the VER test is highly sophisticated and computer assisted it must be infallible. I was recently sent a brain by colleagues in Chicago from a child with oculocerebral dysgenesis. They were very excited because their VER tests showed that stimulation of the left eye only evoked a response from the left hemisphere, and of the right eye only from the right hemisphere. They thought the child must have no chiasma, which would have been truly remarkable! In fact the child had no optic nerves at all. I have no idea what they were recording and neither do they!

Developmental Neurobiology, edited by
Philippe Evrard and Alexandre Minkowski.
Nestlé Nutrition Workshop Series, Vol. 12.
Nestec Ltd., Vevey/Raven Press, Ltd.,
New York © 1989.

Perinatal Cerebral Circulation and Its Pathological Perturbations

Hans Lou

John F. Kennedy Institut, Department of Neuropediatrics, 2600 Glostrup, Denmark

In recent years there has been a growing awareness of the significance of hemodynamic factors in the pathogenesis of perinatal neurologic disorders.

In particular, the "lost autoregulation hypothesis" has received attention as a key to understanding the development of hypoxic-ischemic encephalopathy and periventricular hemorrhage. Under normal conditions the adult, as well as the unstressed newborn, is capable of regulating vascular resistance to obtain a constant cerebral perfusion during relatively wide changes of perfusion pressure. This autoregulation of cerebral blood flow (CBF) is lost in the stressed newborn, exposing the brain to ischemia even during moderate hypotension, and to increased pressure gradient across the capillary wall during moderate hypertension, resulting in increased risk of intracranial hemorrhage (1–3).

This has stimulated interest in defining the factors that regulate cerebral perfusion *in utero* and the stresses surrounding the birth process. Using an animal model, the chronically prepared near-term fetal lamb, the author and Dr. Arnold Tweed examined the autoregulation of CBF *in utero* under normoxic and hypoxic conditions (4). CBF was measured using isotope-labeled 15 μm microspheres 24 to 48 hours after surgical preparations. Seventeen animals were studied, eight considered to be normoxic (ascending aortic O_2 saturation (SaO_2) 57% or higher), and nine spontaneously hypoxic (SaO_2 less than 51%). The fetal hemoglobin averaged 11.5 g/100 ml. CBF autoregulation was assessed in four regions: hemispheres (grey and white matter), basal ganglia, cerebellum, and brain stem. Autoregulation was found to be functionally active in all regions of the normonemic fetus, but was abolished in the mildly hypoxic fetus.

The demonstrated threshold of SaO_2 for impairment of autoregulation of 50% to 60% corresponds to an arterial O_2 concentration of about 3 millimoles/liter, which is similar to the threshold for autoregulation impairment in newborn lambs (5) and adult dogs (6).

This threshold is a little higher than the level required for fetal hypoxic hyperemia (7) in which a hyperbolic relationship between CBF and arterial O_2 concentration has been reported (8).

By partially occluding the umbilical vessels for a period of 1 to 1.5 hr a progressive and severe asphyxia with a final arterial pH of 6.9 was achieved. During this procedure pO_2 changed only slightly (from a mean of 18 mm Hg to 17 mm Hg) whereas pCO_2 increased from a mean of 34 to 60, with a concomitant fourfold increase in cerebral perfusion (up to a cortical blood flow of 5.96 ml/g/min in normotension) indicating that CO_2 is a major determinant of cerebral perfusion *in utero,* as it is after birth.

In this model CBF decreased proportionally to decreases in systemic arterial pressure (9).

It may be concluded from these observations that fetal cerebral perfusion is very labile, and that autoregulation of fetal CBF is a fragile mechanism, apparently due to the relatively hypoxic conditions *in utero.* A minor additional hypoxic insult is sufficient to abolish this protective mechanism. The normal birth process constitutes such an insult, and this may explain why a number of investigators find that vaginally born premature infants are more prone to develop intracranial hermorrhages than prematures born by cesarian section (10,11).

If the hemorrhage penetrates into the ventricular system there is a substantial risk of development of hydrocephalus due to impaired CSF outflow. But the most serious turn of events develops if the hemorrhage spreads into the brain parenchyma. The clinical condition of the infant is likely to deteriorate abruptly in many cases, leading to death. There is some evidence that ischemic lesions of the brain parenchyma precede this development.

In the original series of 19 patients in whom CBS had been measured a few hours after birth, 4 died with clinical signs of hemorrhage verified at autopsy at the ages of 2 to 37 days. In all 4 patients, low values of CBF had been measured immediately after birth. Using continuous EEG recordings and repeated measurements of evoked potentials, flow, and ultrasound scanning, it should be possible to establish whether a low flow state prior to detectable intraparenchymal hemorrhage is accompanied by electrophysiologic signs of ischemic brain dysfunction. Such studies are in progress in our department (Greisen, Lou, and Rosén). The functional state of brain tissue is in fact altered *before* the bleeding, which indicates that the hemorrhage may be interpreted as a hemorrhagic infarction. The hemorrhage itself may, in its turn, aggravate ischemia. Volpe and co-workers have shown with PET scanning that intraparenchymal hemorrhage is surrounded by a zone of severe ischemia (12). This close topical relationship between hemorrhage and ischemia, detected several days after the bleeding, indicates that the hemorrhage in its turn may induce long lasting ischemia. In order to obtain a better understanding of the mechanism, we have, in collaboration with Dr. Lars Edvinsson, examined the effect of blood admixture on the ion composition of mock spinal fluid *in vitro.* It was found that during the first two to three days the K^+ concentration increased dramatically up to about tenfold, depending upon the concentration of blood in the mixture. This level is maintained for at least two weeks. Such a K^+ concentration (about 20–50 meq) has a marked vasoconstrictor effect which could very well be responsible for the perihemorrhagic ischemia. Likewise, it should be mentioned that a similar K^+ concentration is capable of inducing neuronal depolarization and spreading depression. Spreading depression is known to be accompanied by a considerable *increase* in glucose utilization (13).

In summary the following sequence of events may be proposed: Lack of autoregulation and initial hypotension induces ischemic infarction; subsequent increase in blood pressure leads to periventricular hemorrhage which then may spread in infarcted tissue and induce peri-hemorrhagic ischemia, which is aggravated by increased energy demand due to spreading depression.

REFERENCES

1. Lou HC, Lassen NA, Friis-Hansen B. Impaired autoregulation of cerebral blood flow in the distressed newborn infant. *J Pediatr* 1979;94:118–21.
2. Lou HC, Skov H, Pedersen H. Low cerebral blood flow: a risk factor in the neonate. *J Pediatr* 1979;95:606–9.
3. Lou HC, Lassen NA, Friis-Hansen B. Is arterial hypertension crucial for the development of intraventricular haemorrhage in the neonate? *Lancet* 1979;1:1215–7.
4. Tweed WA, Coté J, Pash M, Lou HC. Arterial oxygenation determines autoregulation of cerebral blood flow in fetal lamb. *Pediatr Res* 1983;17:246–9.
5. Coté J, Tweed WA, Lou HC, Gregory GA, Wade J. Impairment and recovery of autoregulation of cerebral blood flow in the newborn lamb. *Pediatr Res* 1986;20:516–22.
6. Höggendal E, Johansson B. Effects of arterial carbon dioxide tension and oxygen saturation on CBF autoregulation in dogs. *Acta Physiol Scand* Suppl 1965;258:27–53.
7. Johnson GN, Palahnink RJ, Tweed WA, Jones MV, Wade J. Regional cerebral blood flow changes during severe fetal asphyxia produced by slow partial umbilical cord compression. *Am J Obstet Gynecol* 1979;135:48–52.
8. Jones PM, Sheldon RE, Peeters LL, Makowski EL, Meschia G. Regulation of cerebral blood flow in the ovine foetus. *Am J Physiol* 1981;235:H162–6.
9. Lou HC, Lassen NA, Tweed WA, Johnson GN, Jones MV, Palahnink RJ. Pressure passive cerebral blood flow and breakdown of the blood-brain barrier in experimental fetal asphyxia. *Acta Paediatr Scand* 1979;68:57–63.
10. Dolfin T, Skidmore MB, Fong KW, et al. Perinatal factors that influence the incidence of subependymal and intraventricular hemorrhage in low birthweight infants. *Syllabus—second special Ross Laboratories conference on perinatal intracranial hemorrhage*. Washington, D.C., December 2–4, 1982.
11. Lou HC, Phibbs RH, Wilson SL, Gregory GA. Hyperventilation at birth may prevent early periventricular hemorrhage. *Lancet* 1982;I:1407.
12. Volpe JJ, Herscovitch P, Perlman JM, Raichle ME. Positron emission tomography in the newborn: extensive impairment of regional cerebral blood flow with intraventricular hemorrhage and hemorrhagic intracerebral involvement. *Pediatrics* 1983;72:589–601.
13. Shinohara M, Pollinger B, Brown G, Rapoport S, Soholoff L. Cerebral glucose utilization: local changes during and after recovery from spreading cortical depression. *Science* 1979;203:188–90.

Developmental Neurobiology, edited by
Philippe Evrard and Alexandre Minkowski.
Nestlé Nutrition Workshop Series, Vol. 12.
Nestec Ltd., Vevey/Raven Press, Ltd.,
New York © 1989.

Positron Emission Tomography in the Study of Regional Cerebral Blood Flow in the Premature Infant with Major Intraventricular Hemorrhage and in the Term Newborn with Asphyxia

Joseph J. Volpe

Division of Neurology, Departments of Pediatrics, Neurology, and Biological Chemistry, Washington University School of Medicine, St. Louis, Missouri 63178

The two major causes of neurological morbidity and mortality related to definable events in the neonatal period are intraventricular hemorrhage (IVH) with hemorrhagic intracerebral involvement in the preterm infant, and hypoxic-ischemic encephalopathy in the asphyxiated term infant. This chapter reviews studies of regional cerebral blood flow (CBF) by positron emission tomography (PET) in these two important groups of infants.

INTRAVENTRICULAR HEMORRHAGE WITH HEMORRHAGIC INTRACEREBRAL INVOLVEMENT IN THE PRETERM INFANT

Periventricular-intraventricular hemorrhage (PVH-IVH) is the most common serious neurological lesion encountered in the premature infant (1). The incidence of PVH-IVH is high, approximately 35% to 45% (2). A recent prospective study by serial real-time ultrasonography in 460 infants with a birth weight below 2,000 gm revealed an incidence of PVH-IVH of 39% (3). Of all patients with PVH-IVH, those with hemorrhagic intracerebral involvement exhibit the highest rates of mortality and neurological morbidity and account for the vast majority of all neurologically impaired infants with PVH-IVH. To prevent this lesion, an understanding of its pathogenesis and basic nature is necessary.

Two possibilities concerning the pathogenesis and basic nature of the hemorrhagic intracerebral involvement with severe PVH-IVH seem most worthy of consideration. First, the intracerebral blood could represent localized extension of blood from the germinal matrix or lateral ventricle into previously normal white matter, or second, the intracerebral blood could represent a component of a larger, primary parenchymal lesion. We reasoned that assessment of regional CBF could provide highly valuable information for the evaluation of these hypotheses. However, until now elucidation of regional CBF in the newborn has not been possible. Positron emission tomography has been recently shown to be highly effective in the study of regional CBF in older patients (4).

In this study, we utilized PET to measure regional CBF in six premature infants with severe IVH and hemorrhagic intracerebral involvement to obtain insight into the basic nature of the parenchymal involvement. The findings demonstrate the value and feasibility of PET for the determination of regional CBF in the newborn with severe IVH and hemorrhagic intracerebral involvement and clarify the basic nature of the parenchymal involvement.

HYPOXIC-ISCHEMIC ENCEPHALOPATHY IN THE ASPHYXIATED TERM INFANT

Hypoxic-ischemic encephalopathy in the term newborn is the most frequently recognized cause of the subsequent nonprogressive motor deficits often grouped under the rubric, cerebral palsy (1). These deficits consist most commonly of spastic weakness of proximal extremities, usually symmetric. The magnitude of the problem of hypoxic-ischemic encephalopathy relates not only to the gravity of the lesions, but also to the relatively high and unchanging prevalence of the encephalopathy (5). Indeed, unlike the decline in neurological sequelae attributable to hypoxic-ischemic encephalopathy in the premature infant with the advent of neonatal intensive care, there has been little or no decrease in such sequelae in the term infant (6).

Further insight into the basic nature and pathogenesis of the major brain injury associated with neonatal hypoxic-ischemic encephalopathy is needed to devise interventions to decrease the high prevalence of the neurological sequelae. Obtaining such insight from neuropathological observations has been difficult because relatively few infants, that is, approximately 10% to 15%, die in the neonatal period, and these as expected represent the most severely affected infants. Diffuse cerebral changes, confirmed by computerized tomography (CT) (7), are common and obscure critical elemental lesions. We reasoned that insight into the basic nature and pathogenesis of the brain injury in surviving infants could be provided by measurements of regional CBF in the acute period of illness. Recently, we have demonstrated the feasibility and value of PET in the study of regional CBF in the newborn (8). Thus, we undertook the present study to measure regional CBF during the acute period of illness in term infants with hypoxic-ischemic encephalopathy and to provide insight into the basic nature and pathogenesis of the associated brain injury.

METHODS

Measurement of Regional Cerebral Blood
Flow by Positron Emission Tomography

Positron emission tomography was performed with the PETT VI tomograph. The design and performance characteristics of this system have been described (9,10). Data are recorded simultaneously from seven slices with a center-to-center separation of 14.4 mm. The in-plane resolution is 11.7 mm. Each PET slice is performed in the horizontal plane parallel to the orbitomeatal line. Head positioning is accomplished with the aid of a vertical laser line, which indicates the level of the lowest PET slice.

For the measurement of regional CBF, an emission scan, 40 sec in duration, is obtained following an intravenous bolus injection of ^{15}O-labeled water, 0.7 mCi/kg, in 0.5 ml of saline. In those studies in which an arterial catheter had been placed for the infant's intensive care, collection of arterial samples was carried out approximately every 5 sec. These samples were weighed and counted and the radioactivity corrected for the physical decay of ^{15}O, as previously described (8). Calibration of the tomograph to obtain the regional isotope concentration in brain from the reconstructed image was carried out as previously described (8).

The scan data and blood curve were analyzed according to the general principles of inert gas exchange, developed by Kety (11) and later embodied in a tissue autoradiographic technique for the measurement of local CBF in laboratory animals (12,13). We have described the details of this analysis (8) and have established the validity of this technique in the adult baboon (14). The correlation between CBF determined by PET, and with ^{15}O-labeled water and standard tracer principles, was excellent. Because of the near linear relationship between local tissue counts and CBF obtained with the PET autoradiographic approach, it is possible to measure accurately relative differences in local blood flows in different brain regions. This is particularly important because the majority of the infants studied herein did not have arterial lines in place and thus absolute blood flow quantitation could not be performed.

The total absorbed radiation dose, in a representative 1 kg subject receiving an intravenous bolus injection of 0.7 mCi of ^{15}O-labeled water, is 63 mrem for the whole body. The critical organs, that is, those receiving the largest radiation exposure, are the brain, heart, kidney, liver, and gastrointestinal tract. These high-flow organs receive 76 mrem.

Other Measurements

Continuous measurements of arterial blood pressure were made from an indwelling umbilical artery catheter. Intracranial pressure was determined at the anterior fontanel with the Ladd monitor. Cranial ultrasonography was performed with an Advanced Technology Laboratories (ATL) sector scanner. Computerized tomography and technetium radionuclide brain scanning were performed by standard techniques.

RESULTS

Intraventricular Hemorrhage with Hemorrhagic Intracerebral Involvement in the Premature Infant

Clinical Features

The birth weights of the six infants studied ranged from 920 to 1,200 gm. Four of the six infants sustained varying degrees of perinatal asphyxia, since their 1 min Apgar scores were 3 or below, and their 5 min scores below 6. Each of these four infants experienced probable intrauterine insults, for example, fetal bradycardia, worsening maternal hypotension, precipitous delivery, and second born of twins. Two infants had large patent ductus arteriosus at the time of the PET study, and all six had severe respiratory distress syndrome. The PET scans were performed on the fifth day of life in two of the infants, on the sixth day in one, on the tenth day in two, and on the seventeenth day in one. The latter infant had a second PET study on the ninetieth day. Four infants expired in the neonatal period.

The cranial ultrasonographic abnormalities are illustrated in a typical case (Fig. 1). The cranial ultrasound scan shows bilateral subependymal hemorrhage and IVH, much more marked on the left, and marked hemorrhagic intracerebral involvement on the left (Fig. 1A). The left sagittal scan (Fig. 1B) demonstrates that the hemorrhagic intracerebral involvement was confined to frontal white matter.

PET Determinations of Regional Cerebral Blood Flow

Each patient exhibited the essential PET findings. These are illustrated in Fig. 2 and include (a) on the side opposite to the intraparenchymal lesion, highest blood flows laterally in the region of adjacent and overlapping frontal-temporal cortex, that is, sylvian cortex, and in some slices, basal ganglia; (b) anteriorly and posteriorly, in the midline, highest blood flows in adjacent, right, and left medial frontal and occipital cortex; and, most significantly, (c) in the hemisphere containing the intraparenchymal blood, decreases in regional blood flow that are much more extensive in distribution that can be accounted for by the locus of the intracerebral blood. Indeed, in the involved left hemispheres marked diminutions of regional CBF are apparent not only anteriorly in frontal white matter, the site of the hemorrhagic intracerebral involvement, but also in posterior cerebral white matter and, to a lesser extent, in frontal-temporal-parietal cortex (especially sylvian cortex).

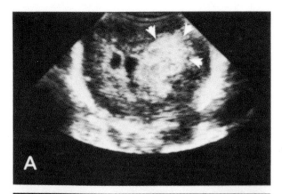

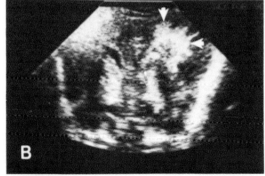

FIG. 1. Ultrasound scans, representative case of intraventricular hemorrhage with hemorrhagic intracerebral involvement in the premature infant. Note in the coronal scans (**A, B**) the region of intraparenchymal involvement on the left *(arrows),* as well as blood in the left lateral ventricle. The relatively limited anteroposterior extent of the intraparenchymal involvement *(arrows)* is apparent in the parasagittal scan (**C**).

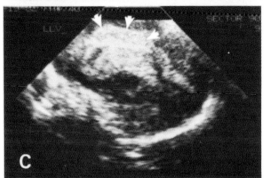

Structural Correlate to the Extensive Impairment of
Cerebral Blood Flow in the Involved Hemisphere

Neuropathological study of three of the cases defined the structural correlate of the extensive impairment of CBF in the hemisphere containing the intraparenchymal hemorrhagic involvement. Thus the blood clot in the left frontal white matter was found to be continuous with extensive nonhemorrhagic softening of the posterior frontal, parietal, and occipital white matter.

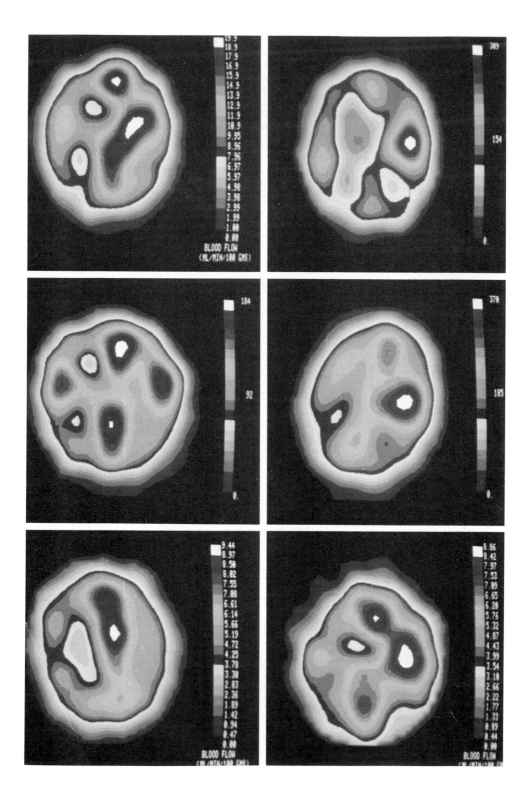

Hypoxic-Ischemic Encephalopathy in the Asphyxiated Term Infant

Clinical Features

The essential clinical features of the 14 infants were characteristic of neonatal hypoxic-ischemic encephalopathy (1). The severity of the asphyxial insults is emphasized by Apgar scores of <4 at 5 min in 11. The likelihood that the Apgar scores reflected depression secondary to intrauterine asphyxia is supported by the findings of fetal distress in 10 of the 12 infants for whom adequate intrauterine data were recorded. One infant sustained a primarily postnatal hypoxic-ischemic event, that is, cardiorespiratory arrest at 4 hr, of unknown etiology.

The neurological features were similar and conformed to the neurological syndrome previously described (1). Eight of the infants experienced neonatal seizures, with onset consistently on the first postnatal day. All infants were treated with phenobarbital (1).

Twelve of the infants exhibited proximal limb weakness. Affection of upper more than lower extremities was consistent (1). The two infants who did not exhibit definite proximal limb weakness also did not exhibit seizures and, on the basis of clinical course, appeared to be the least affected patients in the group.

The PET studies were performed on postnatal days 3 to 5 in twelve infants, on day 7 in one, and on day 20 in one. At the time of the PET studies, all infants had normal blood gases, hematocrit, intracranial pressure, and systemic blood pressure.

PET Determinations of Regional Cerebral Blood Flow

The normal or near normal pattern of regional CBF in the term newborn is apparent in the PET scan obtained from the infant least affected on the basis of clinical findings (Fig. 3A). (For ethical considerations, no clinically normal infants have been studied thus far.) The major PET findings include an external ribbon of relatively higher flows in regions of cerebral cortex. Cerebral blood flow to frontal and parietal cortical regions are approximately 50% higher than to corresponding cerebral white matter. Of the cortical regions, relatively higher flows are especially apparent anteriorly and posteriorly in the midline, in adjacent right and left medial frontal and occipital cortex. Laterally, CBF to adjacent and overlapping frontal-temporal-parietal cortex, that is, sylvian cortex, is approximately 10% higher than CBF to adjacent frontal or parietal cortex. In addition to cerebral cortical regions,

---

FIG. 2. PET scans for each of the six preterm infants with IVH and hemorrhagic intracerebral involvement. The scans represent horizontal sections at slightly different levels of brain. The scale is a linear representation of CBF values, with highest flows at the top and lowest at the bottom. Actual values of CBF were obtained for three cases and thus gray scale numbers are in ml/100 gm/min, as indicated. No arterial line was in place in three infants and the values shown on the scale are relative numbers. In each case the hemorrhagic intracerebral involvement was in the left frontal region.

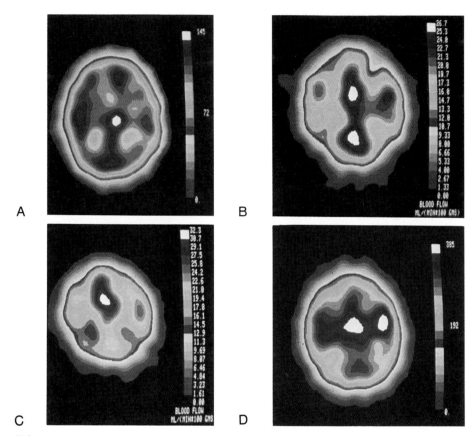

FIG. 3. PET scans for four asphyxiated term infants. See legend to Fig. 2 for orientation of the scans. The least affected infant is shown in **A**. Note the relative decreases in CBF in the parasagittal regions, especially posteriorly, bilaterally, in **B**, **C**, and **D**.

relatively higher flows are also observed centrally, in the region of thalamus and basal ganglia.

The abnormalities of regional CBF in the infants constitute a continuum of deviation from the normal or near normal pattern just described (Fig. 3B–D). The consistent and apparently unifying abnormality was a relative decrease in CBF to parasagittal regions, generally symmetric and more marked posteriorly than anteriorly. The spectrum of this abnormality is apparent in the illustrated PET studies (Figs. 3B–D). In the least affected patients, CBF to posterior parasagittal regions is approximately 25% lower than CBF to sylvian cortex, and in the infants with the most severe affection, parasagittal CBF values are approximately 40% lower than those to sylvian cortex. The relative decreases in parasagittal CBF are slightly less marked in the anterior parasagittal regions. A consistent feature in the affected parasagittal areas is a loss or even reversal of the cortical gray matter versus white matter gradient of regional CBF.

The number of infants who were studied with arterial lines in place and for whom, therefore, absolute values for CBF are available is too small to permit generalizations about the severity of the deviation of parasagittal CBF from normal. In three such infants, the absolute values in the posterior parasagittal regions ranged from 30 to 50 ml/100 gm/min, and in the corresponding sylvian regions, 60 to 80 ml/100 gm/min.

Correlates of the Parasagittal Abnormality in Regional Cerebral Blood Flow

To determine the structural correlates, if any, of the decrease in CBF in parasagittal regions, we initially turned to the CT scan. However, clear topographic correlation of the CT findings with the PET findings was not possible. Thus CT scans obtained within several days of the PET scans showed more diffuse abnormalities, usually diffuse hypodensity of cerebral white matter, as described in previous studies of asphyxiated term infants (7).

We next evaluated correlation with the radionuclide brain scan. Thus far, the two infants evaluated by technetium brain scan have exhibited nearly identical findings (see Fig. 4). A striking pattern of increased uptake of the radionuclide in the parasagittal regions, bilaterally and posteriorly more than anteriorly, was observed. The close correlation of this abnormality with the abnormality of regional CBF is apparent.

Neuropathological correlation of the parasagittal abnormality in CBF was ob-

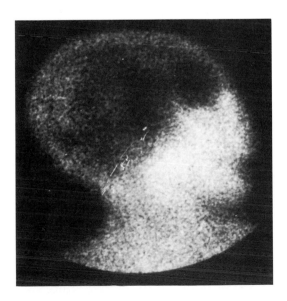

FIG. 4. Technetium brain scan (right lateral view) from asphyxiated term infant. Note the increased uptake of technetium in the parasagittal region, posteriorly more than anteriorly.

tained in the one infant who died. At postmortem examination, softening was apparent in parasagittal parietal cortex bilaterally. Coronal sections of the fixed brain revealed regions of softening in the parasagittal cerebral cortex and subcortical white matter, especially posteriorly. The involvement extended into periventricular white matter. Microscopic sections of the affected areas showed occasional cortical neurons with faintly eosinophilic cytoplasm or pyknotic nuclei and pyknotic nuclei in cerebral white matter; there was no definite tissue reaction, which was not unexpected in view of the short duration of survival. (Similar cellular changes were also observed in the caudate nucleus, ventral pons, and Purkinje cell layer of the cerebellum.)

DISCUSSION

Intraventricular Hemorrhage with Hemorrhagic Intracerebral Involvement in the Premature Infant

The current observations indicate that the hemorrhagic intracerebral involvement in infants with severe PVH-IVH is a component of a larger, primary ischemic lesion. This conclusion is based on consideration of the topography of the abnormality of CBF, shown by PET, and on the nature of the anatomic abnormality, shown by neuropathological study. The lesion involves periventricular white matter and, apparently, frontal, temporal, and parietal cortex, although because of the limits of resolution of PET it remains possible that the lesion involves only white matter. Periventricular white matter is a vulnerable region to ischemic injury in the premature newborn (1). Thus, DeReuck and co-workers have demonstrated the presence of periventricular arterial border zones and end zones, that is, watershed regions, at the sites of occurrence of ischemic neonatal periventricular white matter injury (15). Within the periventricular region, two sites, one anterior and one posterior, are especially likely to be affected by periventricular leukomalacia (16), and in this regard, it is of particular interest that in the infant with the least severe parenchymal involvement, separate anterior and posterior lesions appeared to be present. Our conclusion that the hemorrhagic intracerebral lesion observed in these patients is a component of a primary ischemic lesion is compatible with our own neuropathological observations and those reported by Flodmark et al. (7), who concluded that virtually all of the hemorrhagic parenchymal lesions in their series of preterm infants with severe PVH-IVH were hemorrhagic infarcts. In keeping with this formulation is our demonstration, in the single patient who had a second PET scan, that the relative extent and severity of the decreased CBF in the left hemisphere persisted (data not shown); thus, the ischemia was not a transient acute event, but rather a reflection of a fixed structural lesion.

The etiology and timing of the ischemic injury in our infants remain unclear. The ill preterm infant is considered to be especially susceptible to ischemic cerebral injury, often secondary to systemic hypotension, because of the occurrence of a pressure-passive cerebral circulation (17). In this regard, it is noteworthy that four of six infants experienced perinatal asphyxia, as judged by depressed Apgar scores, and two had a large patent ductus arteriosus, which has been associated with decreased CBF velocity (18). It also remains possible that the ischemic lesion present in the patients was not caused by prior systemic hypotension but rather by the secondary effects of blood in the lateral ventricle, the cerebral parenchyma, or subarachnoid space. Thus, the topography of the lesion is compatible with ischemia in the distribution of the middle cerebral artery. Such a formulation raises the possibility of spasm of this artery, secondary to subarachnoid or intraventricular blood, the former a well-documented event in older patients, or of compression of its branches by local brain swelling.

Why does the intracerebral hemorrhage occur principally anteriorly in a primary parenchymal lesion that also extends far posteriorly? The consistent relation between the laterality of the intraparenchymal blood and the laterality of the more extensive degree of IVH may provide a clue. Thus, as observed in this study of six cases and in our previous ultrasonographic study of 33 cases (3), the hemorrhagic intracerebral component almost invariably occurs on the side of the most marked IVH. This relation raises at least three potential explanations for the anterior placement of the hemorrhage. First, as noted above, the large amount of intraventricular blood could impair venous drainage in the affected hemisphere, and the resulting increased venous pressure, with a propensity for hemorrhage into an infarcted area, would be greatest at the anterior site because of the previously described anatomic peculiarities of the deep venous drainage anteriorly (19). Second, the intracerebral blood may emanate from the anteriorly placed germinal matrix and extend into the periventricular white matter because the latter is infarcted. Third, the intracerebral blood may emanate from the blood-laden lateral ventricle and extend into the infarcted white matter through the external angle of the lateral ventricle because of a combination of pressure effects, related to the large volume of intraventricular blood, and a relative weakness of the ependymal barrier, related to the presence of the anteriorly placed germinal matrix.

Hypoxic-Ischemic Encephalopathy in the Asphyxiated Term Infant

These observations, the first measurements of regional CBF in the term newborn, are of particular importance with regard to the basic nature and probably pathogenesis of the major brain injury in the asphyxiated infant. In addition, the data provide important new information concerning normal regional CBF in the newborn.

Regarding normal regional CBF in the newborn, the data define approximately 50% higher flows to cerebral cortex than to subcortical white matter. It is likely that the true difference between CBF to cerebral cortex and to subcortical white matter is greater than this because of the partial volume averaging effect of the PET technique. Thus, because of the current spatial resolution of PET, 11.7 mm in the image plane, it is not possible to sample pure gray or white matter, and measurements of local tissue radioactivity will receive contributions from both gray and white matter. As a consequence, blood flow is slightly underestimated in cerebral cortex and slightly overestimated in subcortical white matter. In addition to the cortical gray matter–white matter differences, our data indicate that CBF in basal ganglia and thalamus is at least as high as to cerebral cortex. These observations are compatible with regional differences in CBF measured in neonatal animals by tissue autoradiographic techniques (20).

Regarding the major brain injury in the asphyxiated infant, a consistent abnormality has been identified, specifically, a relative decrease in CBF to parasagittal regions, posterior regions being more affected than anterior. A continuum of this abnormality was observed. The absolute severity of the defects in parasagittal CBF is difficult to quantitate precisely because of our lack of normal values for CBF and the relatively small number of the asphyxiated infants in whom absolute values of CBF could be obtained. However, we consider the parasagittal deficits in CBF to be indicative of tissue injury. In support of this conclusion are, first, the findings on the delayed radionuclide brain scans in the two patients studied, the increased uptake of the radionuclide in the parasagittal regions, posteriorly more than anteriorly, correlating closely with the findings on the PET scans; and second, the identification in the single patient studied at postmortem examination of injury to parasagittal cerebral cortex and subcortical white matter, especially posteriorly. It is similarly noteworthy that the few available neuropathological studies of long-term survivors with ''cerebral palsy'' emphasize and illustrate the parasagittal distribution of cerebral cortical and subcortical white matter injury (21,22).

Our CBF findings suggest that parasagittal cerebral injury is an extremely common feature of neonatal hypoxic-ischemic encephalopathy, at least in patients who survive the perinatal insult. Previous studies of asphyxiated term infants by radionuclide brain scans (23,24) showed that this distribution of injury, although the most common single type, nevertheless is demonstrable in only the minority of asphyxiated infants. It is reasonable to speculate that the less marked degrees of disturbance of parasagittal CBF, defined by PET, reflect degrees of tissue injury that would not be detected by radionuclide brain scan. Whether such injury is associated with neurological deficits will require long-term follow-up for resolution.

The pathogenesis of the parasagittal brain injury in these asphyxiated infants is not established by our measurements, but the characteristic parasagittal topography is indicative of ischemia as the principal pathogenetic factor. Thus the parasagittal cerebral injury occurs in the border zones between the end fields of the major cerebral arteries, that is, the anterior, middle, and posterior cerebral arteries. This characteristic topography was defined initially by Meyer in a series of mainly adult patients (one out of his series was an infant who had experienced birth asphyxia) and was related by Meyer to systemic hypotension (25). Experimental support for this watershed concept was provided in the monkey by Brierley and co-workers who reproduced similar parasagittal lesions by producing rapid, profound systemic hypotension while preventing hypoxemia (26). As we observed in our asphyxiated infants, more marked injury was demonstrable in the monkeys in the posterior cerebrum, an observation also made by Brierley and co-workers in affected adult human patients (27).

Our observations emphasize the critical importance of ischemia in the pathogenesis of the brain injury with neonatal hypoxic-ischemic encephalopathy, but do not establish the timing or precise cause of the ischemia. At least one major component of the ischemia may be systemic hypotension in association with the intrauterine asphyxia. Thus, evidence for fetal distress was common in our patients, and the occurrence of systemic hypotension (28), impaired CBF (29), and parasagittal cerebral injury (30) in asphyxiated fetal animals is well-documented. However, the additive role of postnatal hypotension, perhaps in association with difficulties with resuscitation, as evidenced by the depressed Apgar scores, could be considerable. In addition, the possibilities that postnatal hypoxemia, hypercarbia, acidemia, or brain edema could play additive roles in impairing cerebral perfusion, energy metabolism, or both must be considered. Further studies of regional CBF, coupled with the determinations of regional oxygen metabolism, could provide considerable insight into several of these issues. Clearly, PET should be of great value in such subsequent studies.

REFERENCES

1. Volpe JJ. *Neurology of the newborn*. Philadelphia: WB Saunders, 1981.
2. Tarby TJ, Volpe JJ. Intraventricular hemorrhage in the premature infant. *Pediatr Clin N Am* 1982;29:1077.
3. McMenamin JB, Shackelford GD, Volpe JJ. Outcome of neonatal-intraventricular hemorrhage with periventricular echodense lesions. *Ann Neurol* 1984;15:285.
4. Raichle ME. Quantitative *in vivo* autoradiography with positron emission tomography. *Brain Res* 1979;1:47.
5. Brown JK. Infants damaged during birth. In: Hull D, ed. *Recent advances in paediatrics*. London: Churchill Livingstone, 1976:234.
6. Hagberg B, Hagberg G, Olow I. The changing panorama of cerebral palsy in Sweden in 1970 to 1974. II. Analysis of the various syndromes. *Acta Paediatr Scand* 1975;64:193.
7. Flodmark O, Becker LE, Harwood-Nash DC, Fitzhardinge PM, Fitz CR and Chuang SH. Correlation between computed tomography and autopsy in premature and full-term neonates that have suffered perinatal asphyxia. *Radiology* 1980;137:93.
8. Volpe JJ, Herscovitch P, Perlman JM, Raichle ME. Positron emission tomography in the newborn: extensive impairment of regional cerebral blood flow with intraventricular hemorrhage and hemorrhagic intracerebral involvement. *Pediatrics* 1983;72:589.
9. Ter-Pogossian MM, Ficke DC, Hood JT, Yamamoto M, Mullani NA. PETT VI: a positron emission tomograph utilizing cesium fluoride scintillation detectors. *J Comput Tomogr* 1982;6:125.
10. Yamamoto M, Ficke DC, Ter-Pogossian MM. Performance study of PETT VI, a positron computed tomograph with 288 cesium fluoride detectors. *IEEE Trans Nuclear Science* 1982;NS029:529.
11. Kety SS. The theory and applications of the exchange of inert gas at the lungs and tissues. *Pharmacol Rev* 1251;2:1.
12. Landau WM, Freygang WH Jr, Rowland LW, Sokoloff L. The local circulation of the living brain: values in the unanesthetized and anesthetized cat. *Trans Am Neurol Assoc* 1955;80:125.
13. Sakurada O, Kennedy C, Jehle J, Brown JD, Carbin GL, Sokoloff L. Measurement of local cerebral blood flow with iodo[^{14}C]antipyrine. *Am J Physiol* 1978;234:H59.

14. Raichle ME, Martin WRW, Herscovitch P, Mintun M, Markham J. Brain blood flow measured with intravenous $H_2^{15}O$. II. Implementation and validation. *J Nucl Med* 1983;24:790.
15. DeReuck J, Chattha AS, Richardson EB Jr. Pathogenesis and evolution of periventricular leukomalacia in infancy. *Arch Neurol* 1972;27:229.
16. Shuman RM, Selednik LJ. Periventricular leukomalacia. A one-year autopsy study. *Arch Neurol* 1980;37:231.
17. Lou HC, Lassen NA, Friis-Hansen B. Impaired autoregulation of cerebral blood flow in the distressed newborn. *J Pediatr* 1979;94:118.
18. Perlman JM, Hill A, Volpe JJ. The effect of patent ductus arteriosus on flow velocity in the anterior cerebral arteries: ductal steal in the premature newborn infant. *J Pediatr* 1981;99:767.
19. Larroche JC. *Developmental pathology of the neonate*. New York: Excerpta Medica, 1977.
20. Cavazzuti M, Duffy TE. Regulation of local cerebral blood flow in normal and hypoxic newborn dogs. *Ann Neurol* 1982;2:247.
21. Courville CB. *Birth and brain damage*. Pasadena, CA: Courville, 1971.
22. Friede RS. *Developmental neuropathology*. New York: Springer-Verlag, 1975.
23. Volpe JJ, Pasternak J. Parasagittal cerebral injury in neonatal hypoxic-ischemic encephalopathy: clinical and neuroradiologic features. *J Pediatr* 1977;97:472.
24. O'Brien MJ, Ash MJ, Gilday DL. Radionuclide brain scanning in perinatal hypoxia-ischemia. *Dev Med Child Neurol* 1977;21:161.
25. Meyer JE. Uber die lokalisation fruhkindlicher hirschadenin arteriellen grenzebieten. *Arch Psychiatr Nervenkr* 1953;190:328.
26. Brierley JB, Excell BJ. The effects of profound systemic hypotension upon the brain of M. Rhesus: physiological and pathological observations. *Brain* 1966;88:269.
27. Adams JH, Brierley JB, Connor RCR, Treip CS. The effects of systemic hypotension upon the human brain: clinical and neuropathological observations in 11 cases. *Brain* 1966;89:235.
28. Dawes CS. *Foetal and neonatal physiology*. Chicago: Year Book, 1968.
29. Reivich M, Brann AW Jr, Shapiro HM, Myers RE. Regional cerebral blood flow during prolonged partial asphyxia. In: Meyer JS, Reivich M, Lechner H, Eichorn O, eds. *Research on the cerebral circulation*. Springfield, IL: Charles C Thomas, 1972:216–27.
30. Brann AW Jr, Myers RE. Central nervous system findings in the newborn monkey following severe *in utero* partial asphyxia. *Neurology* 1975;25:327.

Developmental Neurobiology, edited by
Philippe Evrard and Alexandre Minkowski.
Nestlé Nutrition Workshop Series, Vol. 12.
Nestec Ltd., Vevey/Raven Press, Ltd.,
New York © 1989.

Discussion for Chapters by Lou and Volpe

Dr. Dubowitz: I agree with Dr. Lou that the primary lesions in large intracranial hemorrhages are ischemic. The demonstration of this is dependent on having a really good 7 MHz ultrasound scanner which allows you to see ischemic lesions preceding the hemorrhage. These can later be seen to involve the ischemic area. You claim that other areas become ischemic following the hemorrhage. We have not found this, although I know Volpe has. We have only seen one case where the infant had a large dose of phenobarbital with a fall in blood pressure. I wonder how often lesions secondary to large hemorrhages are produced by some intervention aimed at preventing the hemorrhage?

Dr. Lou: It is very important to try and sort out which lesions are the result of ischemia and which are the result of the natural course of disease. We have been hesitating for many years trying to decide whether we should use phenobarbital or other types of sedative agents to lessen the effects of stress on these babies, because we have been worried that stress, and even feeding, may cause a rise in blood pressure which would start a hemorrhage. But if ischemia is the primary event, then the use of sedation may *increase* the risk of causing a hemorrhage by reducing perfusion pressure. We have not done any systematic studies on this, but I am very concerned about medication.

Dr. Volpe: I have two points to make about Dr. Dubowitz's question. First, I am not surprised that she did not see any evidence of ischemic lesions in association with areas of hemorrhage using ultrasound; neither do we, either with ultrasound or CT scanning. However, using positron emission tomography (PET) we can show an impressive degree of ischemia posterior to the hemorrhagic lesion. We have neuropathology in a few patients showing tissue injury has occurred. Second, your point about the possible dangers of therapy is very important. In most of these cases ischemic injuries relate primarily to postnatal events. Thus anything we do in the postnatal period in the care of preterm infants must be examined very carefully, including the use of agents which might depress the circulation.

Dr. Caviness: Is it the implication of this hypothesis (that ischemia is an antecedent of intracerebral hemorrhage) that intraventricular hemorrhage has a different pathogenesis from grades 1 through 3?

Dr. Lou: Nobody knows for certain, but I believe that subependymal bleeding, which you see quite often and which is of no consequence, can occur in undamaged brain tissue. However, if you have a large penetrating bleed into the brain parenchyma I suspect very much from present evidence that there has been a preceding infarction. From a practical and prognostic point of view grade 1 hemorrhages should certainly be separated from other bleeds.

Dr. Volpe: I think it is unfortunate that this classification of intracerebral hemorrhage in preterm infants has taken hold so readily. I still feel that we need to distinguish grade 4 hemorrhage, which is the worst degree by whatever name you choose to call it, from an intraventricular hemorrhage. I do not believe that there is an obligatory relationship at all between intracerebral bleeding and intraventricular bleeding. I accept that different amounts of blood within the ventricular system probably deserve different gradings, but I believe that one should separately identify a hemorrhagic cerebral infarct.

Dr. Roig: With regard to seizures, are you suggesting that these are produced locally and that brain edema perhaps has nothing to do with them at this time? I was also surprised at the equality of blood flow distribution between the two sides, particularly the bilateral decrease in blood flow, which seems to go against our clinical experience that many of these patients have asymmetric lesions and clinical signs.

Dr. Volpe: Regarding your first question, we believe that seizures have a variety of effects on the circulation that we have previously been unaware of, but which we must now pay more attention to. We have much less data obtained with PET than with the Doppler technique, but even so one can still determine what happens to anterior cerebral artery flow during seizures using Doppler through the anterior fontanelle. We have studied at least 20 babies during seizures, mostly of the so-called subtle variety, and there is a very consistent increase in blood flow velocity in the anterior cerebral artery during them which appears to be directly related to the seizure-related increase in blood pressure. There is a consistent increase in overall cerebral blood flow, at least if one extrapolates from animal data, which is presumably a central autonomic phenomenon. For this reason we think that seizures pose a considerable threat of initiating germinal matrix hemorrhages.

Regarding the question of why we did not see major asymmetyric lesions in our series, I think this was probably fortuitous. We have now studied 25 or 30 term babies who have been asphyxiated and have identified several with focal cerebral ischemic lesions of the type we can recognize on CT and ultrasound scanning. In our experience these therefore make up a minority of the babies with hypoxic-ischemic encephalopathy. When you look carefully at these patients you find they all have parasagittal injury, so it appears that they not only have border zone lesions but for some reason develop additional focal cerebral infarction as well.

Dr. Minkowski: Since you cannot at present be absolutely sure whether or not ischemia is the primary event in cerebral hemorrhage, I wonder whether you intend to investigate cerebral oxygen consumption and glucose metabolism in addition to your other measurements, since these are now accessible to measurement using positron techniques.

Dr. Volpe: I agree that the proper assessment of the kinds of injury we are dealing with demands the simultaneous measurement of cerebral blood flow, blood volume, and oxygen metabolism. The reason we have not done this yet is primarily that measuring regional oxygen consumption requires considerably longer exposure of the infant to the radionucleotide.

Dr. Lou: It is probable that in the not too distant future we shall be able to measure cerebral oxygen metabolism and blood flow at the cot-side using infrared spectroscopy.

Dr. Dubowitz: Is it possible that the increase in cerebral blood flow due to a convulsion is in compensation for the ischemia which is produced in the brain at such a time, and might therefore even be beneficial?

Dr. Volpe: It is definitely an adaptive response. It has been shown in adult animals to be an attempt to bring glucose and oxygen into a region which requires more fuel because of excessive firing. The rise in blood pressure which occurs is able to cause a local increase in flow because the affected region fails to autoregulate. This is because a shift in cytoplasmic redox state allows a local increase in hydrogen ion concentration and hence local vasodilatation. In the baby, however, this adaptative response may become maladaptive because the circulatory changes may cause problems in vulnerable capillary beds like the germinal matrix.

Dr. Quero: Would you recommend the use of phenobarbital before the appearance of convulsions in patients with severe perinatal asphyxia?

Dr. Volpe: In practice this is what we do with the full-term asphyxiated newborn. If the baby is at term, has clearly documented intrapartum asphyxia, and has a neonatal neurological syndrome that is typical of that disorder, we start that infant on anticonvulsant doses of phenobarbital before the onset of seizures. We recognize, however, that this has never been shown to be beneficial in a controlled trial.

Dr. Ballabriga: Most infants with patent ductus arteriosus (PDA) who have been treated with indomethacin develop hypotension, but I do not think anyone has shown that there is an increased risk of brain damage or hemorrhage.

Dr. Volpe: I am not so sure that PDA is as harmless as it is made out to be. We have studied a large number of babies with PDA using the Doppler technique and have shown that they have impressive decreases in cerebral blood flow velocity. We have also studied several babies before and after ductus closure using PET scanning and have demonstrated that there is a large increase in cerebral blood flow when the duct is closed, up to levels which we now consider to be within the normal range. This suggests that prior to closure of the duct cerebral blood flow may have been low enough to be marginal. This is likely to make the baby particularly vulnerable to other insults which could further compromise the cerebral circulation.

Developmental Neurobiology, edited by
Philippe Evrard and Alexandre Minkowski.
Nestlé Nutrition Workshop Series, Vol. 12.
Nestec Ltd., Vevey/Raven Press, Ltd.,
New York © 1989.

Psychological Factors in Neurological Development

Martin H. Teicher

*Department of Psychiatry, Harvard Medical School, Mailman Research Center and
McLean Hospital, Belmont, Massachusetts 02178*

In exploring the role of psychological factors in neurological development— and by extension—behavior, we tread firmly on the nature–nurture controversy, an arena of debate that has ensnarled many bright minds and often generated great heat but little light. At the present time, with molecular biology in its ascendency, we can readily appreciate and accept the role of the genome in establishing the architectural specificity of the central nervous system (CNS). This has not always been the case. In the early part of this century it was often held that neural connectivity was too complex to be based solely on genetic information. Instead, neuronal processes were posited to grow with little intrinsic control, but those connections that produced functionally appropriate behaviors were selected and maintained through experience (1). This proposition was rejected by the ingenious experiments of Sperry and colleagues, who demonstrated that connections producing nonadaptive behaviors persisted indefinitely and were not necessarily subject to corrective elimination (2). The contribution of experiential factors to neural development enjoyed a modest reawakening with the discovery, in single-unit studies of mammalian visual development, that certain forms of environmental deprivation exert deleterious effects on receptive field organization and neural connectivity (1).

FACTORS AFFECTING NEUROLOGICAL DEVELOPMENT

There is general agreement at the present time that the brain, in its adult form, represents the elaboration of species-specific and individual genetic information through complex spatial and temporal gradients. This process is affected by a host of other factors. Hebb (3) and Tees (4) in their writings on the development of behavior have placed these factors into a useful schema, modified in Table 1 to focus on neural development per se.

In this presentation we will concentrate on the influence of factors IV and VI, though it should be borne in mind that the full range of environmental variables spans factors II through VI.

TABLE 1. *Factors in neurological development*

No.	Class	Source
I	Genetic	Nucleic acids of a fertilized ovum
II	Chemical environment—prenatal	Nutritive or toxic influences in uterine environment
III	Chemical environment—postnatal	Nutritive or toxic influences: food, water, oxygen, drugs, etc.
IV	Sensory-motor environment—constant	Pre- and postnatal experiences normally inevitable for all members of a species
V	Sensory-motor environment—variable	Experiences that vary from one member of a species to another
VI	Traumatic	Physical or experiential factors that tend to destroy cells or disrupt growth; an abnormal class of events to which an animal might conceivably never be exposed

Focal Questions

This chapter focuses on two pressing clinical questions, presented in Table 2, that specify the scope and nature of the problem, but for which only modest and very preliminary data are available. These questions have direct preclinical research analogs that have been explored in greater depth in laboratory animals and serve as a complementary point of reference. This review endeavors to integrate both the salience and relevence of clinical observations with the rigor and control of the laboratory investigation.

TABLE 2. *Focal questions*

Clinical perspective

Can inadequate, inappropriate, or pathological psychological factors impede, arrest, or alter neurological development?

Can an appropriate selection of psychological factors compensate for deficits in an individual's neurobiological endowment or early environment?

Preclinical research perspective

What is the role of sensory-motor experience in normal neurological development? (Does normal neural development depend on sensory-motor experiences, and if so, to what extent and in what ways?)

What are the potential consequences of abnormal sensory-motor experiences on normal neurological development? (Is neural development *sensitive* to alterations or abnormalities in sensory-motor experience, and if so, to what extent and in what ways?)

To what extent and in what ways can alterations in sensory-motor experience influence the outcome of early CNS insult or injury?

NORMAL NEUROLOGICAL DEVELOPMENT—
ROLE OF EXPERIENCE

The first area of inquiry, concerning the dependence of neural development on experiential factors, has been addressed most cogently by G. Gottlieb, who has expanded the theoretical frameworks pioneered by Z.Y. Kuo, T.C. Schneirla, and D.R. Lehrman. Briefly, Gottlieb (5) has postulated that experiential factors can serve three fundamentally different purposes in normal neurological development. These are maintenance, facilitation, and induction.

Maintenance

At the lowest level of effect, maintaining experience serves merely to preserve an already developed state or endpoint. Such a role of experience is readily observed in most sensory systems, and we are aware that long-term sensory deprivation during early neonatal development can lead to atrophy and loss of neural tissue in the sensory system deprived of stimulation (6). Similarly, complete lack of sensory stimulation in the adult can lead to disorientation, hallucinations, and loss of reality testing, dramatically revealing the important role of these factors in maintaining certain of our cognitive faculties.

Facilitation

At the next higher level, facilitating experience assists in the developmental achievement of states or endpoints. However, these experiences are not absolutely necessary, as the development of neural structures or functions eventually occurs even in the absence of the experience, though it may be subpar without it. Facilitation thus regulates the rate of neural development or alters the endpoint in a quantitative fashion.

Both types of facilitating experiences have been observed in the visual cortex. For example, the diameter of cell nuclei and the volume of internuclear material per nuclei peaks at an earlier age in visually experienced mice. However, the visual cortex of dark-reared controls eventually reaches a comparable level on the same parameters, albeit at a slower rate (7). On the other hand, dendritic spine numbers in visual cortex are affected quantitatively by visual experience. Albino rats reared under constant illumination attain and maintain a larger number of dendritic spines in their visual cortex than rats reared in light–dark cycles (8). Moreover, a recent quantitative electron microscopy study revealed that there were (depending on the numerical estimation technique selected) 7% to 16% more synapses per neuron in the occipital cortex of rats raised in pairs from 25 to 55 days than in isolated controls, and 25% to 42% more synapses per neuron in pair-raised rats housed in complex environments (9). The severe delays encountered in the attainment of developmental milestones in some institutionalized children suffering from anaclitic depression may represent a serious clinical analog of the consequence of inadequate facilitatory experience (10).

Induction

Inductive experience, in contrast, signifies those special instances in which the presence or absence of a particular experience, during a critical or sensitive period, completely determines whether or not a given species-typical neural feature will manifest itself later in development. Evidence for this type of function derived from sensory-motor experience in normal development remains mostly theoretical. We are aware of such "canalizing" effects in embryology and developmental neuroendocrinology, where for example the presence or absence of certain gonadal hormones in the perinatal period determine whether the genitalia will be of the male or female type upon maturity (11), or whether sexually dimorphic nuclei in the medial preoptic area of the hypothalamus will mature to male size and form (12).

NEURAL DEVELOPMENT—SENSITIVITY TO DISRUPTION BY ABNORMAL EXPERIENCE

Overall, the vast majority of studies pertaining to the role of experience in normal neural development concentrate on the influence of sensory experience on development of cortical organization. Hubel and Wiesel, in their classic description of receptive field characteristics, addressed this issue in two ways. They first asked whether neurons in the kitten displayed adult binocular properties before eye-opening, and second, whether striate cortical neurons in animals raised with various forms of abnormal visual experience exhibited adult properties. These two approaches yielded somewhat conflicting results. Briefly, it appeared that neurons with adult properties were present before visual experience (13), but that animals raised with abnormal visual experiences did not have a normal distribution of adult properties (14). Hubel and Wiesel interpreted their data as indicating that sensory input does not participate in patterning connections during normal development, but that abnormal visual experience could result in the destruction of normal connections. In short, the binocularity of striate cortical neurons did not *depend* on visual experience, but was *sensitive* to effects of abnormal visual experience.

These principles, derived from studies of binocular interaction, were generally accepted until Hirsch and Spinelli (15) and Blakemore and Cooper (16) reported that orientation specificity of cortical receptive fields was strongly influenced by visual experience. Neuronal distribution studies, conducted mostly in rabbits (1), have clearly suggested that although a vast degree of striate cortical responsiveness is established prior to visual experience, visual experience functions in a facilitative manner, enhancing the specificity of receptive field organization and augmenting the percentage of visually responsive units.

Conceptual Model Predicting Outcome of Sensory Deprivation Studies

More recent studies by Singer (17) and others have produced a fruitful convergence between morphological, physiological, and psychobiological models. Briefly, three factors interact to determine the outcome of neurobiological deprivation studies. These include (a) activity in afferent systems; (b) activity of postsynaptic cortical elements; and (c) a global factor relating to attention or perhaps to general cortical activity during the experience. These three factors interact in explaining and predicting the outcome of most forms of deprivation studies. Their relationship is summarized in Table 3.

In the classic monocular visual deprivation studies, Type 1 and 2 interactions explain the marked enhancement in ocular dominance columns driven by the exposed eye, and the marked diminution in columns connected to the unexposed eye. These types of interactions also explain the result of studies in which subjects are reared in environments with contours of only a single orientation. This environment produces little effect on orientation column systems within layer IV, but massive distortion of columnar systems within nongranular layers. Although cells responding to inexperienced orientations are still present in layer IV and are grouped in regularly spaced bands, activity from these cells is no longer relayed to cells in supra- and infragranular layers. In contrast, activity of layer IV cells, whose orientation preference corresponded to the experienced orientation, is not only relayed to nongranular layers directly above and below the active zone, but spreads tangentially to adjacent cells.

Type 3 interactions are observed, for example, in a monocular visual deprivation study, in which the exposed eye is presented only with flashes of diffuse light, a stimulus unable to activate postsynaptic striate cortex elements. In this case the ocular dominance columns are unaffected. Finally, in the absence of attention or generalized cortical activity, no effects take place. This situation occurs when kittens are paralyzed so that they are no longer interacting with the environment, or when cortical neurons are depleted of norepinephrine by 6-hydroxydopamine, or where unilateral visual neglect is produced by lesions of the medial thalamus. In these instances monocular deprivation fails to seriously alter binocularity (17).

TABLE 3. *Factors affecting cortical connectivity*

Type	Afferent input	Postsynaptic element	Attention[a]	Result
1	Active	Active	+	Enhanced
2	Inactive	Active	+	Diminished
3	Either	Inactive	+	No effect
4	Either	Active	−	No effect

[a]A complex set of factors relating to attention or to generalized cortical activity during the experience.

NEURAL DEVELOPMENT—RELATIONSHIP TO MOTILITY RHYTHMS

At the present time, almost all of the known effects of psychological factors on neurobiological development are limited to the effects of sensory experience. Studies that examine the consequence of more global factors, such as maternal deprivation, handling, and rearing in various size litters or with different species littermates, have often been interpreted in terms of sensory experiences. I would like to introduce the possibility that neurological development is also affected by the expression of motor output, and that we may learn much about neural development by studying motility.

Motility Rhythms in Embryonic Development

Preyer (18), in 1885, was the first embryologist to record that the chick embryo exhibits overt motor activity several days before sensory stimuli become effective in evoking reflexes, thereby implying that efferent (motor) systems begin to function prior to afferent (sensory) systems. Not only was Preyer the first to recognize this phenomenon, but more importantly he clearly recognized the general theoretical implications of this observation for development. Comparative embryological studies have since suggested that spontaneous motility in amphibians and mammals may develop at the same time as reflexive activity, and question whether the activity is truly spontaneous, though this is suggested by deafferentation studies.

One of the most fascinating aspects of this motility, recognized first by Clark and Clark (19), is that it is periodic, waxing, and waning in a somewhat rhythmic fashion. These observations have been expanded in recent years by Hamburger (20) and Corner (21). Generally, these rhythms are somewhat stage specific, but often consist of bursts of activity superimposed on periods of inactivity occurring every few minutes, and modulated by an overall rhythm with a 0.5 to 2 hr periodicity.

Motility Rhythms in Mammalian Development

Richter (22,23) was the first to observe a spontaneous motility rhythm in the neonatal rat, again following a 0.5 to 2 hr periodicity, which he related to gastric contractions. Kleitman (24) recognized a comparable rhythm in the newborn human. Later, he postulated the presence of a basic rest–activity cycle that represented the waking-state manifestation of the rapid eye movement cycle, and which he postulated governed neuronal activity. At the current time, ultradian motility rhythms, with this general form, have been observed in virtually all species studied. They emerge, often as the earliest behavior, in embryonic, larval, or fetal stages (21). They persist into the neonatal period, coexist in some species for a time with circadian cycles, and with age often become much less rhythmic and much more difficult to detect, though they may reappear in old age. This general pattern is illustrated in

Fig. 1 for the albino rat. A subtle ultradian rhythm can be detected in the early neonatal period, though such rhythms reach their greatest intensity during the second to third postnatal week, and lose their salience shortly thereafter (25), often reemerging during senescence (A. Campbell, M. H. Teicher, and R. J. Baldessarini, *unpublished observations*).

Motility Rhythms—A Teleological Hypothesis

Although several studies have demonstrated prominent ultradian motility rhythms in numerous species, no clear hypothesis has been offered regarding the teleological reasons for this universal complex rhythm or pseudorhythm. Based on recent studies, I would like to advance an hypothesis concerning the nature and possible function of these curious rhythms. The first indication of a potential function derives from observations that neuronal sprouting occurs in the embryo during active motility periods (26). This observation dovetails with reports indicating that protein synthesis occurs in cells with a rhythmic periodicity of 0.5 to 4 hr, depending on cell type (27). Thus it appears possible that motility rhythms present early in life are related to neural development and might hinge on the synthesis and elaboration of a protein substance. In short, these modulations may reflect a fundamental neural development rhythm.

Preliminary Data

Some encouraging data in this regard include the discovery that small cortical ablations in adult rats, involving frontal parietal areas, produce a slow (approximately

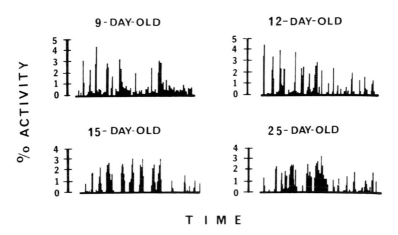

FIG. 1. Twenty-four hour activity profiles from developing rats studied in isolation. Activity was assessed using an extremely sensitive vibrational activity monitor that detected all movements except respiration and slow head motions. Activity is expressed as percent of total activity per 10 min sample interval. (Adapted from ref. 25.)

6 cycles/day), major ultradian rhythm very similar to the prominent ultradian rhythm observed in the 2 week old rat (Fig. 2). This rhythm is present for 1 to 2 weeks and is then replaced by a more rapid and less organized rhythm (28). We suspect that the reemergence of a robust ultradian rhythm occurs during a period of intense neuronal activity resulting in a significant degree of recovery of function (29) and elaboration of potent neuronotropic substances (30) (see also G. Barbin, *this volume*). Similarly, the period of peak ultradian rhythmicity normally observed in developing rodents corresponds precisely with the age range in which isolated stria-

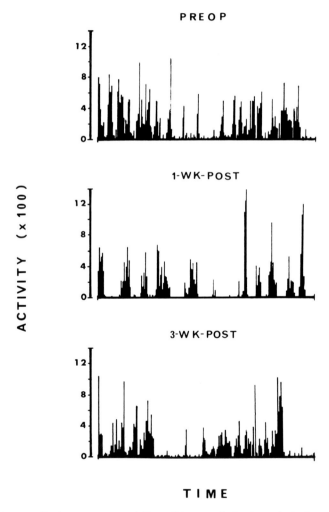

FIG. 2. Activity profile from a representative subject studied prior to lesioning, then 1 and 3 weeks after bilateral ventrolateral aspiration lesion of the cortical area. Activity was assessed at 10 min intervals using computer-interfaced Stoelting Electronic Activity monitors. Data from the first 36 hours only are presented. Note the prominent reorganization of activity into discrete rhythmic bursts during the immediate recovery period. (Adapted from ref. 28.)

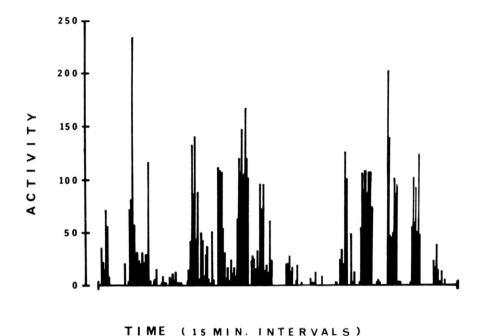

TIME (15 MIN. INTERVALS)

FIG. 3. Electroactigraphy profile from a 55 year old male patient with mild to moderate dementia characterized by a prominent, but not absolute, deficit in incorporation of new memory and a history of prominent alcohol abuse, currently detoxified. Note the strong organization of this activity profile into discrete rhythmic episodes. Activity was sampled at 15 min intervals using a piezoelectric activity monitor with solid-state memory worn on the patient's nondominant wrist. (Adapted from ref. 57.)

tal membrane preparations display prominent neuronotropic activity (31). In short, these rhythms appear to occur during periods of active neuronal organization or reorganization when neuronotropic substances are present.

We have recently observed that humans with acute or progressive cortical lesions display rhythms similar to developing or cortically damaged adult rats. These similarities have been noted in a patient with mild dementia recovering from ethanol withdrawal (Fig. 3), in a patient with a parasagittal meningioma, and in patients with closed head injury (57). These rhythmic disturbances appear to be time limited and change with recovery, as is apparent in a patient 3 months after a right-sided stroke (Fig. 4). Note that the ultradian rhythm is now rapid and the circadian cycle grossly disturbed.

Potential Implications

The hypothesis that motility and motility rhythms are related to neural development may provide a new insight into the observation that many forms of neural insult to the developing brain produce a hyperactivity syndrome. Examples of such

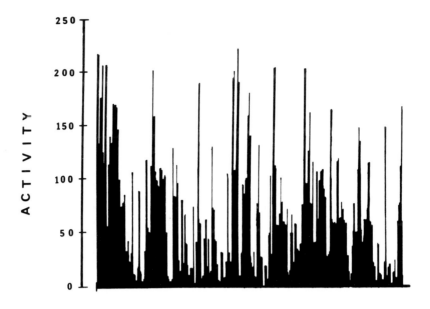

TIME (15 m i n . i n t e r v a l s)

FIG. 4.   Electroactigraph profile from a 70 year old patient recovering from a cerebrovascular accident in the territory of the right middle cerebral artery. Data were obtained approximately 3 months after the stroke when residual deficits were considered to be mild. Activity was sampled at 15 min intervals using a piezoelectric activity monitor with solidstate memory worn on the patient's dominant wrist. Note the near complete loss of circadian rhythmicity in this 48 hr activity profile. (Adapted from ref. 57.)

insults include depletions of any monoamine system: dopamine, norepinephrine, or serotonin; undernutrition; X-irradiation; exposure to ethanol, lead, and mitotic inhibitors; or neonatal viral encephalitis (32–39). All of these forms of CNS damage in developing rats result in a transient period of hyperactivity, which in some cases diminishes following treatment with amphetamine. Hyperactivity in the dopamine-depleted developing rat, often cited as an animal model of minimal brain dysfunction (40), is characterized by the addition of a 6 cycle/day rhythm that remits when the period of hyperactivity ends (M.H. Teicher, R.J. Baldessarini, and B.A. Shaywitz, *unpublished observations*). As noted above, this type of activity rhythm disturbance is seen in other forms of brain damage. We have also found that amphetamine accelerates and attenuates these forms of ultradian rhythms (M.H. Teicher, R.J. Baldessarini, and B.A. Shaywitz, *unpublished observations*).

Conclusions

The most fundamental questions remain unanswered. Are ultradian motility rhythms related at all to neurobiological development? If so, are they simply an external manifestation of what may be occurring at higher levels, or do they serve some role in maintaining or facilitating neurological development? No answers can be given at this time, but they remain important questions. This research may provide new insight into the severe delays produced by single doses of haloperidol on recovery of motor ability in rats with closed head injuries, the ability of "swinging" surrogate mothers to help counteract some of the effects of maternal deprivation, and factors responsible for the abnormal rhythmic movements seen in children with severe neurological disturbances.

RECOVERY FROM NEUROLOGICAL DAMAGE—ROLE OF PSYCHOLOGICAL FACTORS

The concluding theme of this paper centers on a brief discussion of the possibility that the selection of appropriate psychological factors can help compensate for various forms of early brain insult.

Neurological Consequences of Early Undernutrition

Several recent studies have started to ascertain whether environmental enrichment can mitigate some of the neurological consequences of early malnutrition. Katz and Davies (41) and Bhide and Bedi (42), for instance, have reported on the effects of 35 or 80 days of enrichment (including group housing) on malnourished rats (postnatally in the former study, pre- and postnatally in the latter). Briefly, it appears that nutrition and environmental enrichment have different but somewhat overlapping effects on parameters of gross neurological development. The weight and length of the cerebrum may be most markedly affected by undernutrition, while thickness of the occipital cortex may be insignificantly affected. Environmental enrichment appears to have its greatest effect on occipital thickness, and slight but significant effects on cerebrum and hippocampus. No synergy was noted between environment and nutrition, but some additive compensation was noted in undernourished animals subjected to enrichment.

Using rather gross biochemical parameters such as DNA, RNA, and protein content, Crnic (43) found some significant effects of postnatal malnutrition. Enrichment extending through pre- and postweaning periods had no corrective effects on these parameters, but did interact with behavioral measures. In some instances the effect of environmental enrichment partially counteracted the effects of undernutrition, whereas in others it augmented the disturbances. Although the behavioral measures selected were rather primitive, they do illustrate an important point, that environmental complexity and enhanced sensory-motor stimulation may be far more effective in reducing the behavioral sequelae of undernutrition than in actually reversing the fundamental neuropathological alterations. These issues are thoughtfully addressed in clinical populations by A. Ballabriga (*this volume*).

Neonatal Neurotoxic Lesions

A large number of studies in the literature indicate that environmental factors can facilitate recovery from early lesions. A particularly interesting model system centers on the effects of environment and experience on functional recovery of rats with severe permanent depletions of dopamine produced during the neonatal period by the neurotoxin 6-hydroxydopamine (in the presence of norepinephrinergic reuptake blockade to protect norepinephrinergic terminals). This treatment produces a permanent depletion of whole brain dopamine that is extensive in nigrostriatal and mesolimbic projections, but has relatively little effect on short-axoned systems in the hypothalamus (44). This treatment produces a transient period of hyperactivity that commences on about postnatal day 15 (40). The duration and magnitude of the hyperactivity is related to the extent of the depletion and can, with massive depletion, extend well into adulthood (45). Dopamine depletion after day 23 fails to produce hyperactivity (46), and in the adult such depletion produces severe bradykinesia, adipsia, and aphasia, and are usually lethal (47). Several groups, but not all, have found that this developmental hyperactivity can be attenuated by amphetamine

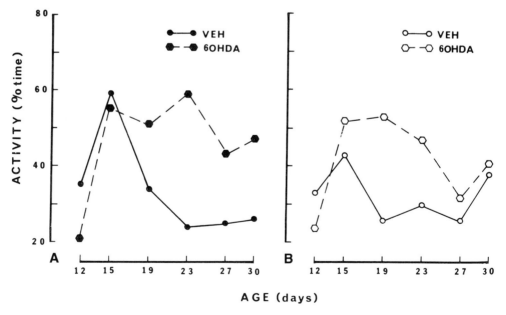

FIG. 5. Alterations in mean activity levels of developing rats raised in either homogeneous litters of vehicle injection controls (VEH) or pups with permanent depletions of forebrain dopamine produced by 6-hydroxydopamine (6OHDA) (**A**), or heterogeneous litters with both dopamine-depleted and control pups (**B**). Note the alterations in age-related activity profiles produced in both control and dopamine-depleted pups as a consequence of the rearing environment. These effects include a decrease in peak activity levels in control pups reared in heterogeneous litters and a persistence of hyperactivity in dopamine-depleted pups raised in homogeneous litters. (Adapted from ref. 51.)

(48,49). It is generally a modest effect that requires careful attention to dose and selection of appropriate measures.

Briefly, we found that appropriate selection of environmental factors could completely eliminate the expression of hyperactivity in rats with neonatal dopamine depletion (50). Thus, testing these pups in the presence of their anesthetized mother, or in homogeneous groupings of treated or control rats, attenuated their activity to normal levels and enabled the depleted pups to habituate their activity in novel environments as rapidly as controls. More important, we were also able to show that environmental experiences during early rearing produced effects that were as dramatic as drug treatments. As seen in Fig. 5, simply rearing depleted animals in mixed litters with normal controls altered the time course of their hyperactivity response and improved performance in simple learning tasks (51). More recently Goldenring, working with Shaywitz (52), discovered that artificially rearing these animals in floating cups in an incubator from days 4 to 18 eliminated the hyperactivity response seen in the standard test paradigm, though depletion effects on learning performance were still present. These environmental modifications do not produce any recovery of dopamine levels per se, which remain depleted. However, it has recently been discovered that there is a considerable amount of serotonergic hyperinnervation that occurs following early lesions (53), and experiential factors may act at this level. Curiously, drugs that modulate the activity of dopamine-depleted pups, including amphetamine and methylphenidate, do so through their effects on serotonergic systems rather than modulation of dopamine or norepinephrine release (54).

CONCLUSIONS

A vast amount of research has been conducted on the effects of sensory experience on cortical development. These experiences serve to maintain cortical development and occasionally to facilitate the rate of development or enhance the degree of attainment. Cortical development is also very sensitive to the consequences of abnormal sensory experiences. The main factors determining the effects of abnormal sensory exposure include activity in afferent pathway, response of postsynaptic elements, and general state of attention or cortical activity. It also appears that rhythmic motility fluctuations occur in almost all species during periods of neural development. These rhythms reemerge in adult mammals during periods of acute neurological insult and may remit following recovery. They are present during the period of hyperactivity in dopamine-depleted rat pups and are responsive to amphetamine administration. The possibility that these motility cycles may reflect an underlying neurological development rhythm is discussed. Finally, some evidence is presented suggesting that environmental enrichment can compensate for some forms of early neurological insult, including various types of malnutrition, and for neonatal dopamine depletions. The mechanisms responsible for such experiential effects remain to be explored.

From the clinical perspective, it does indeed seem possible that abnormal or pathological psychological factors can interfere with normal development, and there is some hope that selection of appropriate environmental factors can compensate, in part, for deficits in neurobiological endowment. This is certainly the hope of programs endeavoring to minimize the damage wrought by trisomy-21, through early environmental enrichment and stimulation (55). Much research is still required to determine whether specific psychological traumas can have discrete effects on neurological development. The recent observations of EEG abnormalities in 77% of the victims of father–daughter incest (56), though complicated (and open to interpretation in many ways), are suggestive, particularly because these patients have a prominent tendency toward dissociative states. However, the key concepts needed to integrate the psychodynamic-ontogenetic models of the previous era with the neuropharmacological models fashionable today may exist within this uncharted and murky region.

ACKNOWLEDGMENT

This work was supported in part by a grant from The Marion Ireland Benton Trust Fund, and by an Ethel Dupont Warren Research Fellowship.

REFERENCES

1. Grobstein P, Chow KL. Receptive field organization in the mammalian visual cortex: the role of individual experience in development. In: Gottlieb G, ed. *Studies on the development of behavior and the nervous system,* vol 3. New York: Academic Press, 1976:155–93.
2. Sperry RW. Embryogenesis of behavioral nerve nets. In: Deltaan RL, Ursprung H, eds. *Organogenesis.* New York: Holt, 1965: 161–86.
3. Hebb DO. *Textbook of psychology,* 3rd ed. Philadelphia: WB Saunders, 1972.
4. Tees RC. Perceptual development in mammals. In: Gottlieb G, ed. *Studies on the development of behavior and the nervous system,* vol 3. New York: Academic Press, 1976:281–326.
5. Gottlieb G. The roles of experience in the development of behavior and the nervous system. In: Gottlieb G, ed. *Studies on the development of behavior and the nervous system,* vol 3. New York: Academic Press, 1976:25–54.
6. Chow KL, Riesen AH, Newell FW. Degeneration of retinal ganglion cells in infant chimpanzees reared in darkness. *J Comp Neurol* 1957;107:27–42.
7. Gyllenstein L, Malmfors T, Norlin ML. Effect of visual deprivation on the optic centers of growing and adult mice. *J Comp Neurol* 1965;124:149–60.
8. Parnavelas JG, Globus A, Kaups P. Continuous illumination from birth affects spine density of neurons in visual cortex of the rat. *Exp Neurol* 1973;40:742–7.
9. Turner AM, Greenough WT. Differential rearing effects on rat visual cortex synapses. I. Synaptic and neuronal density and synapses per neuron. *Brain Res* 1985;329:195–203.
10. Spitz RA. Anaclitic depression. *Psychoanal Study Child* 1946;2:313–42.
11. Goy RW, Bridgson WE, Young WC. Period of maximal susceptibility of the prenatal female guinea pig to masculinizing actions of testosterone proprionate. *J Comp Physiol Psychol* 1964;57:166–74.
12. Arnold AP, Gorki RA. Gonadal steroid induction of structural sex differences in the central nervous system. *Annu Rev Neurosci* 1984;7:413–42.
13. Hubel DH, Wiesel TN. Receptive fields of cells in striate cortex of very young, visually inexperienced kittens. *J Neurophysiol* 1963;26:994–1002.
14. Wiesel TN, Hubel DH. Single-cell responses in striate cortex of kittens deprived of vision in one eye. *J Neurophysiol* 1963;26:1003–17.

15. Hirsch HVB, Spinelli DN. Visual experience modifies distribution of horizontally and vertically oriented receptive fields in rats. *Science* 1970;168:869–71.
16. Blakemore C, Cooper GF. Development of the brain depends on the visual environment. *Nature* 1970;228:477–8.
17. Singer W. Neuronal mechanisms of experience dependent self-organization of the mammalian visual cortex. *Acta Morphol Hung* 1983;31:235–60.
18. Preyer W. *Specielle physiologie des embryo*. Leipzig: Grieben's Verlag, 1885.
19. Clark EL, Clark ER. On the early pulsation of the posterior lymph hearts in chick embryos: their relation to the body movements. *J Exp Zool* 1914;17:373–94.
20. Hamburger V. Some aspects of the embryology of behavior. *Q Rev Biol* 1963;38:342–65.
21. Corner MA. Sleep and the beginnings of behavior in the animal kingdom—studies of ultradian motility cycles in early life. *Prog Neurobiol* 1977;8:279–95.
22. Richter CP. A behavioristic study of the activity of the rat. *Comp Psychol Monogr* 1922;1:1–55.
23. Richter CP. Animal behavior and internal drives. *Q Rev Biol* 1927;2:307–43.
24. Kleitman N. *Sleep and wakefulness*. Chicago: University Chicago Press, 1939.
25. Teicher MH, Flaum LE. The ontogeny of ultradian and nocturnal activity rhythms in isolated albino rats. *Dev Neurobiol* 1979;12:441–54.
26. Kahn JA, Roberts A. The neuromuscular basis of rhythmic struggling movements in embryos of *Xenopus laevis*. *J Exp Biol* 1982;99:197–203.
27. Ya Brodsky W. Protein synthesis rhythms. *J Theor Biol* 1975;55:167–200.
28. Finkelstein S, Teicher MH, Campbell A, Baldessarini RJ. Bilateral ventrolateral cortical lesions slow and accentuate ultradian activity rhythms in rats. *Neurosci Abstr* 1983;9:626.
29. Finkelstein S, Campbell A, Stoll AL et al. Changes in cortical and subcortical levels of monoamines and their metabolites following unilateral ventrolateral cortical lesions in the rat. *Brain Res* 1983;271:279–88.
30. Nieto-Sampedro M, Lewis ER, Cotman CW, et al. Brain injury causes a time-dependent increase in neuronotrophic activity at the lesion site. *Science* 1982;217:860–1.
31. Prochiantz A, Daguet MC, Herbt A, Glowinski J. Specific stimulation of *in vitro* maturation of mesencephalic dopaminergic neurones by striatal membranes. *Nature* 1981;293:570–3.
32. Raskin LA, Shaywitz BA, Anderson GM, Cohen DJ, Teicher MH, Linakis J. Differential effects of selective dopamine, norepinephrine or catecholamine depletions on activity and learning in the developing rat. *Pharmacol Biochem Behav* 1983;19:743–9.
33. Lucot JB, Seiden LS. Effects of neonatal administration of 5,7-dihydroxytryptamine on locomotor activity. *Psychopharmacology (Berlin)* 1982;77:114–116.
34. Loch RK, Rafales LS, Michaelson IA, Bornschein RL. The role of undernutrition in animal models of hyperactivity. *Life Sci* 1978;22:1963–70.
35. Norton S, Mullenix P, Culver B. Comparison of the structure of hyperactive behavior in rats after brain damage from X-irradiation, carbon monoxide and pallidal lesions. *Brain Res* 1976;116:49–67.
36. Branchey L, Friedhoff AJ. Biochemical and behavioral changes in rats exposed to ethanol *in utero*. *Ann NY Acad Sci* 1976;273:140–5.
37. Silbergeld EK, Goldberg AM. Lead-induced behavioral dysfunction: an animal model of hyperactivity. *Exp Neurol* 1974;42:146–57.
38. Rabe A, Haddad RK. Methylazoxymethanol-induced microencephaly in rats: behavioral studies. *Fed Proc* 1972;31:1536–9.
39. Murphree OD, Morgan PN, Jarman R. Learning deficits and activity changes—a partial laboratory model in postencephalitis rats for studies of brain damage. *Cond Relex* 1971;6:30–5.
40. Shaywitz BA, Yager RD, Klopper JH. Selective brain dopamine depletion in developing rats: an experimental model of minimal brain dysfunction. *Science* 1976;191:305–7.
41. Katz HB, Davies CA. The separate and combined effects of early undernutrition and environmental complexity on cerebral measures in rats. *Dev Psychobiol* 1983;16:47–58.
42. Bhide PG, Bedi KS. The effects of a lengthy period of environmental diversity on well-fed and previously undernourished rats. I. Neurons and glial cells. *J Comp Neurol* 1984;227:296–307.
43. Crnic LS. Effects of nutrition and environment on brain biochemistry and behavior. *Dev Psychobiol* 1983;16:129–45.
44. Breese GR, Baumeister AA, McCown TJ, et al. Behavioral differences between neonatal and adult 6-hydroxydopamine treated rats to dopamine agonist: relevance to neurological symptoms in clinical syndromes with reduced brain dopamine. *J Pharmacol Exp Ther* 1984;231:343–54.

45. Miller FE, Heffner TG, Kotake C, Seiden LS. Magnitude and duration of hyperactivity following neonatal 6-hydroxydopamine is related to the extent of brain dopamine depletion. *Brain Res* 1981;229:123–32.
46. Erinoff L, MacPhail RC, Heller A, Seiden LS. Age-dependent effects of 6-hydroxydopamine on locomotor activity in the rat. *Brain Res* 1979;164:195–205.
47. Stricker EM, Zigmond MJ. Brain catecholamines and the lateral hypothalamic syndrome. In: Novin D, Wyrwicka W, Bray G, eds. *Hunger: basic mechanisms and clinical implications*. New York: Raven Press, 1976:19–32.
48. Shaywitz BA, Klopper JH, Yager RD, Gordon JW. Paradoxical response to amphetamine in developing rats treated with 6-hydroxydopamine. *Nature* 1976;261:153–5.
49. Sorenson AA, Vayer JS, Goldberg CS. Amphetamine reduction of motor activity in rats after neonatal administration of 6-hydroxydopamine. *Biol Psychiatry* 1977;12:133–7.
50. Teicher MH, Shaywitz BA, Kootz HL, Cohen DJ. Differential effects of maternal and sibling presence on hyperactivty of 6-hydroxydopamine-treated developing rats. *J Comp Physiol Psychol* 1981;95:134–45.
51. Pearson DE, Teicher MH, Shaywitz BA, Cohen DJ, Young JG, Anderson GM. Environmental influences on body weight and behavior in developing rats following neonatal 6-hydroxydopamine. *Science* 1980;209:715–7.
52. Goldenring JR, Shaywitz BA, Wool RS, Batter DK, Anderson GM, Cohen DJ. Environmental and biologic interaction on behavior: effects of artificial rearing in rat pups treated with 6-hydroxydopamine. *Dev Psychobiol* 1982;15:297–307.
53. Stachowiak MK, Bruno JP, Snyder AM, Stricker EM, Zigmond MJ. Apparent sprouting of striatal serotonergic terminals after dopamine-depleting brain lesions in neonatal rats. *Brain Res* 1984;291:164–7.
54. Heffner TG, Seiden LS. Possible involvement of serotonergic neurons in the reduction of locomotor hyperactivity caused by amphetamine in neonatal rats depleted of brain dopamine. *Brain Res* 1982;244:81–90.
55. Smith L, Hagen V. Relationship between the home environment and sensorimotor development of Down syndrome and nonretarded infants. *Am J Ment Defic* 1984;2:124–32.
56. Davies RK. Incest and vulnerable children. *Sci News* 1979;116:244–5.
57. Teicher MH, Lawrence JM, Barber NI, Finklestein SP, Lieberman H, Baldessarini RJ. Altered locomotor activity in neuropsychiatric patients. *Prog Neuropsychopharmacol Biol Psychiatr* 1986;10:755–61.

DISCUSSION

Dr. Caviness: Do you think that aberrations in ultradian rhythm generation may be relevant to the Sudden Infant Death Syndrome (SIDS)?

Dr. Teicher: Yes. This rhythm is very prominent in the neonate, and it is certainly possible that its suppression could result in respiratory arrest or sudden death. It would be interesting to monitor activity in patients at risk of SIDS to see whether there is a problem with oscillator control. There may be some treatment involving monitoring the frequency of the oscillator or the magnitude of the rhythm that might protect such infants.

Dr. Campagnoni: In your dopamine-depletion experiments why did you treat groups of infant rats? Have you done the experiment on an individual basis?

Dr. Teicher: These animals are depleted of dopamine at least 5 days postnatally. To ensure that they survive long enough to be tested you normally raise them with their mother. We have done artificial rearing studies, placing individual rat pups in cups floating in an incubator and fed on an artificial medium from 4 to 18 days. If you can do such a study successfully you can completely eliminate hyperactivity in the dopamine-depleted rat. Part of this hyperactivity response is the result of environmental contrast—when you take pups from their litter and place them in isolation it normally induces a stress response which triggers profound hyperactivity in the dopamine-depleted animals. However, if they are raised in isolation they do not show this stress response when their environment is changed and you do not see hyperactivity.

Dr. Campagnoni: Why did you anesthetize the mother?

Dr. Teicher: It is best to study the pup's behavior in the absence of maternal behavior. The mother is likely to exert a considerable modulating effect on the pup's behavior, but when she is anesthetized it is the pup's decision rather than hers whether it spends its time next to her or running around the cage. This is analogous to the case of a child with brain dysfunction in whom hyperactivity is often environmentally specific. A hyperactive child may sit quite calmly in your office while his mother complains that he is a terror at school, whereas in the classroom he may be unmanageable.

Developmental Neurobiology, edited by
Philippe Evrard and Alexandre Minkowski.
Nestlé Nutrition Workshop Series, Vol. 12.
Nestec Ltd., Vevey/Raven Press, Ltd.,
New York © 1989.

Nutritional Influences on Neurological Development: A Contemplative Essay

Norman Kretchmer

Department of Nutritional Sciences, University of California, Berkeley, California 94720

Arguments concerned with the impact of malnutrition on neurological development have been a matter of considerable scientific and political interest during the past two decades. These dissensions have not only been heard in clinical and scientific forums but also they have occurred, albeit quite restrained, within the atmosphere of congressional and diplomatic hearing rooms.

The problem of accurate interpretation has been compounded by a desire for the clinician to have a therapeutic panacea, such as "eat well and prevent mental retardation"; the unfair extrapolation of behavioral and neurobiological events that take place in one animal (a rat) to another animal (a human); the failure to recognize the extremes of cellular specialization demonstrated in the brain and the ambition to deal with the complexities of the brain with the same simplicity of analyses accomplished on liver or skin (also a wrong approach in modern cellular biology); and finally to interpret cellular changes utilizing grossly superficial biochemical and anatomic methods as indicative of final performance. Certainly there is a difference between glial cells and neurons and they cannot be homogenized together. Intake of food, whether it is more or less, with an emphasis on overall content or specific nutrients, is a forceful component of the general environment. The critical nature of malnutrition and the effect it may have on the central nervous system have been discussed extensively by Cravioto (1), Dobbing (2,3), and others (4,5). The consideration of the relationship of general malnutrition to neurological development must be carefully defined in context. Is this malnutrition the result of an incomplete protein, or is it a lack of protein as well as energy (i.e., a total lack in calories)? This latter form is a much more common type of malnutrition. It is difficult to visualize the existence of either of these conditions except in the presence of all the ecological complexities that compose poverty. True, people with gastrointestinal disease appear to have generalized malnutrition but lack the multiple additional tragedies of poverty. Needless to say, the unsophisticated concept of malnutrition which presumes that malnutrition affects cell number and cell size, resulting in a "smaller brain" and hence to reduced intellect, is now in disrepute. Dobbing (6) has shown clearly that the premise that cells first multiply and when they finish this proliferation increase in size is not correct. Rather, the phenomena take place in waves and often simultaneously. Please note that in the previous discussion of cell size and number the basic developmental phenomena of migration are not considered, although movement of cells from one position to another is often a necessary preamble to function.

Severe undernutrition unquestionably results in poor progression of growth with early cessation in the development of all organ systems. Usually the growth of the brain is slowed in a pattern similar to general somatic growth. This phenomenon can be associated in the human with intellectual and behavioral deficiencies that can be overcome with planned enrichment programs as shown by Cravioto (1) and Monckeberg (4).

At this point some definitions are in order. A *critical period* is functionally very different from a *vulnerable period*. The former indicates that there is a discrete stage in development when an imposed stimulus is effective. This concept is different from the period of vulnerability, an epoch in the life of the organism when it is vulnerable to external stimuli, for example by all the ecological factors in malnutrition. *Deficit* is used to indicate some lack in the developmental sequence. This term is in contrast to *deficiency* where there is a functional lack of a particular aspect of metabolism. These two, deficits and deficiencies, can result in biochemical or anatomic distortions with functional consequences as pathways or topographies are poorly constructed.

Using this language, it is interesting to view the now classic map of brain growth originally offered by Dobbing (Fig. 1). This chart clearly depicts one of the difficulties of applying data gathered from other animals. When dealing with brain growth and behavioral and neurological development it is absolutely futile. The function of the organism is a mark of the individual nature (culture) of that particular animal, and rat or even subhuman primate data is often not applicable to humans. But basic data on the development of neural membranes, genetic function, or cell–cell interaction can give great insight into a series of fundamental activities.

Malnutrition plus all the associated events can affect the development of the organism. Cravioto (1) suggested that there are three basic models that one can construct to study nutritional effects on performance.

The first is a deprivation model, in which a group that is deprived of a nutrient or nutrients is analyzed for growth and performance. The Dutch famine and the Leningrad siege serve as dramatic human examples. Of course, specific deprivations (e.g., iron and zinc) can be studied and then behavioral performance can be measured, but this model is mostly used in animal studies. The intervention model has many examples: the studies of INCAP, the Bogota study, and the rather abortive, naive study of high and low protein in Harlem. These studies have ethical considerations. If the intervention is supposed to be good, then on what basis can the remainder of the population be deprived of whatever is good? The ecological model is favored at present. In this example there is no deprivation and no intervention in the sense of giving special diets to one group and not the other, but it is a difficult long-

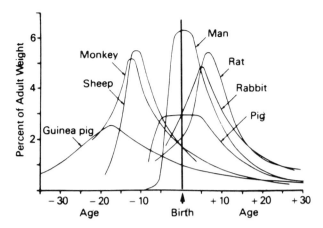

FIG. 1. The brain growth spurts of seven mammalian species expressed as velocity curves of the increase in weight with age. The units of time for each species are as follows: guinea pig, days; rhesus monkey, 4 days; sheep, 5 days; pig, weeks; man, months; rabbit, 2 days; rat, days. Rates are expressed as weight gain as a percentage of adult weight for each unit of time (7).

term model with an appreciation of all the variables (e.g., food, shelter, psychology, infection). This model has shown that children who developed malnutrition before their third birthday will have impaired motor development. Monckeberg and Cravioto have separately shown that with stimulated care these children can be rehabilitated, but the stimulation has to be maintained or they revert to their previous state.

Food can affect neurological development that can be manifested functionally or anatomically, but these functions and structures must be examined carefully and in a developmental context. This approach is considered by the subsequent chapters in this book.

To summarize, neurological development and nutrition are related. Generalized malnutrition is one facet of the composite picture of poverty. Poverty should be called generalized deprivation leading to a complex of functional problems. Simplistic concepts of the undefined cell number and cell size and general retardation in brain and somatic development are no longer acceptable. No panacea, such as giving food, exists to alleviate the whole problem of mental retardation. Rather, the newer methods of cellular and molecular biology can be utilized to understand the function of the neuronal cell. This knowledge coupled with that of genetics can yield particularly pertinent models for the study of specific neurological deficits. Cognitive function demands careful tedious examination of the individual under controlled conditions.

The brain is not an organ that can be dealt with in simple terms using either archaic or modern methods applicable to less complex situations. To understand the true functional relationships of the central nervous system we may need a new biology (8).

REFERENCES

1. Cravioto J. Severe malnutrition and development of motor skills in children. *Ann Nestlé* 1978;44:22–42.
2. Dobbing J. Nutritional growth restriction and the nervous system. *Ann Nestlé* 1978;44:7–21.
3. Dobbing J. Infant nutrition and later achievement. *Am J Clin Nutr* 1985;41:477–84.
4. Monckeberg F. Reviews of several malnourished infants: effect of early sensory-effective stimulation. In: Brozek J, ed. *Behavioral effects of energy and protein deficits*. Washington, DC: DHEW Publications, 1977:121–30.
5. Brozek J. Malnutrition and human behavior. In: *Present knowledge in human nutrition*. Washington, DC: The Nutrition Foundation, 1984:682–92.
6. Dobbing J, Sands J. Vulnerability of developing brain not explained by cell number/cell size hypothesis. *Early Hum Dev* 1981;5:227–31.
7. Dobbing J, Sands J. Comparative aspects of the brain growth spurt. *Early Hum Dev* 1979;3:79–83.
8. Kety SS. A biologist examines the mind and behavior. *Science* 1960;132:1861–70.

Developmental Neurobiology, edited by
Philippe Evrard and Alexandre Minkowski.
Nestlé Nutrition Workshop Series, Vol. 12.
Nestec Ltd., Vevey/Raven Press, Ltd.,
New York © 1989.

Interaction of Alcohol with the Delta-Opioid Receptor

Michael E. Charness, Adrienne S. Gordon, and Ivan Diamond

Ernest Gallo Clinic and Research Center, Department of Neurology, University of California, San Francisco General Hospital, San Francisco, California 94110

Ethanol has both pharmacologic and toxic effects in the developing and mature nervous systems (1). The toxic effects, which are associated with chronic abuse, may depend on ethanol's pharmacologic actions. Ethanol intoxication is characterized by well-known alterations in neurological function and behavior (1). Tolerance develops to many actions of ethanol, and a state of physical dependence follows chronic abuse. These phenomena probably derive from the physical interaction of ethanol with neural cell membranes and the adaptation of these membranes to prolonged ethanol exposure (2,3). Ethanol can induce acute disorder of the membrane lipid bilayer, but after chronic exposure, neural membranes may show several potentially adaptive alterations: increased membrane order; reduced disorder after acute ethanol exposure; and modifications in cholesterol, phospholipid, or fatty acid composition (4–6). Diverse membrane proteins are sensitive to changes in lipid microenvironment; their function may be critically altered both by acute ethanol exposure and by the membrane adaptations that follow chronic abuse. Accordingly, there is great interest in how ethanol affects neurotransmitter receptors and receptor-dependent molecular events, ion channels, and a variety of membrane enzymes that govern neural excitation and synaptic transmission. Investigation of these phenomena has been limited by the heterogeneity of brain cells and the need to use disruptive tissue preparations. We have circumvented some of these difficulties by studying the effects of ethanol in a homogeneous population of intact cultured neural cells. We have reported that in the murine neuroblastoma × glioma hybrid cell line, NG108-15, acute and chronic ethanol exposure causes striking modifications in delta-opioid receptor binding, perhaps reflecting the membrane events responsible for intoxication, tolerance, and the withdrawal syndrome (7).

METHODS AND RESULTS

Delta-opioid binding was measured by incubating a suspension of washed whole cells with [³H]Met-enkephalinamide ([³H]MEA) at 37°C in the presence or absence of 10^{-5} M unlabeled naloxone. A standard filtration assay was employed (8). Specific binding (the difference between binding in the presence or absence of excess cold ligand) was expressed as femtomoles per 10^6 cells. Although a variety of opioid receptor subtypes have been characterized in brain and peripheral tissues, NG108-15 cells express only the delta-opioid receptor subtype (9). Hence, the nonselective opioid peptide radioligand, [³H]MEA, interacted with a single class of high affinity delta receptors.

Our first experiments investigated whether ethanol had any effects on opioid binding to intact neural cells. When ethanol was added to suspended whole cells immediately before [³H]MEA, the specific binding of 2nM [³H]MEA was inhibited $15\% \pm 1$ (SEM) by 100 mM ethanol and $56\% \pm 2$ by 400 mM ethanol. Sucrose (50–500 mM) had no effect on [³H]MEA binding.

Although acute treatment with ethanol reduced opioid binding, cells exposed chronically to ethanol appeared to undergo an adaptive response. Cells cultured for 4 days in 200 mM ethanol were washed and assayed for opioid binding in the absence of ethanol. The binding of 2nM [³H]MEA to these washed cells increased by $75\% \pm 4$ (SEM) over levels in cells from pair-matched controls ($n = 15$, $P < 0.001$, paired t-test).

This increase in opiate binding should reflect changes in one of two fundamental properties of receptors. Chronic exposure to ethanol may have altered the receptor or its milieu, leading to an increase in receptor affinity. Alternatively, the number of binding sites may have increased. Opioid binding was therefore further characterized by Scatchard analysis of saturation isotherms. Cells cultured for 4 days with 100 and 200 mM ethanol showed, respectively, a $40\% \pm 4$ and $85\% \pm 21$ increase in the expression of binding sites. In contrast, receptor affinity was not significantly modified by chronic ethanol exposure (200 mM ethanol:1.70 nM $\pm$ .21 nM; controls:1.60 nM $\pm$ .09 nM). Although chronic ethanol treatment increased opioid receptor expression, there was no change in the potency with which acute ethanol exposure inhibited [³H]MEA binding.

In humans, some tolerance to ethanol may develop over as little as 12 to 24 hr (1). We therefore determined whether the induction of receptor expression by ethanol showed an appropriate time-course to reflect clinical events. Cells were exposed to 200 mM ethanol for 6 to 48 hr, washed free of ethanol and assayed for opioid binding. An increase in opioid binding was first apparent after 18 hr of ethanol exposure; by 24 hr [³H]MEA binding had increased by 47% over levels in control cells. Opioid receptor binding also increased when cells were exposed to lower concentrations of ethanol, but this effect required much longer incubations. For example, when cells were cultured for 13 days in 25 and 50 mM ethanol, opioid binding increased by 50% and 56% respectively, compared to pair-matched control cells. Thus the time required for ethanol to induce opioid receptor expression bore an inverse relationship to the concentration of ethanol employed.

Binding was determined as a receptor concentration per intact cell. It is conceivable that an increase in receptor concentration might reflect a decrease in the surface area of cells, rather than an increase in the number of sites distributed over an unchanged surface area. We therefore measured cellular volume using a logarithmic-scale particle sizer (7). Cell volume did not differ significantly between cells cultured for 24 hr in the presence or absence of 200 mM ethanol. Similarly, effects of ethanol on cell division or growth did not appear to account for opioid receptor up-regulation. Although treatment with 200 mM for 24 hr reduced the number of harvested cells by 10% to 30%, treatment with 25 mM and 50 mM ethanol for 2 weeks did not reduce cell number, yet still induced receptor expression.

Ethanol may exert its primary effects within specific domains of the hydrophobic membrane core (10) either by disordering membrane lipids or by interacting more directly with membrane proteins (11). Alcohols of higher chain length are more lipid soluble than ethanol and reproduce many of ethanol's pharmacologic effects with greater potency (12). If ethanol induces receptor expression as a consequence of its membrane lipid solubility, alcohols of higher chain length might produce more striking responses. Accordingly, cells were cultured for 48 hr with 25 mM ethanol, 25 mM n-propanol, or 25 mM n-butanol. 25 mM ethanol only slightly increased receptor expression during this incubation period; however, 25 mM n-propanol and 25 mM n-butanol each caused large increases in opioid receptor binding, in proportion to the chain length of the alcohols ($r = 0.99$). Thus, the magnitude of opioid receptor up-regulation by various alcohols correlated highly with the lipid solubility of the alcohols.

If increased opioid receptor expression is an adaptive response of cells exposed to ethanol, receptor number should eventually normalize after ethanol withdrawal. Cells were therefore cultured with 200 mM ethanol for 3 to 4 days and then exposed to fresh ethanol-free medium for varying times. Specific [^{3}H]MEA binding remained high during the first 12 hr after ethanol withdrawal and returned to control levels after 24 hr. Thus the adaptive increase in opioid receptor binding induced by ethanol was completely reversible when ethanol was withdrawn.

DISCUSSION

The interaction of ethanol with different opioid receptor subtypes has been studied in animals (13–16). Acute exposure to ethanol *in vitro* reduced the binding affinity of rat brain and neuroblastoma membranes for the relatively selective delta-opioid receptor agonist, D-Ala^2-D-Leu^5-enkephalin (13), whereas chronic administration of ethanol to rats increased the binding affinity of striatal homogenates for this substance (14). In mouse brain, chronic ethanol administration changed the binding interaction of [^{3}H]D-Ala^2-D-Leu^5-enkephalin from two sites of high and low affinity to a single site of intermediate affinity but increased numbers (16). There is also evidence that opioid systems may mediate some behavioral effects of ethanol in humans and animals (17,18). Unfortunately, it is exceedingly difficult to study the molecular mechanisms responsible for these changes in brain preparations.

Cultured neural cells are uniquely suited for studying the regulation and function of specialized proteins such as neurotransmitter receptors. Since the delta-opioid receptor of the NG108-15 cell line undergoes marked changes in the presence of ethanol, it is possible to investigate the cellular and molecular mechanisms that underlie these adaptive responses. We have already learned that receptor up-regulation by ethanol is not a direct consequence of its acute inhibition of receptor binding; rather, this process appears to be regulated by a unique mechanism dependent on protein synthesis. Once inserted in the membrane however, the new receptors are subject to normal physiologic up- and down-regulation.

It is difficult to define the biochemical events which underlie the neurological and behavioral effects of ethanol. The changes in membrane receptor binding we describe may parallel the clinical phenomena of intoxication, tolerance, and the withdrawal syndrome. For example, an acute decrease in receptor binding produced by ethanol could lead to depression of receptor-mediated activity. During continued ethanol exposure the cell membrane may undergo adaptive changes that increase receptor density and restore cellular function. After abrupt withdrawal of ethanol, the increased number of receptors would no longer be inhibited by ethanol, resulting in increased receptor-mediated activity for a short time. Thereafter, the cells would adapt to this change and receptor numbers would return to control levels, restoring cellular homeostasis. The actions of ethanol in cultured cells are also germane to ethanol's interaction with the developing and immature nervous systems. Cyclic AMP regulates neuronal differentiation and synaptogenesis in a variety of systems (19), and opioids in turn regulate the activity of adenylate cyclase in both cultured cells and the brain.

CONCLUSION

Current evidence suggests that ethanol produces its pharmacologic effects by altering the structure and function of neural membranes. Neurotransmitter receptors and receptor-dependent molecular events in the nervous system may therefore be highly sensitive to ethanol. The murine neuroblastoma × glioma hybrid cell line NG108-15 was used to study the acute and chronic interactions of ethanol with intact cells. Ethanol acutely inhibited opioid receptor binding, but after chronic exposure the cells exhibited an apparent adaptive increase in the number of opioid binding sites; this was reversible when ethanol was withdrawn. High levels of ethanol (200 mM) increased opioid binding after 18 to 24 hr; lower concentrations (25–50 mM) produced similar changes after 2 weeks. This model system has great potential for exploring the cellular and molecular mechanisms that underlie ethanol intoxication, tolerance, and the withdrawal syndrome.

ACKNOWLEDGMENT

This work was supported by grants from the United States Public Health Service, (R01 AA06662-01) and the Alcoholic Beverages Medical Research Foundation. M.E. Charness is a recipient of NIAAA Research Scientist Development Award (AA00083-01).

REFERENCES

1. Charness ME, Diamond I. Alcohol and the nervous system. *Current Neurol* 1984;5:383–422.
2. Chin JH, Goldstein DB. Drug tolerance in biomembranes: a spin-label study of the effects of ethanol. *Science* 1977;196:684–5.
3. Rottenberg H, Waring AJ, Rubin E. Tolerance and cross-tolerance in chronic alcoholics: reduced membrane binding of alcohol and drugs. *Science* 1981;213:583–5.

4. Littleton JM, John GR, Grieve SJ. Alterations in phospholipid composition in ethanol tolerance and dependence. *Alcohol Clin Exp Res* 1979;3:50–6.
5. Waring AJ, Rottenberg H, Ohnishi T, Rubin E. Membranes and phospholipids of liver mitochondria from chronic alcoholic rats are resistant to membrane disordering by alcohol. *Proc Natl Acad Sci USA* 1981;78:2582–6.
6. Lyon RC, Goldstein DB. Changes in synaptic membrane order associated with chronic ethanol treatment in mice. *Mol Pharmacol* 1983;23:86–91.
7. Charness ME, Gordon AS, Diamond I. Ethanol modulation of opiate receptors in cultured neural cells. *Science* 1983;222:1246–8.
8. Pert CB, Snyder SH. Opiate receptor: demonstration in nervous tissue. *Science* 1973;179:1011–4.
9. Gilbert JA, Richelson E. Function of delta opioid receptors in cultured cells. *Mol Cell Biochem* 1983;55:83–91.
10. Chin JH, Goldstein DD. Membrane-disordering action of ethanol. Variation with membrane cholesterol content and depth of the spin label probe. *Mol Pharmacol* 1981;19:425–31.
11. Franks NP, Lieb WR. Molecular mechanisms of general anesthesia. *Nature* 1981;300:497–503.
12. Lyon RC, McComb JA, Schreurs J, Goldstein DB. A relationship between alcohol intoxication and the disordering of brain membranes by a series of short-chain alcohols. *J Pharmacol Exp Ther* 1981;218:669–75.
13. Hiller JM, Angel LM, Simon EJ. Multiple opiate receptors: alcohol selectively inhibits binding to delta receptors. *Science* 1981;214:468–9.
14. Pfeiffer A, Seizinger R, Herz A. Chronic ethanol inhibition interferes with delta but not mu opiate receptors. *Neuropharmacology* 1982;20:1229–32.
15. Tabakoff B, Hoffman P. Alcohol interactions with brain opiate receptors. *Life Sci* 1983;32:197–204.
16. Hyncs MD, Lochner MA, Bemis KG, Hymson DL. Chronic ethanol alters the receptor binding characteristics of the delta-opioid receptor ligand, D-Ala^2-D-Leu^5 enkephalin in mouse brain. *Life Sci* 1983;33:2331–7.
17. Blum K, Hamilton MG, Wallace JE. Alcohol and opiates: a review of common neurochemical and behavioral mechanisms. In: Blum K, ed. *Alcohol and opiates.* New York: Academic Press, 1977:203–36.
18. Sinclair JD, Rusi M, Airaksinen MM, Altschuler ML. Relating TIQ's, opiates, and ethanol. In: Bloom F, Barchas J, Sandler M, Usdin E, eds. *Beta-carbolines and tetrahydroisoquinolines.* New York: Alan R Liss, 1982:365–75.
19. Nirenberg M, Wilson S, Higashida H, Rotter A, Kroeger K, Busis N. Modulation of synapse formation by cyclic adenosine monophosphate. *Science* 1983;222:792–9.

DISCUSSION

Dr. Minkowski: Do you have any data which are relevant to the fetal alcohol syndrome? Bloom showed that administration of alcohol to newborn animals causes an enormous increase in endorphines in the hypothalamus and a very marked decrease in dopamine, norepinephrine, and serotonin. What do you think are the likely consequences for the fetal brain?

Dr. Diamond: We have this question in our minds when doing some of this work. The animal models that people have employed have considerable limitations because they depend either on injecting large amounts of ethanol into a small fetus to achieve high intrauterine concentrations or on the creation of systems which result in such an abnormal maternal diet that a lot of change in the brain may occur on its own account (it is very difficult, for example, to ensure that a dam drinks enough alcohol to produce an effect unless her diet is very poor). Nevertheless the changes that you allude to look interesting and important, and can be pursued in cell culture. We think it is going to be possible to identify some of the mechanisms through which alcohol causes abnormal neural function, at the level of both cellular proliferation and differentiation.

Dr. Barbin: What effect does ethanol have on the proliferation rate of the cells in your system? Have you repeated the experiments in a chemically defined medium in order to see whether the presence of serum could have altered the number of receptors on the surface of these cells?

Dr. Diamond: At the concentrations we employ there is little if any effect on replicates, and the growth curves are fairly similar with or without ethanol.

We started out using serum, and the experiments I described were all done with 10% fetal calf serum. We have, however, been able to adapt these cells to grow in completely defined medium, with the same growth curves and responses. If we deplete this medium of insulin or transferrin or selenium we can achieve some degree of growth arrest. We turned to defined medium to avoid the complication of the lipids and critical proteins which are present in serum and which we cannot control for. We have noticed, for example, that the effects of ethanol on some membrane receptors may depend critically on the serum that we use. Thus some serum preparations allow a large response and others do not, suggesting that critical components may have been added in the serum. We can avoid these problems using defined medium.

Dr. Sotelo: One of the problems that bothers me with this type of study is that you are dealing with a genetically homogeneous population of neurons which seem to express the same types of receptors. The brain is heterogeneous though, and alcohol has actions which are more important for some neurons (e.g., Purkinje cells) than others. How close is your beautiful model to reality in the brain?

Dr. Diamond: We think this model is quite close to reality and very useful. If you take the whole brain and look for this kind of response you can find it, but it will be much reduced because you are only sampling a small number of target cells among many that may not respond to the same signal. If you want to take such research further in a whole animal it will be very difficult because the brain is so heterogeneous that the "noise" will be too large. However, if you take a homogeneous population of cells the signal can be amplified to the point where we can have faith in the biological response and use it to go further and deeper in uncovering the specific molecular events which are responsible.

For 30 or 40 years people have been injecting alcohol into animals but we still have very little understanding of the neurobiology of its effects. If you think about it for a moment, you can see the problem: There are hormonal changes produced by alcohol, endocrine changes, respiratory changes, and metabolic changes, with secondary and tertiary effects on different neuronal populations. We feel that our model at least gives us a chance to investigate the primary events in a way we cannot do with the whole brain.

Dr. Lou: It is always puzzling to see how variable is the susceptibility to alcohol intoxication. I wonder if your studies could provide any clues to the reason for this. Have you tried to examine different cell lines for evidence of genetic variability in the response of receptor function to alcohol exposure?

Dr. Diamond: There have been some excellent studies from Scandinavia and the United States which indicate that there are genetic factors in alcoholism, which remain strong even after correcting for socioeconomic problems and so on. We are presently trying to uncover some of the membrane adaptive responses that we think are required to cope with ethanol exposure, with the intention of comparing these responses in alcoholic patients and children at risk of developing alcoholism.

Dr. Campagnoni: Does treatment of your cells with alcohol cause a reduction in protein synthesis, and if so, is there an adaptive recovery during long-term exposure?

Dr. Diamond: We know from other published work that alcohol does affect protein synthesis, but these effects require higher concentrations of alcohol than we have been using. At the concentrations we use we do not see an effect on protein synthesis and the growth curves of the cells are perfectly normal compared with untreated control cells.

Developmental Neurobiology, edited by
Philippe Evrard and Alexandre Minkowski.
Nestlé Nutrition Workshop Series, Vol. 12.
Nestec Ltd., Vevey/Raven Press, Ltd.,
New York © 1989.

Some Aspects of Clinical and Biochemical Changes Related to Nutrition During Brain Development in Humans

Angel Ballabriga

Hospital Infantil Vall d'Hebron, Universidad Autonóma, Barcelona 08035, Spain

A large number of publications during the last 15 years have addressed the question of the influence of nutrition, particularly nutritional deprivation, on brain development. Better knowledge of the role played by the child's social environment and its mutual interactions with nutrition have imposed a revision of the problem. Excellent updates have been published by Dyson and Jones (1), Brozek (2), and Cravioto and Arrieta (3).

Correlations can be established between some chemical markers and certain structural components of the brain. Various determinations at different gestational ages give an idea about the transformations occurring in the developing brain. However, the interpretation of sequential values obtained from different individuals is not free of criticism given the heterogeneity of the series, owing to the different causes of death and to possible postmortem alterations, even after rigorous selection of cases and immediate collection of samples. On the other hand, because of the possibility of survival of infants with very low gestational age in intensive care units, a series of chemical processes of brain growth, normally taking place during intrauterine life, occur during extrauterine life and are directly influenced by postnatal nutrition. Some changes may be irreversible, depending on the timing, the duration, and the intensity of the insult; effects will also vary in different parts of the central nervous system (CNS), for example, the forebrain or cerebellum. However, alterations of the chemical composition of the structures of the CNS do not necessarily correspond to alterations of the function. Nevertheless, in our opinion, analysis of the chemical composition of CNS tissue represents a valid tool for establishing an objective basis for discussion of the problem.

ENCEPHALIC GROWTH

In order to assess the influence, if any, of undernutrition, the precise patterns of normal development must serve as background. Before presenting biochemical data, consideration is first given to the simplest used by Dobbing (4) to define his concept of the brain-growth spurt, that is to say, increase of the weight of the cerebrum. In a study of 90 carefully selected brains of human newborns who died on the first day of life, the weight of the brain was related to gestational age, as was the weight of the cerebellum in 44 cases. The weight of both cerebrum and cerebellum increase exponentially Whereas the weight of the cerebellum increases almost 12-fold between 20 and 40 weeks of gestation, the weight of the cerebrum increases only 5-fold during the same period. The average velocity of growth of the cerebellum is more than double that of the cerebrum during the second half of intrauterine life in humans.

When the data are plotted on a semilogarithmic scale (logarithm of the weight vs gestational age, the slopes of the regression lines, approximately 1.5 times steeper for cerebellum than for cerebrum, reflect the faster growth of the former. After birth growth slows progressively in both organs after 3 months and particularly after 6 months. Even so, there is a tendency for growth of the forebrain to slow before that of the cerebellum. In our study, the ratio of brain weight to body weight shows a quadratic parabolic profile with a downward slope, where the ratio does not decrease until a body weight of approximately 2,000 g is reached, though there are large individual variations. The curvilinear regression is significant at $p<0.001$. Thus, it seems that during the first part of gestation the relative growth of the brain is faster than that of the body until the fetus weighs approximately 2 kg. This corresponds to an average gestational age of 33 weeks. From that time on the cerebral growth, although remaining very active, is slower than the growth of body weight, and as a consequence the ratio brain weight/body weight starts to decrease.

However, the same index for the cerebellum (cerebellum weight/body weight $\times 100$), instead of following a linear or parabolic curve with a downward slope, follows an ascending line, again with large individual variations. The growth of the cerebellum during the last 3 months of intrauterine life is so rapid that it may even be faster than that of the body, and the index increases linearly during the second half of gestation. The selection of material for these "normal" data should be made very carefully, bearing in mind that presence of cerebral edema, generally a complication of anoxia, can cause an increase of up to 10% in the water content of the brain (5).

In Brown's series (6), the weight of the brain in malnourished infants was lower, in absolute terms, than in the nonmalnourished, but the brain weight/body weight index was slightly higher in malnourished infants, suggesting a degree of brain sparing. In the series of Naeye et al. (7) the weight of the brains of newborns from underweight mothers with low weight gain during pregnancy appeared to be relatively spared in comparison with the weight of other organs. In our cases the brain weight versus body weight ratio is higher in malnourished infants, although absolute values of brain weight and DNA content with respect to gestational age can be lower. This does not necessarily imply a correlation with function.

The occipitofrontal head circumference is an accurate measure of intracranial volume even if in abnormally shaped skulls the relation between the values can differ

(8). An extremely close correlation exists between intracranial volume and brain size (9). The brain weight and its protein content increase hyperbolically when compared with head circumference but linearly when compared with the theoretical cranial volume calculated from the head circumference (10). The increase in occipitofrontal head circumference correlates well with the growth of the intracranial volume of the brain. Reductions in head circumference in relation with malnutrition have been widely reported (11–14). The head circumference decreased by an average of 13.2% in 33 cases with marasmus described by Undurraga (15). In the study of Lloyd-Still (16), severe malnutrition up to the age of 1 to 3 months reduced brain weight by 18% and head circumference by 4.1%. Rosso et al. (17), in cases of severe marasmus, found a reduction in brain weight and head circumference of 30% and 9%, respectively, and in children of less than 2 years of age these authors described reductions of 52% and 12%, respectively.

Head circumference and brain weight correlate well during normal growth, less well in mild malnutrition, and not so well in severe forms of malnutrition where brain weight is reduced more than the cranial circumference (16–18). In the study by Stoch and Smythe (11) the difference between mean values of head circumference has increased over the 10 year period of observation in comparison with the controls, while the difference in mean height values has decreased. However, the significance of head circumference measurements has been questioned (19). Some authors point out that children presenting with stunting also show arrest of the head circumference (13,20) and that the size of the brain can also be affected. Monckeberg (14), in a report on 14 Chilean children with marasmus diagnosed between 1 and 5 months of life, showed that 3 to 6 years later, even if weight and height were normal, head circumference was reduced. Thus there is a relation between infant undernutrition, suboptimal head circumference, and suboptimal brain growth, but this by no means implies functional consequences.

It has been suggested that in human beings total DNA in the brain is correlated with head circumference (21). In the monkey, the relationship between brain DNA and head circumference is best demonstrated by a quadratic expression (22). Relatively minor undernutrition during a very short period of human brain growth can cause a reduction of the final volume of the brain (23). However, it does not seem possible to establish a close correlation between the growth of the brain, the number of cells, and the head circumference, and none of these can be directly correlated with intelligence.

BIOCHEMICAL CHANGES IN THE BRAIN DURING DEVELOPMENT IN RELATION TO NUTRITION

The DNA content in the brains of 9 infants who died of malnutrition has been found to be severely reduced compared to values obtained in normally nourished infants who died due to other causes, although the protein content per cell was unchanged. The number of glial cells is most affected when malnutrition occurs during the first 2 years of life (24).

In the study of Chase et al. (25) on 6 small-for-gestational-age infants and 10 appropriate-for-gestational-age infants, the cerebellum was very intensely affected during intrauterine development in the small-for-date group, with a 35% reduction of the DNA content and 19% in the cerebrum–brain stem fractions. Cerebroside-sulfatide content was significantly reduced in the small-for-date brains but values of phospholipids, cholesterol and gangliosides did not decrease. Galactolipid-sulfotransferase activity in the brain of small-for-date infants was also reduced. These findings suggest a decreased myelin content in the brain. A reduction of the DNA content in the cerebrum of small-for-date infants was reported by Sarma and Rao (26) whereas values in the other regions did not differ from control values. No decrease was observed in the total content or in the concentration of glycolipids, although the values of cholesterol were notably low in the brain. Fox et al. (27) analyzed the brains of three malnourished infants who died at 4, 12, and 22 months; the lipid composition of myelin isolated from the brains was normal but the content of cerebrosides and plasmalogens in white matter was reduced. Thus malnutrition seems to cause a decreased deposition of normal myelin. Myelin lipids and gangliosides during early human brain development have been studied in our laboratory in normal and undernourished infants (28,29).

Plasmalogens can probably be considered as a marker for myelin. Plasmalogens in the cerebrum of four marasmic infants who died between 10 weeks and 4.5 months of age were decreased, the severity of the reduction being directly related to the severity of the nutritional insult. The concentration of plasmalogens was about 80% of control values. In the cerebellum plasmalogen concentration was also decreased. Cerebral ganglioside level was slightly lower than control values. Total gangliosides were decreased in the cerebellum. Gangliosides were not as affected as the plasmalogens; this is explained by the lower speed of accretion of gangliosides in the cerebrum and by sparing mechanisms preserving the more important structures. Summarizing, the results suggest that in the human, myelinogenesis during the perinatal period is probably more vulnerable in the forebrain than in the cerebellum. These four marasmic infants showed a diminished concentration of cerebral galactolipids (Table 1) while cerebellar galactolipids were normal. These findings suggest that myelinogenesis is extremely vulnerable in the forebrain during the perinatal period.

TABLE 1. *Galactolipid concentration (μmol per g of wet tissue) in cerebrum (FB) and cerebellum (CL) of four postnatally undernourished infants*

Birth	Age	FB	CL
Full term	10 weeks	0.806	4.65
Full term	10 weeks	1.31	4.18
Full term	3 months	1.68	4.40
36 weeks of gestation	4.5 months	1.88	4.53

The four infants were born with a normal nutritional status and became marasmic in the postnatal period.

FATTY ACIDS AND BRAIN DEVELOPMENT

Previous studies (30–33) present the patterns of fatty acids during brain development in relation to gestational age; these patterns serve as references. Fatty acids in the brain are either synthesized in other parts of the organism or obtained from diet and transported to the brain, or they are synthesized inside the brain. The constancy of the fatty acid pattern of ethanolamine phosphoglycerides (EPG) in brain membranes is remarkable; this pattern is probably necessary for normal impulse propagation in the neurons (34).

There is general agreement that dietary fatty acids influence the fatty acid composition of most tissues (35–41) but there is still some controversy as to whether the

TABLE 2. *Normal values of fatty acids in ethanolamine phosphoglycerides (EPG) and choline phosphoglycerides (CPG) in liver and brain*

Fatty acid	Liver EPG	Liver CPG	Brain EPG	Brain CPG
	Mean values obtained from 6 cases with a gestational age of 37 weeks, dying during the first day of life			
14:0	—	0.46 ± 0.07	—	2.39 ± 0.46
16:0	19.34 ± 2.94	36.52 ± 1.34	6.23 ± 0.36	50.42 ± 0.80
16:1	0.76 ± 0.22	3.57 ± 1.07	0.51 ± 0.12	6.27 ± 0.61
18:0	23.57 ± 2.55	11.40 ± 1.52	26.71 ± 1.49	9.13 ± 0.86
18:1	6.23 + 1.31	17.24 ± 2.66	7.98 ± 0.41	22.42 ± 0.61
18:2	4.86 ± 1.64	9.21 ± 2.62	0.45 ± 0.12	0.67 ± 0.16
18:3 + 20:1	0.22 ± 0.06	0.15 ± 0.04	0.39 ± 0.05	0.38 ± 0.08
20:3w9	0.24 ± 0.15	0.19 ± 0.10	0.77 ± 0.31	0.17 ± 0.05
20:3w6	1.49 ± 0.21	2.01 ± 0.57	1.12 ± 0.17	0.60 ± 0.13
20:4w6	22.10 ± 1.84	13.06 ± 1.91	16.98 ± 0.58	5.27 ± 0.48
22:4w6	1.68 ± 0.76	0.24 ± 0.04	14.85 ± 1.00	0.78 ± 0.09
22:5w6	1.20 ± 0.50	0.31 ± 0.12	4.56 ± 0.85	0.25 ± 0.11
22:5w3	0.58 ± 0.21	0.26 ± 0.07	0.54 ± 0.21	Tr
22:6w3	17.72 ± 3.50	5.39 ± 1.66	18.90 ± 1.06	1.24 ± 0.19
	Mean values obtained from 6 cases after parenteral nutrition			
14:0	—	0.25 ± 0.09	—	2.17 ± 0.68
16:0	15.99 ± 1.86	32.17 ± 1.40	5.70 ± 0.56	49.09 ± 2.08
16:1	0.52 ± 0.21	2.27 ± 0.56	0.57 ± 0.14	6.20 ± 0.85
18:0	25.32 ± 1.90	12.12 ± 1.34	26.62 ± 0.98	9.07 ± 1.36
18:1	8.43 ± 0.70	15.55 ± 0.78	7.66 ± 0.80	22.24 ± 1.28
18:2	15.06 ± 3.75	23.97 ± 3.29	0.59 ± 0.22	1.63 ± 0.37
18:3 + 20:1	0.20 ± 0.11	Tr	0.37 ± 0.14	0.44 ± 0.10
20:3w9	0.25 ± 0.11	0.18 ± 0.16	1.17 ± 1.06	0.23 ± 0.24
20:3w6	0.74 ± 0.28	1.08 ± 0.52	1.19 ± 0.32	0.74 ± 0.27
20:4w6	22.28 ± 3.86	9.17 ± 2.01	17.65 ± 0.85	5.51 ± 0.37
22:4w6	1.13 ± 0.19	0.19 ± 0.06	14.10 ± 1.57	0.85 ± 0.24
22:5w6	0.66 ± 0.20	0.16 ± 0.06	5.19 ± 1.04	0.33 ± 0.08
22:5w3	0.56 ± 0.22	0.18 ± 0.09	0.67 ± 0.25	Tr
22:6w3	8.86 ± 2.37	2.70 ± 0.62	18.51 ± 1.63	1.46 ± 0.22

Values are expressed as % (weight) ± SE of total fatty acids.

fatty acid composition of phosphoglycerides in the brain can be modified by altering the fat intake. Important changes in fatty acid composition of brain EPG have been observed in rats with low essential fatty acid (EFA) diets (42,43). In experimental studies in rats with low EFA diets for three generations, Svennerholm et al. (44) found a reduction of cerebrosides and an increased brain content of 20:3(n-9) and 22:5(n-6). However, the question remains whether the nature of lipids deposited in the brain, particularly EFA, during the first months of life depend on the quantities of linoleic acid that are ingested. According to Widdowson (45) this seems rather unlikely. Studies (46) with different diets containing different quantities of linoleic acid show that during the first month of life, the quantity of linoleic acid contained in the lipid stroma of red cells can be very rapidly influenced by modifying the quantities of linoleic acid ingested, although apparently the permeability and function of the membrane are not influenced. However, the composition of fatty acids in the brain seems to resist dietary modifications strongly, for example when faced with an overload in linoleic acid, as occurs when fat is given intravenously during total parenteral nutrition in newborns (47). We have found only one significant difference in the content of linoleic acid in choline phosphoglycerides (CPG) compared to values considered normal in the brain, whereas variations are prominent in the liver and other organs (Table 2). The study of the fatty acid patterns in EPG and CPG of cerebrum and cerebellum in our small-for-date and postnatally malnourished newborns during the first 3 months of life do not demonstrate any significant modification (48).

NEUROLOGICAL FINDINGS RELATED TO NUTRITIONAL DISTURBANCES

Apathy and irritability are present as well as poor motivation and environmental unresponsiveness. Motor function is characterized by a certain degree of clumsiness. Echoencephalographic studies (49) have shown a reversible increase in the size of the lateral ventricles in kwashiorkor. Abnormalities of variable degree in brain transillumination have also been reported (50,51), and motor nerve conduction velocity (51) was reduced to a moderate degree and returned to normal values after recovery. Waking EEG rhythms (52,53) and evoked potentials (54) can show reversible alterations. In infants older than 4 months, malnourished from birth, a great number of sinus pauses increasing during quiet sleep has been described (55).

Some spectrographic investigations of crying in infants with marasmus show alterations similar to those observed in children with brain damage (56). In kwashiorkor crying analysis is normal. Lester (57), studying the crying of malnourished infants with a real time spectrum analyzer, found a higher pitch, lower amplitude, longer duration, and longer latency to the next signal compared with normal infants. The apathy of the child with malnutrition carries a reduction of his capacity to respond to stimulation and at the same time can cause a change in attitude of the mother faced with this type of reaction and consequently a reduction of the interaction of the mother with her child. As in experimental animals (58), malnutrition in early life functionally isolates the developing infant from the immediate environment.

After recovery the evolution of psychological development will depend on the intensity and duration of the episode of malnutrition, the persistence or not of a poor food intake, and the influence of social environment and particularly the degree of stimulation. Early malnutrition seems to have a greater effect than later malnutrition (59), although in one study no association was found between the intellectual level of subjects and the age at which they had been admitted with severe malnutrition during the first 2 years of life (60). Changes are found in intersensory integration and language abilities, with low values for perceptual tests and for abstract reasoning, lack of attention, easy distractibility, poor memory, poor motivation, emotional lability, and reduced social skills; there are also changes in orientational response and decreased motor skills such as coordination, strength, agility, and balance. There is little or no response to affective contacts and a reluctance to follow moving objects visually. Malnutrition reduces the child's activity level, thus limiting the ability to utilize the environment and to respond to it (61). Canosa et al. (62) suggest that differences of performance level in the malnourished are owing to their reduced ability to concentrate on a given task. Some authors (63) find the verbal function more affected than the nonverbal; on the other hand, one should bear in mind that language ability, and more particularly vocabulary, is very sensitive to social differences. Thus malnutrition interferes with normal cognitive development, sometimes resulting in a permanent cognitive retardation.

THE EFFECTS OF EARLY CHILDHOOD MALNUTRITION ON LATER INTELLECTUAL AND MOTOR DEVELOPMENT

The later intellectual and motor development of infants previously affected by early childhood malnutrition is still the subject of much controversy, due in part to the enormous difficulty in distinguishing between nutritional factors and all the other socioeconomic and cultural factors that influence development. Thus results from different studies are sometimes contradictory.

Hoorweg and Stanfield (64) in Kampala studied 20 controls and 60 children between 11 and 17 years of age, who presented with protein-energy malnutrition (PEM) between 8 and 27 months. Environmental variables were also studied. They concluded that PEM exerts a permanent impairment of intellectual ability and motor development, but they also showed that many variables are involved in this process. The school age group of 37 cases studied by Birch et al. (65) had suffered from kwashiorkor between 6 and 30 months of age; siblings and classmates were used as controls. The developmental quotient (full scale WISC IQ) in the malnourished children was 68.5 and 81.5 in the controls; verbal and performance differences were also observed. However, one should always bear in mind that long periods of hospitalization can have a depressive effect on development. The group of 14 children with marasmus between 1 and 5 months of age studied by Monckeberg (14) between 3 and 6 years of age showed a very important language retardation; the damage was considered permanent.

Cabak and Najdamvic (66) studied children aged 7 to 14 years who had presented with malnutrition between 4 and 24 months. When they were examined, the degree of somatic development was normal but the IQ was below normal; however, the social background of the families was different. In the study of Lloyd-Still (67) the socioeconomic factors have been very well accounted for. Groups of patients with cystic fibrosis who had presented severe episodes of malnutrition were compared with healthy siblings; a certain degree of intellectual deficit was observed between 2 and 5 years after the episode of malnutrition but it did not persist later on. In these cases the long periods of hospitalization and separation from the family which can play a role must also be borne in mind. The study of Evans et al. (68) concerning 14 cases examined at a mean age of 8.9 years, with siblings as controls, failed to show significant differences of nonverbal IQ. It has been suggested (69) that nutrition contributes especially to verbal intelligence and environmental stimulation to nonverbal scores.

Richardson et al. (70) studied children aged 6 to 10 years who had had severe malnutrition in the first 2 years of life. Previously malnourished children who were tall and had a good social background had an 11 points higher IQ than control children who were short with an unfavorable social background. The group with previous malnutrition, unfavorable social background, and short stature had an IQ 9 points below nonmalnourished children.

Champakam et al. (71) have demonstrated that the cognitive function of children aged 8 to 11 years who had presented with malnutrition during some periods in the first 3 years of life was affected. Likewise, Stoch and Smythe (11) observed a marked disturbance of visual motor perception in 17 out of 20 children between 15 and 18 years of age who had been affected by severe undernutrition in early life. Nonverbal scores were higher than the verbal in these children. The authors considered that there was evidence of irreversible intellectual impairment. Chase and Martin [72] observed a lower developmental quotient in 19 children who had presented with undernutrition during the first year of life when compared 3 to 4 years later with a group of normal children. Children with undernutrition of longer duration were more severely affected. Language development was very poor. The group of infants of less than 6 months of age with undernutrition studied by Cravioto and Robles (73) 3 to 4 months after the acute phase presented low performance scores in adaptive behavior. Fitzhardinge and Steven (74) studied 96 children with severe intrauterine undernutrition and followed up during a minimum of 5 years, of whom 25% showed evidence of minimal brain dysfunction. Speech defects featuring immaturity of reception and expression were present in 33% of boys and 26% of girls.

Other studies failed to show a relation between malnutrition and impairment of intellectual development. Observations in the Netherlands after the period of starvation at the end of World War II showed that in pregnant women who suffered important caloric restrictions, there was a reduction of fetal growth (75), but as shown 20 years later (76–78) no mental retardation was associated with gestations occurring during the famine; nutritional deprivation in these cases was not directly associated with an adverse home environment. The longitudinal study by Sheffer et al. (79) deals with mental development of 17 Jamaican children who had presented PEM, compared with 20 normal controls. Evaluation was performed 24 months later using the Caldwell Inventory of Home Stimulation, and scores were similar in both groups. The authors concluded that the mothers of the malnourished group were poor but had good mother–child relationships and that the ecology of malnutrition differs in different cultures. Hansen et al. (80) showed that a single episode of kwashiorkor in infants after the age of 10 months does not affect long-term brain development if the environment is acceptable. Liang et al. (81), in Indonesia, studied 107 children from 12 to 15 years of age belonging to families of low socioeconomic status and including 46 children with preceding malnutrition. The lowest IQ values were associated with previous malnutrition. Survivors of severe malnutrition studied 2 to 5 years after recovery by Cravioto (82) and compared with controls of the same ethnic group of similar economical condition and with equal quality and quantity of stimulation showed lower performances with regard to motor skills. Galler et al. (83) studied the academic performance of 129 children aged between 5 to 11 years who had presented with marasmus during the first year of life, compared with 129 controls. Previous malnutrition influenced behavior and, to a lesser degree, IQ.

Retrospective studies are very difficult to interpret. The diagnosis of malnutrition, its intensity, and its duration are sometimes difficult to evaluate; some controls might also have been malnourished or could have had different social backgrounds. Differences in the mother's educational background can also be of importance, and it is almost impossible to account for the effects of early disturbances of mother–infant interactions. The length of the follow-up may also play a role, since differences tend to disappear with time. Interactions between nutritional and social determinants of cognitive development may be different in boys and girls (84). On the other hand, scoring systems used in preschool children are often unsatisfactory predictors of later intelligence scores. At the same time, tests designed to be used in industralized countries are not applicable to other countries with different cultures, since all tests reflect the skills and concepts of a particular culture (85) and are consequently inappropriate for others.

ARE THE CONSEQUENCES OF NUTRITIONAL INSULT IRREVERSIBLE?

There seems to be no general answer to this question. Catch-up growth depends on environmental conditions (86). Adequate postnatal nutritional and environmental rehabilitation can correct the greater part of the functional and nutritional deficiencies in small-for-dates infants, although biochemical alterations probably occur in the brain. To cause a permanent deficit in these cases, the combination of a severe prenatal insult at a particular time and postnatal deprivation appear to be necessary. In postnatal malnutrition, particularly in early life, the effects seem to be more severe. Early marasmus probably has a greater effect on learning and behavior than protein deficiency, and there was no catch-up growth of the head circumference after rehabilitation in marasmic children studied in Ethiopia (87). Infants presenting with marasmus during the first months of life seem to show permanent brain damage with an average IQ below that of children of low socioeconomic status (14). In a longitudinal study of the head circumference in 32 small-for-dates infants, Brandt (88) demonstrated that in 15 cases catch-up occurred up to the end of the 18 month study period. Adequate nutrition can produce parallel changes in head circumference and radiological findings (89), and catch-up growth in head size can even occur years after severe malnutrition. Evans (19) suggested that catch-up can occur at any time, though Stoch and Smythe (11) do not share this opinion. The possibilities of catch-up will depend for a large part on the mutual interactions between various aspects of rehabilitation. In various groups of marasmic children receiving the same dietary treatment, the group receiving extra stimulation improved more rapidly (90). The best results are obtained when combining psychological and nutritional rehabilitation (91). Korean children with antecedents of malnutrition adopted by American families before the age of 3 years and studied by Winnick (92) obtained IQ scores equal to American children after 6 years or more.

CONCLUSIONS

The effects of nutritional deprivation on CNS development depend on the timing, duration, and severity of the nutritional insult. In any case, great caution is necessary in making interspecies comparisons; the animal model of malnutrition is possibly far from being free of psychosocial contamination (93). The CNS is relatively protected against nutritional insult, and although the brain may stop growing and certain biochemical changes may be produced, functional alterations are less clear and seem to be observed in smaller mammals rather than in humans. Malnutrition probably needs to reach a certain threshold of intensity and duration in order to alter brain development, and more particularly in order to alter functional development. For this reason, longitudinal studies are preferable to cross-sectional ones. It is impossible in humans to separate nutrition from other factors that can affect intelligence, since malnutrition is a multifactorial problem. The social background, the combination of poor nutrition, and lack of environmental stimulation interfere with cognitive development, sometimes resulting in definitive impairment. Factors such as availability of nutrients (in terms of quantity as well as of quality), diseases that can affect directly or indirectly the dietetic intake, infections, and prenatal and postnatal socioeconomic factors interact and combine. All these factors, depending on their intensity, timing, and duration, condition the prognosis.

REFERENCES

1. Dyson SE, Jones DG. Undernutrition and the developing nervous system. *Progr Neurobiol* 1976;7:171–96.
2. Brozek J. Nutrition, malnutrition and behaviour. *Annu Rev Psychol* 1978;29:157–77.
3. Cravioto J, Arrieta R. *Nutricion, desarrollo mental, conducta y aprendizaje.* Mexico, DIF: Instituto Nacional Ciencias y technologia de la salud del niño, 1982.
4. Dobbing J. Vulnerable periods in developing brain. In: Davison AN, Dobbing J, eds. *Applied neurochemistry.* Oxford: Blackwell, 1968:287–316.
5. Anderson MJ. Increased brain weight/liver weight ratio as a necropsy sign of intrauterine undernutrition. *J Clin Pathol* 1972;25:867–71.
6. Brown RE. Decreased brain weight in malnutrition and its implications. *East Afr Med J* 1965; 42:584–95.
7. Naeye RL, Blanc W, Paul C. Effects of maternal nutrition on the human fetus. *Pediatrics* 1973; 52:494–503.
8. Buda FB, Reed JC, Rabe EF. Skull volume in infants. Methodology, normal values and application. *Am J Dis Child* 1975;129:1171–4.
9. Bray PF, Shields WD, Wolcott GJ, Madsen JA. Occipitofrontal head circumference an accurate measure of intracranial volume. *J Pediatr* 1969;75:303–5.
10. Winick M, Rosso P. Head circumference and cellular growth of the brain in normal and marasmic children. *J Pediatr* 1969;74:774–8.
11. Stoch MB, Smythe PM. 15-Year developmental study on effects of severe undernutrition during infancy on subsequent physical growth and intellectual functioning. *Arch Dis Child* 1976;51:327–36.
12. Chase HP, Canosa CA, O'Brien D. Nutrition and biochemical maturation of the brain. In: *Nutrition, growth and development. Modern problems in paediatrics.* Basel: Karger, 1975:14:110–18.
13. Graham GG. Effect of infantile malnutrition on growth. *Fed Proc* 1967;26:139–43.
14. Monckeberg F. Effect of early marasmic malnutrition on subsequent physical and psychological development. In: Scrimshaw N-S, Gorden JE, eds. *Malnutrition, learning and behaviour.* Cambridge, MA: The MIT Press, 1968:267–9.
15. Undurraga O, Manterola A, Segure T. Efectos de la desnutrición infantil precoz y grave sobre el crecimiento del craneo. *Vol Med Hosp Infant* 1977;34:571.
16. Lloyd-Still JD. *Malnutrition and intellectual development.* Lancaster, PA: MTP Press, 1976.
17. Rosso P, Hormazabal J. Winick M. Changes in brain weight, cholesterol, prospholipid and DNA content in marasmic children. *Amer J Clin Nutr* 1970;23:1275–9.
18. Usher RH, McLean F. Normal fetal growth and significance of fetal growth retardation. In: Davis JA, Dobbing J, eds. *Scientific foundations of paediatrics.* London: Heinemann, 1974:69–79.
19. Evans DE, Moodie AD, Hansen JDL. Kwashiorkor and intellectual development: a 10-year follow-up study. *S Afr Med J* 1971;45:143–56.
20. Ambrosius DK. El comportamiento del peso de algunos organos en niños con desnutricion de tercer grado. *Bol Med Hosp Infant Mex* 1961;18:47.
21. Winick M, Rosso P. The effect of severe early malnutrition on cellular growth of human brain. *Pediatr Res* 1969;3:181–4.
22. Cheek DB, Mellits DE, Hill DE, Holt AB. Mathematical appraisal of biochemical determinants of brain growth. In: Cheek DB, ed. *Fetal and postnatal cellular growth. Hormones and nutrition.* New York: John Wiley, 1975:55–97.
23. Davies PA, Davis JP. Very low birth weight and subsequent head growth. *Lancet* 1970;II:1216–9.
24. Dobbing J. Infant nutrition and later achievement. *Nutr Rev* 1984;42:1–7.
25. Chase HP, Welch NN, Dabiere CS, Vasan NS, Butterfield LJ. Alterations in human brain biochemistry following intrauterine growth retardation. *Pediatrics* 1972;50:403–11.
26. Sarma MK, Rao KS. Biochemical composition of different regions in brains of small-for-date infants. *J Neurochem* 1974;22:671–7.
27. Fox JH, Fishman MA, Dodge PR, Prensky AL. The effect of malnutrition on human central nervous system myelin. *Neurology* 1972;22:1213–6.
28. Martinez M. Myelin lipids and gangliosides during early human brain development in normal and undernourished infants. In: *Proceedings of the sixth European congress of perinatal medicine.* Stuttgart: Georg Thieme, 1978;174–81.
29. Martinez M. Myelin lipids in the developing cerebrum, cerebellum and brain stem of normal and undernourished children. *J. Neurochem* 1982;39:1684–92.

30. Martinez M, Conde C, Ballabriga A. Some chemical aspects of human brain development. II. Phosphoglyceride fatty acids. *Pediatr Res* 1974;8:93–102.
31. Martinez M, Conde C, Ballabriga A. A chemical study on prenatal brain development in humans: nutrition, growth and development. *Mod Probl Paediatr* 1975;14:100.
32. Ballabriga A, Martinez M. A chemical study on the development of the human forebrain and cerebellum during the brain growth spurt period. II. Phosphoglyceride fatty acids. *Brain Res* 1978;159:363–70.
33. Martinez M, Ballabriga A. A chemical study on the development of the human forebrain and cerebellum during the brain growth spurt period. I. Gangliosides and plasmalogens. *Brain Res* 1978;159:351–62.
34. Karlson J. Effects of different dietary levels of essential fatty acids on the fatty acid composition of ethanolamine phosphoglycerides in myelin and synaptosomal plasma membranes. *J Neurochem* 1975;23:101–7.
35. Klenk E, Oette K. Über die natur der in den leberphosphatiden auftretenden C20 und C22 polyensäuren bei verabreichung von Linol und linolen-säure an fetfrei ernährten Ratten. *Hoppe-Seylers Z Physiol Chem* 1960;318:86.
36. Hansen AE, Stewart RA, Hughes G, Söderhjelm L. The relation of linoleic acid to infant feeding. *Acta Paediatr Scand* Suppl 1962;137:1–41.
37. Mohrhauer H, Holman RT. Alteration of the fatty acid composition of brain lipids by varying levels of dietary essential fatty acids. *J Neurochem* 1963;10:523.
38. Mendy F, Hirtz J, Berret R, Rio B, Rossier A. Etude de la composition en acides gras polydésaturés des lipides sériques de nourrisons soumis à des régimes différents. *Ann Nutr Aliment* 1968;22:267–85.
39. Olegard R, Svennerholm L. Fatty acid composition of plasma and red cell phosphoglycerides in full term infants and their mothers. *Acta Paediatr Scand* 1970;59:637–47.
40. Ballabriga A, Martinez M, Gallart-Catalá A. Composition of subcutaneous fat depot in prematures in relationship with fat intake. *Helv Paediatr Acta* 1972;27:91–8.
41. Ballabriga A, Martinez M. Aorta fatty acids in the newborn period. *Pediatr Res* 1974;8:131, abstract.
42. Alling C. *Essential fatty acid malnutrition and brain development.* Göteborg: University of Göteborg, 1974;1–31.
43. Paoleti R, Galli C. Effect of essential fatty acid deficiency on the central nervous system in the growing rat. In: *Lipids, malnutrition and the developing brain (Ciba Found Symp).* 1972;121–40.
44. Svennerholm L, Alling C, Bruce A, Karlsson I, Sapia O. Effects on offspring of maternal malnutrition in the rat. In: *Lipids, malnutrition and the developing brain (Ciba Found Symp).* 1972;141–57.
45. Widdowson FM. Artificial milks and their effects on the composition of the infant. In: Wilkinson AW, ed. *Early nutrition and later development.* London; Pitman Medical, 1976:71–8.
46. Ballabriga A, Martinez M. Changes in erythrocyte lipid stroma in the premature infant according to dietary fat composition. *Acta Paediatr Scand* 1976;65:705–9.
47. Ballabriga A, Martinez M. Changes in organ chemical composition during parenteral nutrition. In: *Problemi attuali di nurizione in pediatria.* Milano: Sapil, 1975;115–25.
48. Ballabriga A, Martinez M. Some aspects of biochemical brain development with relation to nutrition. In: *Proceedings of the sixth European congress of perinatal medicine,* Vienna, 1978:159–74.
49. Vahlquist B, Engsner G, Sjögren I. Malnutrition and size of the cerebral ventricles. *Acta Paediatr Scand* 1971;60:533–9.
50. Rozovski NJ, Novoa SF, Abarzua FJ, Monckeberg BF. Cranial transillumination in early and severe malnutrition. *Br J Nutr* 1971;25:107–11.
51. Vahlquist B. Early malnutrition and brain development. *Acta Paediatr Hung* 1972;13:309–22.
52. Engel R. Abnormal brain wave patterns in kwashiorkor. *Electroencephalogr Clin Neurophysiol* 1956;8:489.
53. Valenzuela RH, Hernandez-Peniche J, Macias R. Clinical electroencephalographic and physiological aspects of recuperation of the undernourished child. *Gac Med Mex* 1959;89:651.
54. Barnet AB, Weiss IP, Sotillo MV, Ohlrich ES, Shkurovich MZ, Cravioto J. Abnormal auditory evoked potentials in early human malnutrition. *Science* 1978;201:450–2.
55. Salzarulo P, Fagiolo I, Salomon F, Ricour C. Developmental trend of quiet sleep is altered by early human malnutrition and recovered by nutritional rehabilitation. *Early Hum Dev* 1982;7:257–64.
56. Juntunen K, Sirviö P, Miehelsson K. Cry analysis in infants with severe malnutrition. *Eur J Pediatr* 1978;128:241–6.

57. Lester BM. Spectrum analysis of the cry sounds of well-nourished and mal-nourished infants. *Child Dev* 1976;47:237–41.
58. Levitsky DA, Massaro TF, Barnes RH. Maternal malnutrition and the neonatal environment. *Fed Proc.* 1975;35:1583–6.
59. Cravioto J. Appraisal of the effect of nutrition on biochemical maturation. *Am J Clin Nutr* 1962;11:484.
60. Hertzig ME, Birch HG, Richardson SA, Tizard J. Intellectual levels of school children severely malnourished during the first two years of life. *Pediatrics* 1972;49:814–24.
61. Christiansen N, Voori L, Mora JO, Wagner M. Social environment as it relates to malnutrition and mental development. In: Cravioto J, et al, eds. *Early malnutrition and mental development.* Uppsala: Almquist and Wiksell, 1974.
62. Canosa CA, Salomon JB, Klein RE. The intervention approach: the Guatemala study. In: Moore WM, Silverberg MM, Read MS, eds. *Nutrition, growth and development of North American indian children.* Washington, DC: DHEW Publications, 1972; no. 26.
63. Barrera Moncada G. *Estudios sobre alteraciones del crecimiento y del desarrollo psicologico del sindrome pluricarencial (Kwashiorkor).* Caracas: Editora Grafos. 1963.
64. Hoorweg J, Paget Stanfield J. The effects of protein energy malnutrition in early childhood on intellectual and motor abilities in later childhood and adolescence. *Dev Med Child Neurol* 1976;18:330–50.
65. Birch HG, Piñeiro C, Alcalde E, Toca T, Cravioto J. Relation of kwashiorkor in early childhood and intelligence at school age. *Pediatr Res* 1971;5:579–85.
66. Cabak V, Najdanvic R. Effect of undernutrition in early life on physical and mental development. *Arch Dis Child* 1965;40:532–4.
67. Lloyd-Still JD, Wolff PH, Hurwitz I, Shwachman H. Studies on intellectual development after severe malnutrition in infancy in cystic fibrosis and other intestinal lesions. In: *Proceedings of the ninth international congress of nutrition.* Basel: Karger, 1975;2:357–64.
68. Evans DE, Bowie MD, Hansen JDL, Moodie AD, van der Spuy HIJ. Intellectual development and nutrition. *J Pediatr* 1980;97:358–63.
69. Waterlow JC, Cravioto J, Stephen JML. Protein malnutrition in man. Clinical and social aspects. *Adv Protein Chem* 1960;15:138.
70. Richardson SA, Birch HG, Ragbeer C. The behaviour of children at home who were severely malnourished in the first 2 years of life. *J Biosoc Sci* 1975,7.255–67.
71. Champakam S, Sirkantea SG, Gopalan C. Kwashiorkor and mental development. *Am J Clin Nutr* 1968;21:844–52.
72. Chase HP, Martin HP. Undernutrition and child development. *New Engl J Med* 1970;282:933–9.
73. Cravioto J, Robles B. Evolution of adaptative and motor behavior during rehabilitation from kwashiorkor. *Am J Orthopsychiatry* 1965;35:449.
74. Fitzhardinge PM, Stevens FM. The small for date infant. Later growth patterns. *Pediatrics* 1972;49:671–81.
75. Smith C. The effect of wartime starvation in Holland upon pregnancy and its product. *Am J Obstet Gynecol* 1947;53:599–608.
76. Stein ZA, Susser M, Saenger G, Marolla F. Nutrition and mental performance. *Science* 1972; 178:708–13.
77. Stein Z, Susser M, Saenger G, Marolla F. Intelligence test results of individuals exposed during gestation to World War II famine in the Netherlands. *Tijdschr Soc Geneeskd* 1973;50:766–75.
78. Stein ZA, Susser MW. Prenatal nutrition and mental competence. In: Lloyd-Still JD, ed. *Malnutrition and intellectual development.* Lancaster, PA: MTP Press, 1976.
79. Sheffer ML, Grantham McGregor SM, Ismail SJ. The social environment of malnourished children compared with that of other children in Jamaica. *J Biosoc Sci* 1981;13:19–30.
80. Hansen JDL, Freesemann C, Moodie AD, Evans DE. What does nutritional growth retardation imply? *Pediatrics* 1971;47:299.
81. Liang PH, Hie TT, Jan OH, Glok LT. Evaluation of mental development in relation to early malnutrition. *Am J Clin Nutr* 1967;20:1290–4.
82. Cravioto J. Severe malnutrition and development of motor skills in children. *Ann Nestlé* 1980; 44:22–41.
83. Galler JR, Ramsey F, Solimano G. The influence of early malnutrition on subsequent behavioral development. III. Learning disabilities as a sequel to malnutrition. *Pediatr Res* 1984;18:309–13

84. Klein RE, Freeman HE, Kagan J, Yarbrough C, Habicht J-P. Is big smart? The relation of growth to cognition. *J Health Soc Behav* 1972;13:219–25.
85. Vernon PE. Measurements of learning. In: Scrimshaw NS, Gordon JE, eds. *Malnutrition, learning and behavior*. Cambridge, MA: MIT Press, 1968:486–96.
86. Graham GC, Adrianzen B. Growth, inheritance and environment. *Pediatr Res* 1971;5:691–7.
87. Engsner G, Belete S, Sjögren I, Vahlquist G. Brain growth in children with marasmus. A study using head circumference measurement, transillumination and ultrasonic echo ventriculography. *Ups J Med Sci* 1974;79:116–28.
88. Brandt IL. Normwerte für den opfumfang vor und nach dem regulären Geburtstermin bis zum Alter von 18 Monaten. Absolutes Wachstum und Wachstumsgeschwindigkeit. *Monatsschr Kinderheilkd* 1976;124:141–50.
89. Dodge PR, Prensky AL, Feigin RD. *Nutrition and the developing nervous system*. St. Louis: Mosby, 1975.
90. Yatkin US, McLaren DS, Kanawati AA, Sabbagh S. Effect of undernutrition in early life on subsequent behavioural development. In: *Proc Int Congr Pediatr* 1971;2:71.
91. Lopez I, de Andraca I, Colombo M. Relevance of psychological rehabilitation in severe malnutrition. *Ann Nestlé* 1985;43(1):31–41.
92. Winick M, Katchadurian K, Harris RC. Malnutrition and environmental enrichment by early adoption. Development of adopted Korean children differing greatly in early nutritional status is examined. *Science* 1975;190:1173–5.
93. Levine S, Wiener S. A critical analysis of data on malnutrition and behavioral deficits. In: Schulman J, ed. *Adv Pediatr* 1976;22:113–36.

DISCUSSION

Dr. Volpe: Do you think that the effects of malnutrition and of the disturbed environment are additive, or do you think they could be synergistic, the effect of both being greater than you would expect from the two added together?

Dr. Ballabriga: This is very controversial. For instance, the infants studied by Monckeberg in Chile appeared to show that malnutrition *per se* caused long-term developmental changes, whereas those studied by Richardson in Jamaica showed just the contrary—his studies indicated that social factors were very important right from the start. The problem is that from an experimental point of view it is only possible to study one factor at a time in isolation. Take the experience of the Dutch population during World War II. During the Dutch famine pregnant women were surviving on 700 kcal/day, leading to a marked increase in the number of abortions and a reduction in birth weight. When infants born during this period were studied 20 years later there were no identifiable deficiencies. Interpretation is very difficult because there is the possibility that the most severely affected infants all died and that an excellent level of mother–child interaction in this particular population prevented serious consequences for the remainder. In underdeveloped countries it is impossible to separate nutritional deficiencies from other environmental deficiencies. It is perhaps for this reason that Richardson found social factors to be fundamental; maybe it is only in cases of really catastrophic nutrient deficiency that the problem becomes irreversible.

Dr. Diamond: Do you have any information on the possible roles of parasitic disease and other types of infection in the interpretation of the effects of malnutrition? These disorders themselves produce marked effects on the nervous system.

Dr. Ballabriga: We tend not to consider infectious diseases and parasitic infestations because they are phenomena that are very difficult to evaluate or control. Of course infants in such circumstances also have impaired immune responses, and there is synergism between worsening malnutrition and increasing numbers of infectious episodes. It is very difficult to identify which plays the more important role.

Dr. Minkowski: Long-term follow-up is always very difficult because so many factors interfere. What do you think about using siblings as controls? Is this a good way to avoid some of the confounding factors?

Dr. Ballabriga: I cannot answer that question.

Dr. Dubowitz: In relation to studies on siblings, would you like to comment on Stoch's studies in South Africa where she has a sibling control group and a 17-year follow-up?

Dr. Ballabriga: Stoch and her group have published three different papers in the last 10 years. The view of this group is very pessimistic about the long-term outcome of malnutrition, although there are some cases of good individual improvement. It is very difficult to make generalizations. You can always pick out individual cases, but in every family the interaction between mother and child is unique and results in very many completely different situations, even within the same family.

Dr. Dubowitz: I thought that in Stoch's latest follow-up she found smaller differences among the sibling index and control cases than she did in the early follow-up reports. Am I wrong?

Dr. Ballabriga: No, but outcome very much depends on the severity of the original deficiency. Between kwashiorkor at one end of the scale and subclinical biochemical deficiency at the other there is a wide range, and within this range each individual case has a very different prognosis depending on the duration and intensity of nutrient deficiency. Thus results may be quite different from one study to another.

Dr. Goyens: We know severe zinc deficiency during a short but critical time in pregnancy can modify immunocompetence in mice for two generations. Are there any arguments that the same could be true for neurobiological development?

Dr. Ballabriga: We have studied the zinc, manganese, and copper content of the human brain at different gestational ages in relation to its DNA content. The evolution of the three minerals is quite different. Uptake and storage of zinc is faster than the other two, presumably because zinc is incorporated in a particular series of developing metalloenzymes, but there is no particular indication that zinc deficiency at this stage in development results in impaired brain growth or function.

Dr. Lou: Do you think we can learn anything from studies done in developed countries on children who were seriously malnourished in early life because of pyloric stenosis, cystic fibrosis, and so on?

Dr. Ballabriga: Yes I do. There is at least one interesting study on children with cystic fibrosis, treated and followed up over a long period. These children have completely normal mental development, but only when their families care for them well in a psychological sense. Any reduction in their abilities can be accounted for by environmental factors connected with their chronic relapsing disease. In such children there is clear evidence of deficiency of polyunsaturated fatty acids reflected in the composition of the aortic wall, but no apparent repercussions on brain development.

Dr. Bourre: In nutritional terms I would say that premature infants are more vulnerable than full-term infants in the postnatal period, because they may be exposed to fatty acid deficiencies for a longer time. Neural membrane turnover of fatty acids is extremely slow, at least one or two orders of magnitude slower than in other organs. Thus if you incorporate the right molecule in the membrane *in utero* you will keep the molecule for a very long time and you will need a long period of postnatal undernutrition before any defect is likely to appear in the membranes.

Dr. Ballabriga: There is one surprising thing in the human infant, which is the fact that alterations in the concentrations of polyunsaturated fatty acids are very much more rapid than in the adult. For example, the composition of subcutaneous fat changes to reflect an altered dietary intake of linoleic acid in about 10 days. In the adult it takes 3 to 4 months. In erythrocyte lipid stroma phosphoglycerides change immediately to reflect dietary changes, but without any apparent alteration in clinical condition. Nevertheless there are infants in many countries who have been fed milk with low linoleic acid content for prolonged periods without any apparent effect on behavior or neurological development. There may well be a critical limit below which adverse clinical effects occur, but it seems that the margin between the appearance of biochemical changes and the appearance of clinical changes is very wide.

Developmental Neurobiology, edited by
Philippe Evrard and Alexandre Minkowski.
Nestlé Nutrition Workshop Series, Vol. 12.
Nestec Ltd., Vevey/Raven Press, Ltd.,
New York © 1989.

Experimental Studies on the Effect of Early Malnutrition on the Norepinephrinergic System Projecting to the Cerebral Cortex

*Rubén Soto-Moyano, *A. Hernández, *H. Pérez, *S. Ruiz, and †J. Belmar

*Institute of Nutrition and Food Technology (INTA), University of Chile, and †Department of Cell Biology, Catholic University of Chile, Santiago 11, Chile

It is generally accepted that the higher functions of the central nervous system are closely related to association areas of the cerebral cortex. This notion is based on considerable evidence obtained from studies mainly performed in freely moving monkeys. Electrophysiological studies in this animal species have revealed a relationship between the discharges of cortical parietal neurons and voluntary movements (1,2) and also that the response of these neurons can be behaviorally modified (3). These results support previous behavioral studies which indicate that posterior parietal lobe lesions induce clear-cut deficiencies in the acquisition and performance of tasks involving sensory discrimination (4). Comparable studies have also demonstrated that lesions of the prefrontal cortex (PFC) cause deficits in cognition, emotional reaction, and social interaction (5–7).

Since the early reports indicating that perinatal malnutrition induces lower intellectual performance in humans (8–12) and lower scores in learning tasks in animals (13–15), considerable efforts have been devoted to the study of the organic change induced by malnutrition on brain structures, which could provide the anatomical basis for the cognitive deficits.

Morphological studies have revealed that early malnutrition results in alterations in the cerebral cortex, such as decreased cortical thickness, reduced dendritic length, diminished number of dendritic spines, lower cellular density, and decreased synapse–neuron ratios (16–20). Other studies (21) have shown that protein deprivation induces a curtailment of the dendritic development of multipolar and fusiform cells within the locus coeruleus (LC). This nucleus has been demonstrated to be responsible for the norepinephrinergic innervation of the neocortex (22). In addition, the out-of-phase development of dendritic spines in the LC and in the nucleus raphe dorsalis (responsible for the serotonin innervation of the neocortex) does not take place in protein-deprived animals (21,23,24), suggesting that the reciprocal inhibitory interactions between these nuclei (25) are probably disrupted by malnutrition. The physiological relevance of this structural change must be evaluated bearing in mind that dendritic networks and synaptic contacts constitute the anatomical basis of the higher functions of the central nervous system.

Neurochemical studies have shown that maternal protein restriction in the rat results in increased concentration of norepinephrine (NE) and serotonin (5-HT) in various regions of the pup brain. These studies also showed that NE and 5-HT remain elevated if dietary protein restriction is continued after weaning (26). It has also been reported that intrauterine growth retardation, after ligation of the artery and vein supplying one uterine horn in pregnant rats, results in long-lasting elevation in 5-HT levels in the forebrain of pups (27). The functional implications of the increased brain monoamine concentrations reported in malnutrition remain unclear. No correlation has been found between these changes and electrophysiological and behavioral disturbances. This is interesting in view of the assertion that changes in the levels of biogenic amines are found in several affective disorders (28). Moreover, experimental studies in laboratory rodents and nonhuman primates have shown that norepinephrinergic hyperactivity is associated with some anxiety states, such as fear and profound alterations in attentiveness and vigilance to physiologically relevant stimuli (29). In humans, increased NE levels have been associated with deficits in attention and information processing (30).

Electrophysiological studies utilizing electrical stimulation of the parietal association area of the rat cerebral cortex have shown that prenatal or postnatal malnutrition decrease cortical excitability and diminish the ability of cortical neurons to follow repetitive stimulation (31,32). These effects, which persist in adult animals (33), indicate functional alterations of the axodendritic synapses mediating direct cortical evoked responses. Similar excitability and fatigability disturbances have been found in studies in the PFC of rats submitted to early malnutrition (34). In addition it has been reported that the spontaneous firing rate of neurons of layers III to V of the rat frontal cortex is lowered by protein malnutrition occurring during development (35), and that prenatal protein malnutrition significantly decreases the low-frequency power content in the EEG obtained from the frontal cortex during slow-wave sleep in rats less than 3 weeks of age. In these animals rapid-eye-movement (REM) sleep time is reduced and time spent in aroused waking is increased (36).

It can be assumed then that the behavioral disorders found in malnutrition could be caused, in part, by alterations at the cortical level and to subcortical structures that modulate the activity of the cerebral cortex. Cortical alterations have been confirmed by the research reviewed above. The presence of subcortical lesions has not received conclusive support.

Since the LC norepinephrine system has been implicated in higher integrative functions (23) and since it strongly modulates cortical neuronal activity (37), we studied the long-term effects of early protein-energy malnutrition in the rat on the development of norepinephrinergic projections to the PFC.

Male and female Wistar rats were studied within the following dietary treatment groups: a control group comprising 10 separate litters of 8 pups per dam; and a malnourished group also comprising 10 separate litters but with 18 pups per dam. Malnutrition resulted from competition for maternal milk during lactation. Throughout gestation and lactation, all dams were fed the standard pelleted stock diet providing 200 g protein/kg. After weaning at 21 days of age, the pups were maintained on this same diet fed *ad libitum*. The body weight of the pups was measured periodically.

Electrophysiological procedures. At 21, 30, 45, 70, and 100 days of age the animals were anesthetized with 100 mg/kg of α-chloralose intraperitoneally and placed in a Horsley-Clarke stereotaxic apparatus modified for use in rats. A single intramuscular dose of 1.5 mg/kg of D-tubocurarine was injected as muscle relaxant and adequate ventilation was maintained by means of a respirator pump. After exposure of the frontal lobe of one cerebral hemisphere, bipolar stimulation of the LC was carried out using stainless steel coaxial electrodes. The following de Groot coordinates were used to approach LC stereotactically in animals older than 45 days: *A* −2.0, *L* 0.8, and *V* −3.5 (in mm). For younger animals, these coordinates were corrected according to the method proposed by Valenstein et al. (38). Locus ceruleus stimulation consisted of single rectangular electrical pulses of 350 μA, 0.1 msec duration, and 0.25 Hz. Evoked responses were conventionally recorded from the PFC, between de Groot coordinates *A* 9.5 to 10.5, and *L* 1.0 to 2.0 (in mm). Recordings were amplified (8,000–10,000 Hz bandwidth), displayed on an oscilloscope and digitized at a rate of 1000/sec with an A/D converter interfaced to a microcomputer. They were also stored on magnetic tape for retrieval and averaging. Body temperature and expired CO_2 were monitored and remained within normal limits throughout the experiments. To confirm the correct placement of the stimulating electrodes, an electrolytic lesion was induced after completion of the electrophysiological procedures by passing an anodal current of 1 mA for 20 sec. Histologic sections of the area were then evaluated. Animals were killed by perfusing a 10% formalin solution through the heart, and the brains were removed and weighed. Twenty additional animals were used to determine brain weight on days 8 and 15.

Neurochemical methods. Normal and malnourished animals were divided into three groups and killed by decapitation at ages 21, 45, and 100 days. The brains were rapidly removed and cooled on ice. The frontal lobes were dissected and about 200 mg of cortex was obtained. Determinations were made on pooled tissue from three rats. This was weighed and homogenized in 0.32 M sucrose buffered at pH 7.2 with 1 mM potassium phosphate. Aliquots were precipitated with 0.4 N perchloric acid and precipitates were centrifuged at 1000 g and 4°C for 15 min. Supernatants were absorbed on alumina and the eluates were used for spectrofluormetric determination of NE according to Campuzano et al. (39). Internal standards were used in each NE determination. The acid precipitated was dissolved in 1.0 N NaOH and assayed for proteins according to Lowry et al. (40), using serum albumin as the standard.

RESULTS AND DISCUSSION

Protein-energy malnutrition in suckling pups resulted in decreased body weight of the pups, with the maximal deficit observed at weaning. Afterwards catch-up growth occurred. However, at 100 days of age a significant body weight deficit persisted (Fig. 1A). The brain weight of the pups showed a similar trend (Fig. 1B).

This reduction in body and brain weights reflects the changes caused by malnutrition during early development. In rats, the sucking period corresponds to the period of the brain growth spurt. Disruption of brain growth results in permanent disturbances of brain development (41). Our observations are in agreement with previous data by others indicating a persistent reduction of brain weight throughout adulthood, even when *ad libitum* feeding is restored (41,42).

Norepinephrine measurements showed that nutritional restriction in pups increased the concentration of this neurotransmitter in the PFC. This effect was more evident at 21 days of age. Despite the fact that differences in NE content between normal and deprived animals tended to decrease during prolonged follow-up, they still remained significant at 100 days of age (Fig. 2). Similar increases have previously been reported in larger brain regions, such as the telencephalon, diencephalon, midbrain, pons-medulla, and cerebellum (26). One possible factor underlying these results may be the increase in tyrosine hydroxylase activity observed in the brain of perinatally malnourished rats (43). Whether other metabolic presynaptic impairments such as disorders of storage, release, uptake, or degradation may contribute to these increased NE levels remains to be determined.

Figure 3 shows the average of 10 responses evoked by LC stimulation in the PFC of a normal and a protein-energy-deprived 45 day old rat. It consisted of an early positive–negative potential followed by a later one of varying shape. At 30, 45, 70, and 100 days of age, protein-energy malnutrition significantly reduced the peak-to-peak amplitude of the positive–negative early response, the effect being most marked at 45, 70, and 100 days of age (Fig. 4). At weaning, early responses in mal-

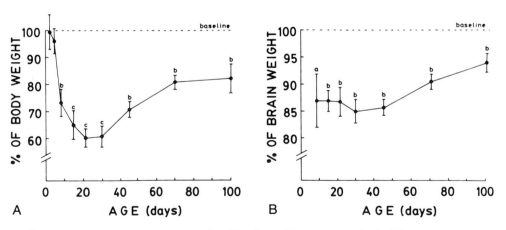

FIG. 1. Effect of protein-energy malnutrition in suckling pups on body (**A**) and brain (**B**) weights. Results are expressed as the percentage of body and brain weights observed in the control group (baseline). Values are means ± SE. Malnourished versus control animals: a, $P<0.025$; b, $P<0.005$; c, $P<0.001$ (Student's *t*-test).

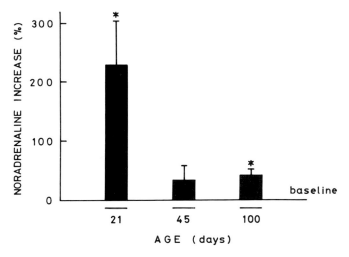

FIG. 2. Norepinephrine (NE) levels in the prefrontal cortex of rats submitted to protein-energy malnutrition during lactation. Results are expressed as percentages of the mean values observed in the control group (baseline). Values are means ± SE. Malnourished versus control animals: *, P<0.05 (Student's t-test).

nourished rats were reduced compared to normal animals, but the differences were not statistically significant (P>0.05).

Amplitudes of PFC-evoked responses elicited by LC stimulation were found to be decreased in the malnourished animals. This effect could depend on metabolic derangements and/or structural alterations of the NE system projecting to the neocortex. The first alternative is supported by the increased concentration of NE observed in the PFC of protein-energy-deprived rats. On the basis of data indicating that electrical stimulation of the LC exerts both inhibitory and excitatory influences on cortical neuronal activity (37), one could surmise that the cortical cells responsible for the evoked potential may be directly inhibited by the elevated NE level or through the excitation of inhibitory neurons. Recent electrophysiological investigations have shown that protein malnutrition during development diminished the ability of cortical neurons to follow repetitive stimulations (32,33) and lowered the spontaneous firing rate of neurons of layers III to V of the rat frontal cortex (35). It has also been

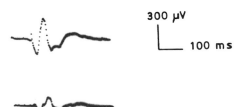

300 μV

100 ms

FIG. 3. Responses evoked by electrical stimulation of the locus ceruleus in the prefrontal cortex of the rat (45 days old). *Upper trace:* normal rat; *lower trace:* protein-energy-deprived rat. Each trace is the average of 10 responses. Malnutrition reduces the peak-to-peak amplitude of the positive–negative early response.

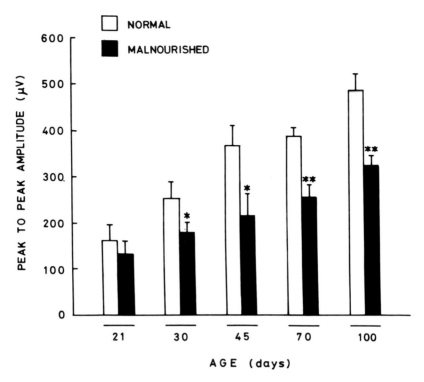

FIG. 4. Ontogenic development of prefrontal evoked responses elicited by electrical stimulation of the locus ceruleus in normal and protein-energy-malnourished rats, from weaning to 100 days of age. Values are mean peak-to-peak amplitudes of responses ± SE. Malnourished versus control animals: *, $P<0.05$; **, $P<0.005$ (Student's t-test).

reported that single NE fibers enter layer VI of the cortex and branch at all levels to undergo extensive collateralization (22). Taking into account these considerations, the hypothesis that the elevated NE level found in malnutrition could result in increased inhibition of cortical cells appears plausible. Nevertheless, this topic deserves further investigation. The second hypothesis, suggesting morphological alterations of norepinephrinergic projections to the PFC produced by malnutrition, has not been investigated. According to Mason and Fibiger (44) norepinephrinergic innervation of the neocortex originates from scattered cells located throughout the LC except in the ventral part. These neurons are presumably fusiform cells (45). As protein deprivation induces a curtailment of dendritic development of fusiform cells within the LC in the rat (21), one cannot rule out the possibility of alterations at their terminal axon arborization in the PFC. It has been argued that the topography of NE innervation is induced by the structure being innervated (22). Since malnutrition imposed during development alters the morphology of the cerebral cortex (14), the existence of an abnormal cortical NE innervation is possible.

Electrophysiological and neurochemical parameters were altered at all ages in malnourished rats. This indicates that nutritional restriction in pups results in long-term functional derangements of the NE system projecting to the PFC.

Central norepinephrinergic systems have been implicated in several higher brain functions, such as learning acquisition and extinction (46–48), long-term memory (49), and sleep-waking behavior (50). Since most of these behaviors exhibit long-lasting derangements after early malnutrition (13,14), the results presented here could provide functional evidence linking structural changes and behavioral disturbances.

REFERENCES

1. Hyvarinen J, Poranen A. Function of the parietal associative area 7 as revealed from cellular discharges in alert monkeys. *Brain* 1974;97:673–92.
2. Mountcastle VB, Lynch JC, Georgopoulos A, Sakata H, Acuna C. Posterior parietal association cortex of the monkey: command functions for operations within extrapersonal space. *J Neurophysiol* 1975;38:871–908.
3. Robinson DL, Goldberg ME. Sensory and behavioral properties of neurons in posterior parietal cortex of the awake, trained monkey. *Fed Proc* 1978;37:2258–61.
4. Pribram KH. On the neurology of thinking. *Behav Sci* 1959;4:265–87.
5. Brown RM, Crane AM, Goldman PS. Regional distribution of monoamines in the cerebral cortex and subcortical structures of the rhesus monkey: concentrations and *in vivo* synthesis rates. *Brain Res* 1979;168:133–50.
6. Butter CM, Snyder DR. Alterations in adversive and aggressive behaviors following orbital frontal lesions in rhesus monkeys. *Acta Neurobiol* 1972;32:525–65.
7. Franzen EA, Myers RE. Neural control of social behavior: prefrontal and anterior temporal cortex. *Neuropsychologia* 1973;11:141–57.
8. Monckeberg F. The effect of malnutrition on physical growth and brain development. In: Prescott JW, Read MS, Coursin DB, eds. *Brain function and malnutrition*. New York: John Wiley, 1975:15–39.
9. Celedón JM, De Andraca I. Psychomotor development during treatment of severely marasmic infants. *Early Hum Dev* 1979;3:267–75.
10. Cravioto J, DeLicardie E. Nutrition, mental development and learning. In: Falkner F, Tanner JM, eds. *Human growth*, vol 3. *Neurobiology and nutrition*. New York: Plenum Press, 1979:481–511.
11. Resnick O, Morgane PJ, Hasson R, Miller M. Overt and hidden forms of chronic malnutrition in the rat and their relevance to man. *Neurosci Biobehav Rev* 1982;6:55–75.
12. Colombo M, De Andraca I, López I. Desnutrición severa en el niño. Desarrollo psicomotor, neurológico y conducta. In: Celedón JM, ed. *Nutrición e inteligencia en el niño*. Santiago: Editorial Universitaria, 1983:73–121.
13. Smart J. Early life malnutrition and later learning ability: a critical analysis. In: Oliverio A, ed. *Environment and intelligence*. Amsterdam: Elsevier/North Holland, 1977:215–35.
14. Morgane PJ, Miller M, Kemper T, et al. The effects of protein malnutrition on the developing central nervous system in the rat. *Neurosci Biobehav Rev* 1978;2:137–230.
15. Celedón JM, Colombo M. Desnutrición y capacidad de aprendizaje: Análisis crítico. *Rev Chil Nutr* 1981;9:189–97.
16. West CD, Kemper TL. The effect of a low protein diet on the anatomical development of the rat brain. *Brain Res* 1976;107:221–37.
17. Cordero ME, Díaz G, Araya T. Neocortex development during severe malnutrition in the rat. *Am J Clin Nutr* 1976;29:358–65.
18. Salas M, Díaz S, Nieto A. Effects of neonatal food deprivation on cortical spines and dendritic development of the rat. *Brain Res* 1974;73:139–44.
19. Leuba G, Rabinowicz T. Long-term effects of postnatal undernutrition and maternal malnutrition on mouse cerebral cortex. I. Cellular densities, cortical volume and total numbers of cells. *Exp Brain Res* 1979;37:283–98.

20. Warren MA, Bedi KS. Synapse-to-neuron ratios in the visual cortex of adult rats undernourished from about birth until 100 days of age. *J Comp Neurol* 1982;210:59–64.
21. Díaz-Cintra S, Cintra L, Kemper T, Resnick O, Morgane PJ. The effects of protein deprivation on the nucleus locus coeruleus: a morphometric Golgi study in rats of three age groups. *Brain Res* 1984;304:243–53.
22. Levitt P, Moore RY. Noradrenaline neuron innervation of the neocortex in the rat. *Brain Res* 1978;139:219–31.
23. Moore RY. The reticular formation: monoamine neuron systems. In: Hobson JA, Brazier MAB, eds. *The reticular formation revisited*. New York: Raven Press, 1980:67–81.
24. Morgane PJ, Kemper T, Cintra L, Díaz-Cintra S. Out-of-phase development of dendritic spines in locus coeruleus and nucleus raphe dorsalis in rats of three age groups. *Dev Brain Res* 1982;4:487–90.
25. Kostowski W, Samanin R, Vareggi SR, Marc V, Garattini S, Valselli L. Biochemical aspects of the interaction between midbrain raphe and locus coeruleus in the rat. *Brain Res* 1974;82:178–82.
26. Stern WC, Miller M, Forbes WB, Morgane PJ, Resnick O. Ontogeny of the levels of biogenic amines in various parts of the brain and in peripheral tissues in normal and protein malnourished rats. *Exp Neurol* 1975;49:314–26.
27. Chanez C, Priam M, Flexor MA, et al. Long lasting effect of intrauterine growth retardation on 5-HT metabolism in the brain of developing rats. *Brain Res* 1981;207:397–408.
28. Kety S. Brain amines and affective disorders. In: Ho BT, MacIsaac WM, eds. *Brain chemistry and mental disease*. New York: Plenum Press, 1971:237–44.
29. Charney DS, Redmond DE. Neurobiological mechanisms in human anxiety. Evidence supporting central noradrenergic hyperactivity. *Neuropharmacology*. 1983;22:1531–6.
30. van Kammen DP, Antelman S. Impaired noradrenergic transmission in schizophrenia? *Life Sci* 1984:34:1403–13.
31. Soto-Moyano R, Ruiz S, Pérez H, Carrillo R, Hernández A. Effect of prenatal malnutrition on cortical reactivity of the rat parietal association area. *Int J Neurosci* 1981;13:99–102.
32. Pérez H, Ruiz S, Hernández A, Soto-Moyano R. Effect of early undernutrition on reactivity of the rat parietal association area. *Exp Neurol* 1983;82:241–4.
33. Pérez H, Ruiz S, Hernández A, Soto-Moyano R. Long-term effects of early undernutrition on reactivity of the rat parietal association cortex. *Neurosci Lett* 1984;48:103–7.
34. Hernández A, Ruiz S, Pérez H, Soto-Moyano R. Effect of early malnutrition on dynamic properties of axodendritic synapses in the rat prefrontal cortex. *J Neurobiol* 1985;16:389–93.
35. Stern WC, Pugh WW, Resnick O, Morgane PJ. Developmental protein malnutrition in the rat: effect on single-unit activity in the frontal cortex. *Brain Res* 1984;306:227–34.
36. Bronzino JD, Austin K, Siok CJ, Cordova C, Morgane PJ. Spectral analysis of neocortical and hippocampal EEG in the protein malnourished rat. *Electroencephalogr Clin Neurophysiol* 1983; 55:699–709.
37. Olpe HR, Glatt A, Laszlo J, Schellenberg A. Some electrophysiological and pharmacological properties of the cortical noradrenergic projection of the locus coeruleus in the rat. *Brain Res* 1980;186:9–19.
38. Valenstein T, Case B, Valenstein ES. Stereotaxic atlas of the infant rat hypothalamus. *Dev Psychobiol* 1969;2:75–80.
39. Campuzano HC, Weilkerson JE, Horvath SM. Fluorimetric analysis of epinephrine and norepinephrine. *Anal Biochem* 1975;64:578–87.
40. Lowry OH, Rosebrough NJ, Farr AL, Randall RJ. Protein measurement with the Folin phenol reagent. *J Biol Chem* 1951;193:265–75.
41. Dobbing J, Sands J. Vulnerability of developing brain. IX. The effects of nutritional growth retardation on the timing of the brain growth-spurt. *Biol Neonate* 1971;19:363–78.
42. Winick M. Malnutrition and the developing brain. In: Plum F, ed. *Brain dysfunction in metabolic disorders*, vol 53. New York: Raven Press, 1974:253–63.
43. Shoemaker WJ, Wurtman RJ. Perinatal undernutrition: accumulation of catecholamines in rat brain. *Science* 1971;171:1017–9.
44. Mason ST, Fibiger HC. Regional topography within noradrenergic locus coeruleus as revealed by retrograde transport of horseradish peroxidase. *J Comp Neurol* 1979;187:703–24.
45. Swanson LW. The locus coeruleus: a cytoarchitectonic, Golgi and immunohistochemical study in the albino rat. *Brain Res* 1976;110:39–56.

46. Anlezark GM, Crow TJ, Greenway AP. Impaired learning and decreased cortical norepinephrine after bilateral locus coeruleus lesions. *Science* 1973;181:682–4.
47. Mason ST, Iversen SD. Learning in the absence of forebrain noradrenaline. *Nature* 1975;258: 422–4.
48. Amaral DG, Foss JA. Locus coeruleus lesions and learning. *Science* 1975;188;377–8.
49. Dismukes RK, Rake AV. Involvement of biogenic amines in memory formation. *Psychopharmacologia* 1972;23:17–25.
50. Morgane PJ, Stern WC. Chemical anatomy of brain circuits in relation to sleep and wakefulness. In: Weitzman E, ed. *Advances in sleep research,* vol 1. New York: Spectrum Publications, 1974: 1–131.

Developmental Neurobiology, edited by
Philippe Evrard and Alexandre Minkowski.
Nestlé Nutrition Workshop Series, Vol. 12.
Nestec Ltd., Vevey/Raven Press, Ltd.,
New York © 1989.

Brain Development and Nutrition

N. Herschkowitz

Department of Pediatrics, University of Bern, 3010 Bern, Switzerland

Two questions regarding brain development and nutrition are of particular importance: How long does brain development (i.e., growth and differentiation) continue? and What are the effects of malnutrition on neurotransmitter systems? Many
of the research data available today are derived from animal experiments, and the
limitations of animal studies are well known. However, knowledge gained from
these animal experiments has led to significant research on humans. The knowledge
of the effects of malnutrition on brain development in humans will certainly increase
thanks to new noninvasive techniques such as nuclear magnetic resonance imaging,
permitting longitudinal studies of the metabolism and development of structures in
the human brain.

BRAIN DEVELOPMENT

For operational reasons it is useful to divide brain development in humans and in
rats into four periods.

First Period

In humans this extends between the 8th and 32nd week of gestation, and in rats
from the 3rd day of gestation until birth. This period is characterized by neuroblast
proliferation and migration, and aggregation of neurons to form primary layers.
There are distinct regional differences in the period of neuroblast proliferation. During this period the formation of the first synapses takes place. These are probably ca-
techolaminergic initially and later serotonergic. The final number of neurons is not
attained by the end of this period. In humans the first major neuroblast proliferation
takes place between 10 and 18 weeks of gestation (1,2). Despite contrary dogma it
is very likely that neuroblast proliferation continues much longer, at least in some
areas. In the rat the number of neurons in the dentate granular layer increases stead-
ily until at least 1 year of age (3).

From 18 weeks of gestation, there is an intensive proliferation of glial cells. It is
difficult to determine when the number of human brain cells reaches a plateau. In

the cerebellum this occurs at about 15 months, by which time the forebrain has only about 65% of its "adult" cell number, which is reached at about 4 years. In this period the cellular density in the human forebrain decreases, partly due to growth of cells but also due to cell death. At 24 weeks of gestation there are 5,000 cells per unit volume, dropping to 2,000 cells per unit volume at 32 weeks (4). Myelination is already taking place in the human spinal cord at 17 weeks and reaches a first plateau around the end of the first period of brain development.

Second Period

In humans this extends between the 32nd week of gestation and birth; the second period in rats is from birth until 10 days of age. This period is characterized by intensive brain growth. Factors contributing to brain growth are mainly cell migration, cell differentiation, and proliferation of glial cells (astrocytes and oligodendrocytes). The cytoarchitecture is further developed. Myelination begins in the brain.

Third Period

In humans this extends between birth and 2 years of age; the third period in rats is between 11 and 20 days of age. This is a period of intensive brain growth and differentiation. Adult brain weight is attained at about 2 years. Thus roughly 5/6 of brain growth takes place postnatally. The cytoarchitecture of the brain layers is basically established. This is the period of intensive neuronal differentiation with formation of dendrites and synapses. It is also the period of intensive activity of the oligodendrocytes leading to myelinogenesis in the central nervous system. Myelination slows down at the end of this period.

Experiments in mouse brain cell cultures give new insight into the regulation of oligodendrocyte proliferation (5). The postnatal development of mouse brain oligodendrocytes *in vivo* and in culture can be compared under proper conditions. *In vitro* the number of oligodendrocytes, identified by immunological markers, reaches a plateau at 14 days, by which time the rate of proliferation has slowed from 26% on day 7 to 10% per day. If oligodendrocytes are completely destroyed on day 14 by complement-dependent cytotoxicity, their number reaches 60% of the normal number 7 days later. These newly appearing oligodendrocytes show a proliferation rate of 25% compared to 10% in the normal controls. These results indicate that precursors of oligodendrocytes are still present in 14-day-old cultures and that proliferation can be induced at a higher rate than in undisturbed controls. Under these experimental conditions there is, therefore, a clear indication that regeneration can occur when the high proliferation rate has slowed down under normal conditions.

Fourth Period

In humans this extends from 2 years of age; the fourth period in rats is from 20 days of age onwards. When this period ends remains to be determined. Brain growth slows down, but differentiation is still active, especially with regard to the formation of the synaptic network. Until recently, this phenomenon was supposed to persist only until about 5 years of age in man. However, it has been shown that in normally aging humans the density and length of dendrites of the neurons in the parahippocampal region increase significantly from 50 to 80 years (6). In presenile dementia, density and length of dendrites decreases during this period. These findings indicate that neuronal differentiation may persist much longer than previously thought (7).

It used to be thought that there was a period of fast myelination in man until about 2 years of age, followed by slow myelination until about 20 years. However, animal experiments indicate that myelination in rats (with a life span of 2 years) does not stop at about 40 days but continues until at least one year of age. Not only should quantitative aspects be taken into account when considering brain development, but also age-dependent changes in the composition of structures. Newer findings show that the number of neurons in certain brain areas is increasing, that myelination continues for a much longer period than previously thought, and that differentiation of neurons in humans takes place for up to 80 years. Development and regression might be a lifelong process, differing from region to region. Nutrition could therefore be of importance to brain development for a much longer period than previously thought. Although brain development later in life may be less intensive than during the first 4 years, it may nevertheless continue to influence human behavior.

If some brain regions develop for longer periods these regions might also be vulnerable for longer periods. But persistence of structural development also implies possibilities for regeneration. Thus we arrive at a concept where brain development, in the widest sense of the word, is a lifelong process during which the brain is vulnerable to exogenous factors such as nutrition but also retains the capability for repairing damage.

NUTRITION AND BRAIN DEVELOPMENT

The effect of nutrition on myelination has been extensively investigated in the past. Less attention has been given to the effect of nutrition on neurons (8). However, numerous studies have shown important effects of undernutrition on neurons, such as retarded neuropil development (9), decreased dendritic arborizations (10), decrease in the size and density of presynaptic endings (11), and a decrease in the number of synapses per unit area (12). There are indications that in the long term nutrition affects the structural and functional development of these systems. Nutrition may also directly affect neurotransmitter (NT) metabolism in the brain and hence affect behavior. Recent work has shown that food intake can directly affect NT synthesis in the brain (13,14). If brain NT synthesis is modified by changes in food intake, it must be influenced by precursor availability. NT synthesis is precursor dependent if the following four requirements are met (13,14): (a) Precursor levels in plasma must depend on intakes; (b) the brain must not be able to synthesize as much of the precursor as it needs; (c) a low affinity transport system must mediate uptake across the blood–brain barrier; and (d) a low affinity enzyme must catalyze the key step converting the precursor into the neurotransmitter, and its activity may not be under feedback control.

These criteria are met for the synthesis of acetylcholine, catecholamines, and serotonin, which are dependent on the availability of choline, tyrosine, and tryptophan, respectively (15). Most of the basic research in this field has been done in the rodent brain and will be briefly reviewed. At birth, activity of enzymes involved in NT synthesis is relatively low, and the number of sites for NT uptake as well as of receptors is also relatively small. They increase during the first 3 to 4 weeks after birth. During this period of intensive brain growth, including myelination and synaptogenesis, both systems show a very high metabolic activity and are therefore particularly dependent on adequate nutrition. Thus myelinogenesis and synaptic development might thus both be affected by inadequate nutrition with possible consequences on behavior.

Acetylcholine

Whole brain acetylcholine (ACh) is reduced in undernourished animals. However, undernutrition does not cause irreversible defects in ACh synthesis and storage (16), as levels return to normal when a normal diet is reintroduced. Undernourished suckling rats initially show reduced choline acetyltransferase (ChAT) activity. But total brain ChAT activity becomes normal by day 21 despite continuing nutritional deprivation. Low ChAT activity persists in olfactory bulbs and in the hypothalmus but normalizes after five weeks of nutritional rehabilitation. ChAT activity in the brain stem does not recover, indicating more severe damage in this region. In contrast, no reduction of ChAT activity is observed in the brain stem when undernutrition starts after weaning, indicating the crucial importance of the time of exposure. It is not known whether the reduction of enzyme activity is due to reduced enzyme synthesis, increased enzyme turnover, structural changes of the enzyme protein, or modifications of activators or inhibitors.

Animals undernourished until weaning and then given a normal diet for one week show a significant reduction of cholinergic muscarinic receptor binding in the corpus striatum and hypothalamus, a slight increase in the midbrain, and no changes in the cerebral cortex and cerebellum (15). These changes are due to alterations in the concentrations of binding sites and not to changes in the affinity of receptors. No data are available on the possible functional effects of these modifications.

Catecholamines

Dopamine concentration in the brain is reduced in early malnutrition, mainly in the corpus striatum (17). Nutritional rehabilitation seems to normalize dopamine content. Undernutrition in adult rats has no effect on brain dopamine content.

Early undernutrition reduces norepinephrine concentration in the brain stem and telencephalon (18). Several months of normal diet can reverse this deficit. Since undernutrition does not affect the supply of the precursor (tyrosine) for catecholamine synthesis and since *in vivo* conversion of tyrosine to dopamine is enhanced and tyrosine hydroxylase activity is elevated in cases of undernutrition (19), the reduction of the content of catecholamines does not seem to be due to deficient synthesis but to enhanced turnover.

Early undernutrition in rats reduces the number of catecholamine receptors in adult life but not their affinity characteristics (20). Dopamine receptors in the corpus striatum are reduced in animals that have been undernourished before weaning. This finding might explain the reduced response to apomorphine (a direct dopamine receptor agonist) observed in rats when protein-malnourished during postnatal development (21).

Serotonin synthesis is related to brain tryptophan content. In undernutrition free tryptophan concentration in serum is increased, probably because of increased competition of nonesterified fatty acids for binding sites on albumin and because of the reduction of serum albumin concentration. Thus the pool of tryptophan that can enter the brain is increased (21,22). Concomitantly the activity of tryptophan hydroxylase in brain is increased in undernutrition. Both factors can explain why serotonin concentration is elevated in the brain of undernourished animals. The content of 5-hydroxyindolacetic acid (a serotonin metabolite) is also increased in the brain of undernourished animals, indicating an increased turnover of serotonin (24). Thus undernutrition seems to increase serotonin synthesis as well as its release. Increased concentrations of serotonin and of its metabolites are mainly observed in the diencephalon and in the brain stem. This seems also to be the case in short-term fasting (24). These experiments do not prove that serotonic transmission is increased. Nevertheless, one could question whether the apathy observed in undernourished animals is due in part to the increased serotonin content of the brain, and whether a comparable mechanism also operates in undernourished humans, in whom apathy is a major problem.

Newborn pups born to dams fed an isocaloric, low protein diet (8% casein instead of the normal 25%) prior to mating and throughout gestation may have normal body and brain weights but show alterations in serotonin metabolism in the central and peripheral nervous system and abnormal spontaneous activity of single neurons in the frontal cortex (25). These changes seem to be irreversible and are not affected by cross-fostering at birth with dams fed on a 25% casein diet. In this model normal growth does not correlate with normal brain development. Similar results have been obtained in small-for-gestational-age rats born to mothers fed an isocaloric 6% casein diet, nursed by dams also fed a 6% casein diet (26).

Food intake can influence the synthesis of neurotransmitters and serotonin, since it affects plasma concentrations of amino acids which share with tryptophan the same transport system into the brain. There has been speculation that diet, particularly the carbohydrate-to-protein ratio, may directly influence the flux of NT precursors to the brain and hence the level of NT synthesis (27). This could have an influence on such functions as appetite, sleep, level of aggression, and so on. It is not known whether prolonged periods of altered diet could affect behavior in the long term and in this way disturb the normal interactions with the environment. These interactions by themselves can affect development. Doerner (28) compared the ratio of plasma tryptophan to neutral amino acids (valine, isoleucine, phenylalanine, and tyrosin) in formula-fed and breast-fed infants. In formula-fed infants the ratio of tryptophan to neutral amino acids was significantly lower due to an increase in the concentration of the neutral amino acids. The authors conclude that this might lead to a decreased entry of the precursor tryptophan into the brain and thus to a decrease in serotonin synthesis, with possible consequences such as developmental obesity and/or permanent changes of mental capacity. It is evident that these conclusions are purely speculative and need further research.

GABA

Dietary restrictions cause a reduction in the activity of the GABA synthesizing enzyme glutamic acid decarboxylase (GAD) in all brain areas except the cerebellum and brain stem (29). The enzyme activity becomes normal with time, even with a restricted diet. The findings suggest that development of GAD activity is delayed and not arrested (30).

GABA receptor binding is significantly increased in undernutrition, especially in the cerebral cortex, corpus striatum, midbrain, and hypothalamus. The changes in receptor binding are probably due to an increase in the number of receptors and not to alterations in their affinity (8). Using a different model of undernutrition it has been shown that undernutrition enhances the binding of GABA by increasing the availability of high affiity sites and the number of low affinity receptors.

These studies suggest that undernutrition decreases the production of some endogenous inhibitors that normally mask the high affinity sites. These could be GABA-modulin or GABA itself (8). No data are yet available showing any functional consequences of these apparent receptor modifications.

In summarizing the various findings regarding neurotransmitter synthesis, turnover, and binding, one must bear in mind that experimental results depend on the type of under- or malnutrition, the timing of dietary alterations, and the species studied. However, a general pattern is emerging, suggesting that undernutrition reduces the activity of cholinergic and GABAergic systems in the developing brain, whereas the activity of catecholamine and serotonin systems increases. This selective effect on brain neurotransmitter activity might have several functional consequences, but none is yet established. Many of the neurochemical disturbances described so far normalize when dietary intakes return to normal, even after the period of intensive brain development.

CONCLUSION

Recent research suggests that brain development (growth and differentiation) lasts much longer than previously thought. This is particularly true of structural and biochemical differentiation in distinct brain areas. Structural and biochemical brain development in humans needs to be carefully studied and possible correlations with the development of behavior evaluated.

There are indications that regeneration at a cellular level may take place in the central nervous system of rodents. Regeneration may be due to increased differentiation or increased proliferation of precursor cells or both. Future research should address the question of cellular regeneration processes in the human brain.

Nutrition affects the structural and biochemical development of neurotransmitter systems and myelin. Functional consequences of these structural and biochemical changes need to be evaluated.

Food intake has a direct influence upon the synthesis of neurotransmitters such as acetylcholine, catecholamines, and serotonin. These neurotransmitters seem to have direct effects on behavior. Possible effects of food intake on human behavior such as appetite, sleep, aggressivity, and arousal need to be studied. Fine but distinct alterations in food intake may perhaps affect brain development or be used in a therapeutic way to correct abnormal brain development.

ACKNOWLEDGMENT

This work was supported by grant 3.493.083 from the Swiss National Research Foundation, a grant from the Swiss Multiple Sclerosis Society, and a grant from the Swiss Foundation for Encouragement of Research in Mental Retardation.

REFERENCES

1. Molliver ME, Kostovic I, Van der Loos H. The development of synapses in cerebral cortex of the human fetus. *Brain Res* 1973;50:403–7.
2. Dobbing J, Sands J. Timing of neuroblast multiplication in developing human brain. *Nature* 1970;226:639–40.
3. Bayer SA. Neurons in the rat dentate gyrus granular layer substantially decrease during juvenile and adult life. *Science* 1982;216:890–2.
4. Rabinowicz T. Morphological features of the developing brain. In: Brazier MAB, Coceani F, eds. *Brain dysfunction and infantile febrile convulsions*. New York: Raven Press, 1973:1–23.
5. Bologa L, Z'Graggen A, Rossi E, Herschkowitz N. Differentiation and proliferation: two possible mechanisms for the regeneration of oligodendrocytes in culture. *J Neurol Sci* 1982;57:419–39.
6. Kaplan MS, Hinds JW. Neurogenesis in the adult rat: electron microscopic analysis of light radioautographs. *Science* 1977;197:1092–4.
7. Huttenlocher PR. Synaptic density in human frontal cortex. *Brain Res* 1979;163:195–205.
8. Telang S, Fuller G, Wiggins R, Enna SJ. Early undernutrition and [³H]y-Aminobutyric acid binding in rat brain. *J Neurochem* 1984;43:640–5.
9. Cragg B. The development of cortical synapses in early starvation in the rat brain. *Brain* 1972; 95:143–50.
10. Hammer R. The influence of pre- and postnatal undernutrition on the developing brain stem reticular formation: a quantitative Golgi study. *Dev Brain Res* 1981;227:191–207.
11. Shoemaker WJ, Bloom FE. Effect of undernutrition on brain morphology. In: Wurtman RJ, Wurtman JJ, eds. *Nutrition and the brain*. New York: Raven Press, 1977, 132–147.
12. Gambetti P, Gambetti A, Rizzuno N, Shafer B, Gontas B. Quantitative and intrastructural study of rat cerebral cortex. *Exp Neurol* 1974;4:464 73.
13. Wurtman RJ, Fernstrom JD. Control of brain monoamin synthesis by diet and plasma amino acids. *Am J Clin Nutr* 1975;28:638–47.

14. Gadisseux P, Ward JD, Young HF, Becker DP. Nutrition and the neurosurgical patient. *J Neurosurg* 1984;60:219–32.
15. Wiggins RC, Fuller G, Enna SJ. Undernutrition and the development of brain neurotransmitter systems. *Life Sci* 1984;35:2085–94.
16. Kulkarni AB, Gaitonde BB. Effects of early undernutrition and subsequent rehabilitation on acetylcholine levels in rat brain. *Experientia* 1982;38:377–8.
17. Shoemaker WJ, Wurtman RJ. Effect of perinatal undernutrition on the metabolism of catecholamines in the rat brain. *J Nutr* 1973;103:1537–47.
18. Hisatomi K, Niiyama Y. Effect of postnatal undernutrition on the catecholamine and serotonin contents of suckling rat brain. *J Nutr Sci Vitaminol (Tokyo)* 1980;26:279–92.
19. Kalyanasundaram S, Ramanamurthy PSV. Effect of undernutrition on tryptophan and tyrosine hydroxylases in the developing rat brain. *J Neurochem* 1981;36:1580–2.
20. Keller EA, Munaro NI, Orsinger OA. Perinatal undernutrition reduces alpha and beta adrenergic receptor binding in adult rat brain. *Science* 1982;215:1269–70.
21. Leahy JP, Stern WC, Resnick O, Morgane PJ. A neuropharmacological analysis of central nervous system catecholamine systems in developmental protein malnutrition. *Dev Psychobiol* 1978;11:361–70.
22. Miller M, Leahy JP, Stern WC, Morgan PJ, Resnick O. Tryptophan availability: relation to elevated brain serotonin in developmentally protein-malnourished rats. *Exp Neurol* 1977;57:142–57.
23. Miller M, Resnick O. Tryptophan availability: the importance of prepartum and postpartum dietary protein on brain indoleamine metabolism in rats. *Exp Neurol* 1980;67:298–314.
24. Fuenmayor LD, Garcia S. The effect of fasting on 5-hydroxytryptamine metabolism in brain regions of the albino rat. *Br J Pharmacol* 1984;83:357–62.
25. Resnick O, Miller M, Forbes W, Hall R, Kemper T, Bronzino J, Morgane PJ. Developmental protein malnutrition: influences on the central nervous system of the rat. *Neurosci Biobehav Rev* 1979;3:233–46.
26. Resnick O, Morgane PJ. Ontogeny of the levels of serotonin in various parts of the brain in severely malnourished rats. *Brain Res* 1984;303:163–70.
27. Fernstrom JD. Dietary precursors and brain neurotransmitter formation. *Annu Rev Med* 1981;32:413–25.
28. Doerner G, Bewer G, Lubs H. Changes of the plasma tryptophan to neutral amino acids ratio in formula-fed infants: possible effects on brain development. *Exp Clin Endocrinol* 1983;82:368–71.
29. Rajalakshmi M, Paramesvaran M, Telang SR, Ramakrishnan CV. Effects of undernutrition and protein deficiency on glutamate dehydrogenase and decarboxylase in rat brain. *J Neurochem* 1974;23:129–33.
30. Patel AJ, DeVecchio M, Atkinson DJ. Effect of undernutrition on the regional development of transmitter enzymes: glutamate decarboxylase and choline acetyltransferase. *Dev Neurosci* 1978;1:41–53.

Subject Index

A

Acatalasemia
  biochemical defects in, 67–68
  clinical features of, 67
Accessory olive projections, in cerebellum, 156–159
Adenylate cyclase, 5-HT effect, 172,173,174
Age
  brain lipid composition and, 186–187
  brain weight and, 262–263
  differentiation and, 299
  fatty acid synthesis and, 130
  for myelination, 113,187–188
  myelin lipids and, 191–192
  of neural pruning, 8
Alcohol
  delta-opioid receptor binding and, 265–268
  dependence, 265,268
  effects of, 265,268,270
  FAS and, 24,26,269
  membrane effects, 265,266–268,270
  neuronal growth and, 9
  opioid system and, 267
  pial-glial barrier disorders and, 18
D-Amino acid oxidase
  adaptive changes in, 83
  biological significance of, 81–82
  of cerebellum, 80–81
  MAM effect, 80–81
  reactions catalyzed by, 81–82
  in reeler mice, 82–83
Anencephaly, CSF obstruction in, 28,30
Arachidonic acid
  biosynthesis, 138
  human brain level, 137
Aromatic amino acid decarboxylase (AADC), in neurons in culture, 176–178,179
Astrocytes
  in development, 3
  function of, 1,111
  GFAP and, 3
  RCGs and, 23
Autophagy, of glial processes, 23,26
Axons, pruning of, 8

B

Behavior
  cerebral malformations and, 13–15
  in nutritional disturbances, 276,287–288, 293,301–302,303
  neurological development and, 243–244
  parietal lobe lesions and, 287

Biparietal diameter
  in polymicrogyria, 33
  in prenatal hydrocephalus, 29–30
  ultrasound determination of, 29–30,33
Blood-brain barrier
  fatty acid transport and, 133
  in Refsum's disease, 137
Brain
  cervonic acid and, 140
  development, 11,12–15,75–77,263,272
  DNA content, 273
  EFA deficiency, 139–141,275–276
  fatty acids, 131–132,139–140,275–276
  galactolipid content, 274
  gestational age and, 272
  growth, 172
  head circumference and, 272–273
  5-HT trophic effect, 171–172,174–179
  human, 187–198,263,271–280
  linoleic acid, 139
  linolenic acid, 137,139,276
  in malnutrition, 272–274,276–278
  membranes of, 143–144
  mother's weight and, 272
  myelination, 187–190,298,299
  plasmalogens, 186–187,190–191,274
  PUFA of, 137,141–143
  weight at birth, 272
  weight in development, 262–263,272–273
Brun's layer, see Subpial granular layer

C

cDNA
  for mouse MBPmRNA, 99,101,102,103–106
  sequencing of, 102,103–106
Cerebellar cortex
  autoradiographic studies, 156–157
  development, 3–5,156,163–164
  differentiation, 5–7
  olivocerebellar projections of, 155–161
  organization of, 155,166–167
  Purkinje cells of, 3–4,155,164–167
  of rat, 155–167
  spinocerebellar topography of, 160–163
Cerebellum
  D-amino acid oxidase activity of, 80–81
  development, 164–167,187–190,191
  galactolipids of, 188–189,274
  growth, 272
  lipid levels in, 187
  MAM effect on, 80–81
  myelination in, 187–190,191

305